Qualitative Research in Nursing
Second Edition

Immy Holloway
Stephanie Wheeler

D0507929

Blackwell
Science

First edition published 1996
Reprinted 1997, 1998, 2000
Second edition published 2002
Reprinted 2003, 2004

Library of Congress Cataloging-in-Publication Data is available

ISBN 0-632-05284-8

A catalogue record for this title is available from the British Library

Set in 10/13pt Sabon
by DP Photosetting, Aylesbury, Bucks
Printed and bound by Replika Press Pvt. Ltd., India.

The publisher's policy is to use permanent paper from mills that operate a sustainable forestry
policy, and which has been manufactured from pulp processed using acid-free and elementary
chlorine-free practices. Furthermore, the publisher ensures that the text paper and cover board
used have met acceptable environmental accreditation standards.

For further information on Blackwell Publishing, visit our website:
www.blackwellpublishing.com

Contents

Foreword

In the foreword for the first edition in 1996 I wrote that this book will become a 'must have' on the reading lists of those teaching qualitative methods. I can confidently say the same of this second edition. Holloway and Wheeler have struck an excellent balance between updating and expanding some areas of their book, whilst retaining all of the features which made it such an attractive book in the first place.

In particular it is good to see that they have again steered clear of the potential problem for research texts when methods discussions are transported from their original disciplinary homes – in this case anthropology and sociology. The subtleties of methodological debate can be lost when the practicalities of research methods are unhitched from their epistemology and philosophical foundations. In the capable hands of these authors we get no such violence done to the discussion of methods.

The inclusion of the legal aspects of the ethical discussion is a welcome addition as are the new chapters on narrative inquiry and action research. Other improvements on the first edition include a reorganisation of some of the material to give fuller coverage of some areas and giving less prominence to others, for example feminist research (qualitative methods by another name for some of us), thereby achieving a balanced approach to their discussion of methods.

Holloway and Wheeler have confronted some of the difficult debates in qualitative methods and have included clear discussions of a variety of similar approaches where distinctions are difficult to draw. This feature of the book will make it attractive to experienced researchers as well as newcomers to qualitative methods.

Press on ... this is a very good read.

Kath M. Melia
Chair of Nursing Studies
University of Edinburgh

Preface

This is the second edition of our book. In the six years since it was first published, qualitative research has become much more sophisticated, and more and more texts have been written and edited. We have learnt much in the intervening years, and some of this is reflected in the book. The chapters have been rewritten and updated although we have not changed ideas and examples that still seemed appropriate and valid. We have, however, added new examples and references.

We have added two new chapters, one on action research and one on narrative inquiry, as these approaches are becoming more frequent in qualitative research. The ethics chapter has been updated to include legal aspects. Problematic issues have been integrated into relevant chapters rather than in a separate section as before. Although each approach has its own style of analysis, we have also added a chapter on data analysis, including a discussion about computer-aided analysis and attempted to update the references fully.

The reference lists at the end of each chapter are rather long and contain both significant and less important articles and books. We have tried to include classic texts as well as up-to-date books and articles on each area of qualitative research so that nurses and midwives can go to the sources and find out about different approaches. This, and our wish to give all the sources used, is the reason for the extensive referencing.

The initial purpose of the book and its intended readership has stayed the same as it was six years ago. This book is intended for a number of groups:

(1) Undergraduates, especially mature students, who have nursing and midwifery experience
(2) Preregistration nursing and midwifery students with some appreciation of research methods
(3) Postgraduates who undertake a qualitative research project and wish to revisit the procedures and strategies of qualitative research, in particular MSc or MA students
(4) Research students who wish to have a quick revision of research approaches before going on to more detailed and sophisticated texts

(5) Nursing and midwifery professionals who are carrying out research in clinical or educational settings

The aim of this book is to provide nurses and midwives with both theoretical understanding and practical knowledge of the qualitative research process. To achieve this, we have not only explained practical procedures but also the theoretical concepts that underlie qualitative research, as researchers often undertake projects in a vacuum without considering the theoretical basis of their research and the origins of the approaches they use. We realise that novice researchers might find some of the issues rather complex, and we have tried to make the processes explicit. This accounts for the variation in length and complexity in the different chapters of the book.

Overview of the book

The book is divided into four parts. In Part One, the first chapter of the book describes the salient features of qualitative inquiry and explains its position in the wider framework of research. In the following chapter we outline the steps in the research process from the initial stages of formulating the research question to writing a proposal. Access and entry to the setting and participants are discussed. The third chapter deals with ethical requirements that must be fulfilled and the philosophical and legal frameworks on which they are based. Chapter 4 is devoted to the nature and importance of supervision in qualitative research.

Part Two gives an overview of and practical guidelines for data collection. In Part Three we discuss the major research approaches in greater detail and briefly outline others. The issues of validity and reliability, and the criteria of trustworthiness and authenticity seen as alternatives in qualitative research, are also debated. Part Four is devoted to data analysis, including the use of computers, and the completion of a project. The last chapter of the book gives guidelines for writing up the research. The glossary is intended to give a quick explanation of some of the terms used.

How to read this book

Students need not read the whole book from start to finish, although this will help them to understand the nature of qualitative research. It is essential however for those who are undertaking a research project to study Chapters 1, 2, 3, 4, 12 and 13. In addition they should read the chapter on their chosen approach. References at the end of each chapter provide guidance for further reading.

We hope that the book will help researchers in nursing and midwifery to understand the different approaches, to present a proposal and write the research report. Doing research is a challenging and demanding activity. We hope you will also enjoy it.

The authors

This book is the work of authors who complement each other in knowledge and expertise. Professor Immy Holloway, Reader in Health Studies, has a special interest in grounded theory and ethnography, and in the practicalities of doing and writing up research. She is a sociologist of health and illness. Stephanie Wheeler, who has a nursing and health visiting background, is a specialist in healthcare ethics and law and chair of the local research ethics committee. Both work in the Institute of Health and Community Studies at Bournemouth University and have organised a number of conferences in qualitative research for health and social care. They have also published widely in the area of qualitative research.

Acknowledgements

We would like to thank Griselda Campbell and Beth Knight, our editors at Blackwell Publishing, for their support and patience. Jacky Griffith reviewed the text, and we are very grateful for her comments and constructive advice, which has been invaluable.

We are also indebted to a number of other people:
Our colleagues and friends
Les Todres who is always willing to help and advise
Jan Walker with whom we often discuss issues in research
Kate Galvin, for her support and encouragement
The colleagues who have read and commented on various chapters in the book
Last but not least, our students from whom we have learnt so much over the years

This book is dedicated to our mothers

Irmgard Peters 1904–2000
Mavis Wheeler 1927–2001

PART ONE

Introduction to Qualitative Research

CHAPTER 1

The Nature of Qualitative Research: Development and Perspectives

This chapter is an attempt to trace the background of qualitative research, its development and its main features. It also focuses on some epistemological and methodological issues. The aim is to put the more pragmatic and practical sections in the book into a theoretical and methodological context.

Qualitative research is a form of social inquiry that focuses on the way people interpret and make sense of their experiences and the world in which they live. In the words of Atkinson *et al.* (2001: 7) it is an 'umbrella term', and a number of different approaches exist within the wider framework of this type of research. Most of these have the same aim: to understand the social reality of individuals, groups and cultures. Researchers use qualitative approaches to explore the behaviour, perspectives, feelings and experiences of people and what lies at the core of their lives. Specifically, ethnographers focus on culture and customs, grounded theorists investigate social processes and interaction, while phenomenologists consider the meanings of experience and describe the life world. Qualitative methodology is also useful in the exploration of change or conflict. The basis of qualitative research lies in the interpretive approach to social reality and in the description of the lived experience of human beings.

Qualitative and quantitative approaches: underlying philosophies

Social reality can be approached in different ways, and researchers will have to select between varieties of research approaches. While often making a choice on practical grounds, they must also understand the philosophical ideas on which it is based.

The initial choice is not easy. Approaches to social inquiry consist not only of the procedures of sampling, data collection and analysis, but they are based on particular ideas about the world and the nature of knowledge which sometimes reflect conflicting and competing views about social reality. Some of these positions towards the social world are concerned with the very nature of reality and existence (*ontology*). From this, basic assumptions about knowledge arise. *Epistemology* is the theory of knowledge and is concerned with the question of what counts as valid knowledge. *Methodology* refers to the principles and ideas on which researchers base their procedures and strategies (*methods*). To assist in understanding the background to the interpretive/descriptive approach, the following section provides a discussion of epistemological and methodological ideas.

Several sets of assumptions underlie social research; they are often referred to as the *positivist* and the *interpretivist* paradigms (Bryman, 2001). Conflict and tension between different schools of social science have existed for a long time. In the positivist approach, the focus was on the methods of natural science that became a model for early social sciences such as psychology and later sociology. Interpretivists stressed that human beings differ from the material world and the distinction between humans and matter should be mirrored in the methods of investigation. Qualitative research was critical of the natural science model. Many researchers hold a 'separatist' position and believe the worldviews of qualitative and quantitative researchers to be completely incompatible. They reject a mix of the two (Murphy and Dingwall, 2001).

Social scientists continue to raise the paradigm debate in spite of the warning by Atkinson (1995) that simplistic polarisation between positivist and qualitative inquiry will not do. He criticises the use of the concept of the term *paradigm* and the 'paradigm *mentality*'. Nurse researchers, too, accuse nursing of unwarranted 'paradigmatic thinking' and maintain that it restricts rather than extends knowledge (Thorne *et al.*, 1999). Nevertheless, qualitative researchers are defensive of their methodologies and tend to develop arguments against other approaches. Indeed, they often follow the same path of which they accuse quantitative researchers (Darbyshire, 1997), namely to be critical of other approaches and uncritical of their own perspective.

It is important to describe and trace the development of ideas so that novice researchers are able to identify the roots of the different approaches.

The natural science model: positivism, objectivism or naturalism

From the nineteenth century onwards, the traditional and favoured approaches to social and behavioural research were quantitative. Quantitative research has its base in the positivist and early natural science paradigm that has influenced social science throughout the nineteenth and the first half of the twentieth century.

Positivism is an approach to science based on a belief in universal laws and insistence on objectivity and neutrality (Thompson, 1995). Positivists follow the natural science approach by testing theories and hypotheses. The methods of natural – in particular physical – science stem from the seventeenth, eighteenth and nineteenth centuries. Comte (1798–1857), the French philosopher who created the terms 'positivism' and 'sociology', suggested that the emerging social sciences must proceed in the same way as natural science by adopting natural science research methods.

One of the traits of this type of research is the quest for objectivity and distance between researcher and those studied so that biases can be avoided. Investigators searched for patterns and regularities and believed that universal laws and rules or law-like generalities exist for human action. They thought that findings would and should be generalisable to all similar situations and settings. Behaviour could be predicted, so they believed, on the basis of these laws. Even today many researchers think that numerical measurement, statistical analysis and the search for cause and effect lie at the heart of all research. They feel that detachment and objectivity are possible, and that numerical measurement results in objective knowledge. In this positivist approach, researchers control the theoretical framework, sampling frames and the structure of the research. This type of research seeks causal relationships and focuses on prediction and control.

Popper (1959) claimed falsifiability as the main criterion of science. The researcher formulates a hypothesis – an expected outcome – and tests it. Scientists refute or falsify hypotheses. When a deviant case is found the hypothesis is falsified. Knowledge is always provisional because new incoming data may refute it. There has been criticism of Popper's ideas (for instance by Feyerabend (1993)) but the debate cannot be developed here. It is discussed in philosophy of science texts.

The positivist approach develops from a theoretical perspective, and a hypothesis is often, though not always, established before the research begins. The model of science adopted is hypothetico-deductive; it moves from the general to the specific, and its main aim is to test theory. The danger of this approach is that researchers treat perceptions of the social world as objective or absolute and neglect everyday subjective interpretations and the context of the research.

Nineteenth-century positivists believed that scientific knowledge can be proven and is discovered by rigorous methods of observation and experiments and derived through the senses. Chalmers (1999) argues against a simplistic view of science as knowledge deriving from sense perception only. Even natural scientists – for instance biologists and physicists – do not necessarily agree on what science is and adopt a variety of different scientific approaches. Social scientists too, use a number of approaches and differ in their understandings about the nature of science. Scientific knowledge is difficult to prove and is not merely derived from the senses. The search for objectivity may be futile for scientists. They can strive for it, but their own biases and experiences intrude. Science, whether natural or social science, cannot be 'value free', that is, it cannot be fully objective as the values and background of the researchers affect the research.

The paradigm debate

In the 1960s the traditional view of science was criticised for its aims and methods by both natural and social scientists. The new and different evolutionary stance taken within disciplines such as biology and psychology had gone beyond the simplistic positivist approach. Qualitative researchers go further still. Lincoln and Guba (1990), for instance, argue that a 'paradigm shift' occurred – in line with the ideas of Kuhn (1962, 1970).

Kuhn's thinking has had great impact on the paradigm debate. 'Normal science', with its community of scholars, he asserts, proceeds through a series of crises that hinder its development. Earlier methods of science are questioned and new ways adopted; certain theoretical and philosophical presuppositions are replaced by another set of assumptions taking precedence over the model from the past. Eventually, one scientific view of the world is replaced by another. Although Kuhn wrote mainly about the physical sciences, writers have used his work to draw analogies with the shift in the ideas of social science. Kuhn's (1962:162) definition of paradigm is 'entire constellation of beliefs, values, techniques, and so on, shared by the members of a given community'.

A paradigm then consists of theoretical ideas and technical procedures that a group of scientists adopt and which are rooted in a particular worldview with its own language and terminology. Kuhn has been extensively criticised (Fuller, 2000) but the critique cannot be developed here.

Social researchers today often claim that a 'paradigm shift' in social science has occurred – in the same way in which Kuhn discussed it – that a whole worldview is linked to the new paradigm. They attack the positivist stance for its emphasis on social reality as being 'out there', separate from the individual and maintain that an objective reality independent of the people under study is difficult to grasp. Quantitative research, in all its variations, is useful and valuable, but it is sometimes seen as limited by qualitative researchers, because it neglects the participants' perspectives within the context of their lives.

The controlled conditions of traditional approaches sometimes limit practical applications. This type of research does not always or easily answer complex questions about the nature of the human condition. Researchers using these approaches are not inherently concerned about human interaction or feelings, thoughts and perceptions of people in their research but with facts, measurable behaviour and cause and effect.

> Quantitative approaches are important and solve many types of research problem. Qualitative research is appropriate for different types of questions.

It must not be forgotten that natural scientists, too, have criticised the sometimes mechanistic natural science view of the world, and some sociologists began to see it as socially constructed and defined. However, one could argue, that there has not been a 'scientific revolution' with a new paradigm. Many, such as Atkinson (1995) and Thorne et al. (1999) challenge the notion of paradigm shift and believe that the debate is a simplification of complex issues.

The interpretive/descriptive approach

The interpretive or interpretivist model and descriptive research have their roots in philosophy and the human sciences, particularly in history, philosophy and anthropology. The methodology centres on the way in which human beings make sense of their subjective reality and attach meaning to it. Social scientists approach people not as individual entities who exist in a vacuum but explore their world within the whole of their life context. Researchers with this worldview believe that understanding human experiences is as important as focusing on explanation, prediction and control. The interpretive/descriptive model has a long history, from its roots in the nineteenth century to Dilthey's philosophy, Weberian sociology and George Herbert Mead's social psychology.

The interpretivist view can be linked to Weber's *Verstehen* approach. Philosophers and historians such as Dilthey (1833–1911) considered that the social sciences need not imitate the natural sciences; they should instead emphasise empathetic understanding. Understanding in the social sciences is inherently different from explanation in the natural sciences. Weber was well aware of the two approaches that existed in the nineteenth century (this was the time of the *Methodenstreit* – the conflict between methods). The concept of *Verstehen* – understanding something in its context – has elements of empathy, not in the psychological sense as intuitive and non-conscious feeling, but as reflective reconstruction and interpretation of the action of others. Weber believed that social scientists should be concerned with the interpretive understanding of human beings. He claimed that meaning could be found in the intentions and goals of the individual.

Weber argued that *understanding* in the social sciences is inherently different from *explanation* in the natural sciences, and he differentiates between the nomothetic, rule-governed methods of the latter and idiographic methods that are not linked to the general laws of nature but to the actions of human beings. Weber believed that numerically measured probability is quantitative only, and he wanted to stress that social science concerns itself with the qualitative. We should treat the people we study, he advised, 'as if they were human beings' and try to gain access to their experiences and perceptions by listening to them and observing them. Although Weber did not have a direct impact on early qualitative researchers (Platt, 1985), contrary to the beliefs of some social scientists, he did however influence the sociologist Schütz and ethnomethodology, as well as later writers such as Denzin and Douglas, and his ideas have helped shape the qualitative perspective through them. Sociologists developed further the interpretive perspective that initially stemmed from the writings of Mead, Weber, Schütz and others in the early twentieth century. Phenomenology as a qualitative research approach is based on philosophy in the nineteenth and early twentieth centuries, in particular the ideas of the mathematician and philosopher Husserl (1859–

1938), and Heidegger (1889–1976) who focus on ontological questions of meaning and lived experience.

Qualitative researchers claim that the experiences of people are essentially context-bound, that is, they cannot be free from time and location or the mind of the human actor. Researchers must understand the socially constructed nature of the world and realise that values and interests become part of the research process. Complete objectivity and neutrality are impossible to achieve; the values of researchers and participants can become an integral part of the research (Smith, 1983); researchers are not divorced from the phenomenon under study. This means reflexivity on their part; they must take into account their own position in the setting and situation, as the researcher is the main research tool. Language itself is context-bound and depends on the researchers' and informants' values and social location. Detailed replication or duplication of a piece of research is impossible because the research relationship, history and location of participants differ from study to study.

Qualitative methodology is not completely precise, because human beings do not always act logically or predictably. Investigators in qualitative inquiry turn to the human participants for guidance, control and direction throughout the research. Structure and order are, of course, important for the research to be scientific. The social world, however, is not orderly or systematic; therefore it is all the more important that the researcher proceeds in a well structured and systematic way.

The historical background

Qualitative research has its roots in anthropology, philosophy and sociology. It was first used by anthropologists and sociologists as a method of inquiry in the early decades of the twentieth century, although it existed in a non-structured form much earlier; researchers tried to find out about cultures and groups a long time before then – both in their own and foreign settings – and told stories of their experiences. In the 1920s and 1930s, however, social anthropologists such as Malinowski (1922) and Mead (1935), and sociologists of the Chicago School, such as Park and Burgess (1925), adopted more focused approaches. At that time qualitative research was still relatively unsystematic and journalistic (and much of it is now seen as unscientific). Researchers reported from the field – the natural settings they studied, be they foreign places or the slums and street corners of their own cities – by observing and talking to people about their lives.

Since the 1960s qualitative research has experienced a steady growth, starting with the emergence of approaches from a symbolic interactionist perspective (Becker *et al.*, 1961) and the development of grounded theory (Glaser and Strauss, 1967). Filstead (1970) edited a volume of readings on qualitative research. Publications in ethnography such as Spradley's books (1979, 1980) also gave impetus to this type of approach. Sociologists and anthropologists carried out most of the research while academics and professionals in the education and healthcare fields adapted these approaches for their own areas. Earlier journalistic methods were abandoned because they were seen to lack rigour. In psychological phenomenology, Giorgi (1985) and Colaizzi (1978), among others, developed phenomenological research approaches rooted in the ideas of Husserl.

Much work originated in North America. The journal *Qualitative Sociology* was first published in 1978, and the *International Journal for Qualitative Studies in Education* in 1988. In 1994, Denzin and Lincoln edited the comprehensive *Handbook of Qualitative Research*, now in its second edition (2000). In Britain, qualitative research became fashionable through its use in educational sociology in the 1970s and 1980s (for instance, Delamont, 1976; Burgess, 1985; and the text by Hammersley and Atkinson (1983) of which a second edition was published in 1995). At that time health professionals in particular saw qualitative research as a type of inquiry appropriate and relevant to their work (Webb, 1984; Field and Morse, 1985; Leininger, 1985; Melia, 1987), and in the 1980s and 1990s this work grew rapidly (for instance, Morse, 1991, 1994; Smith, 1992; Benner, 1994; Morse and Field, 1996; Streubert and Carpenter, 1996, 1999). These are only a few of the many textbooks in education and nursing about qualitative research. In medicine, qualitative approaches are becoming respectable but have not yet been wholly accepted as an alternative form of research. However, a book edited by Crabtree and Miller (1992, 1999) and a series of articles in the *British Medical Journal* by sociologists compiled in a small volume (Mays and Pope, 1996, 1999) explained its use and made doctors more conscious of qualitative research, and the book edited by Greenhalgh and Hurwitz (1998) is important. Significantly, the World Health Organisation also published an overview of 'the concepts and methods used in qualitative research' (Hudelson, 1994). Murphy *et al.* (1998) published an extensive review of the literature in qualitative research in the area of health technology assessment.

The attention of British psychologists turned to qualitative research when Nicholson (1991) prepared a report for the Scientific Affairs Board of the British Psychological Society that urged a wider use of qualitative research (Richardson, 1996). In Britain, the first major general text about qualitative psychological research appeared in 1994 (Banister *et al.*, 1994). Books on specific approaches in psychological inquiry, such as discourse analysis, were published from the 1980s onwards (for instance, Potter and Wetherell, 1987; Potter, 1996). A special issue of the journal of the British Psychological Society was devoted to qualitative research (*The Psychologist*, special issue, 8, 3). Smith *et al.* (1995) and Richardson (1996) edited texts that encompassed discussions of both theoretical and practical aspects of qualitative research.

Researchers who take these approaches do not always use the term 'qualitative research'; they adopt different labels. Some call it naturalistic inquiry (Lincoln and Guba, 1985), field research (Burgess, 1984; Delamont, 1992), case study approaches (Stake, 1995; Travers, 2001) interpretive (or sometimes interpretative) research (Bryman, 2001). Others seem to use the term ethnography as an overall name for much qualitative research, for instance Hammersley and Atkinson (1995). The latter highlight the lack of a 'hard and fast distinction between ethnography and other sorts of qualitative inquiry' (p. 2) and stress the diversity of qualitative approaches on the one hand and the epistemological and methodological similarities on the other. Although there are differences between qualitative approaches (Creswell, 1998), it is sometimes difficult to find clear distinctions between them even though they can be important. All qualitative research, however, focuses on the lived experience, interaction and language of human beings.

The methodology – the underlying rationale and framework of ideas and theories – determines approaches, methods and strategies to be adopted. Qualitative researchers choose a variety of approaches and procedures to achieve their aims. These include ethnography, grounded theory, phenomenology, conversation analysis, discourse analysis and cooperative inquiry among others. Some forms of social inquiry such as action research, and feminist approaches generally, though not always, use qualitative methods and techniques.

The characteristics and aims of qualitative research

Different types of qualitative research have common characteristics and use similar procedures while differences in data collection and analysis do exist.

The following elements are part of most qualitative approaches

- The data have primacy; the theoretical framework is not predetermined but derives directly from the data
- Qualitative research is context-bound, and researchers must be context sensitive
- Researchers immerse themselves in the natural setting of the people whose thoughts and feelings they wish to explore
- Qualitative researchers focus on the *emic* perspective, the views of the people involved in the research and their perceptions, meanings and interpretations
- Qualitative researchers use 'thick description': they describe, analyse and interpret
- The relationship between the researcher and the researched is close and based on a position of equality as human beings
- Data collection and data analysis generally proceed together, and in some forms of qualitative research they interact

The primacy of data

Researchers usually approach people with the aim of finding out about them; they go to the participants to collect the rich and in-depth data that may become the basis for theorising. The interaction between the researcher and the participants leads to the generation of concepts, which are a product of the 'research act' (Denzin, 1989b). The data themselves generate new theoretical ideas, they help modify already existing theories or uncover the essence of phenomena. It means that the research design cannot be strictly predefined before the start of the research. In other types of research, assumptions and theories lead to hypotheses which are tested; sampling frames are imposed, while in qualitative research data have priority. The theoretical framework of the research project is not predetermined but based on the incoming data.

This approach to social science is, initially at least, inductive. Researchers move from the specific to the general, from the data to theory or description. They do not impose ideas or follow assumptions but give accounts of reality as seen by others. They must be open minded though they cannot help having some 'hunches' about what they may find, especially if they are familiar with the setting.

While some qualitative research is concerned with the generation of theory (Glaser and Strauss, 1967), many researchers do not achieve this; others, such as phenomenologists, do not wish to do so but focus on a phenomenon. They usually do provide description or the interpretation of participants' experiences, describing 'the characteristics and structure of the phenomenon' under study (Tesch, 1991: 22). Qualitative research is not static but developmental and dynamic in character; the focus is on *process* as well as outcomes.

Contextualisation

Researchers must be sensitive to the context of the research and immerse themselves in the setting and situation. The context of participants' lives or work affects their behaviour, and therefore researchers have to realise that the participants are grounded in their history and temporality. Researchers have to take into account the total context of people's lives. The conditions in which they gather the data, the locality, the time and history are all important. Events and actions are studied as they occur in everyday, 'real life' settings. It is important to respect the context and culture in which the study takes place. If researchers understand the context, they can locate the actions and perceptions of individuals and grasp the meanings that they communicate. In a broader sense, the context includes the economic, political and cultural framework.

Immersion in the setting

Qualitative researchers use the strategies of observing, questioning and listening, immersing themselves in the 'real' world of the participants. This may generate descriptions of a culture (Hammersley and Atkinson, 1995). It helps to focus on process, that is, on the interactions between people and the way they construct, or change, rules and situations. Qualitative inquiry can trace progress and development over time, as perceived by the participants.

For the understanding of participants' experiences, it is necessary to become familiar with their world. When professionals do research they are often part of the setting they investigate and know it intimately. This might mean that they could miss important issues or considerations. To be able to examine the world of the participant, researchers must not take this world for granted but should question their own assumptions and act like strangers to the setting as 'naïve' observers. They 'make the familiar strange' (Delamont and Atkinson called their 1995 book *Fighting Familiarity*). Immersion might mean attending meetings with or about informants, becoming familiar with other similar situations, reading documents or observing interaction in the setting. This can even start before the formal data collection phase, but it means that researchers immerse themselves in the culture they study.

Most qualitative research investigates patterns of interaction, seeks knowledge about a group or a culture or explores the life world of individuals. In clinical, social care or educational settings this may be interaction between professionals and clients or relatives, or interaction with colleagues. It also means listening to people and attempting to see the world from their point of view. The research can be a macro- or microstudy – for instance it may take place in a hospital ward, a classroom, a residential home, a reception area or indeed the community. The culture does not just consist of the physical environment but also of particular ideologies, values and ways of thinking of its members. Researchers need sensitivity to describe or interpret what they observe and hear. Human beings are influenced by their experiences; therefore qualitative methods encompass processes and changes over time in the culture or subculture under study.

The 'emic' perspective

Qualitative approaches are linked to the subjective nature of social reality; they provide insights from the perspective of participants, enabling researchers to see things as their informants do; they explore 'the insiders' view'. Anthropologists and linguists call this the *emic perspective* (Harris, 1976). The term was initially coined by the linguist Pike in 1954. It means that researchers attempt to examine the experiences, feelings and perceptions of the people they study, rather than imposing a framework of their own that might distort the ideas of the participants. They 'uncover' the meaning people give to their experiences and the way in which they interpret them, although meanings should not be reduced to purely subjective accounts of the participants as researchers search for patterns in process and interaction, or the invariant constituents of the phenomenon they study.

Qualitative research then, is based on the premise that individuals are best placed to describe situations and feelings in their own words. Of course, these meanings may be unclear or ambiguous, and they are not fixed; the social world is not frozen in a particular moment or situation but dynamic and changing. By observing people and listening to their accounts, researchers seek to understand the process by which participants make sense of their own behaviour and the rules that govern their actions. Taking into account their informants' intentions and motives researchers gain access to their social reality. Of course, the report individuals give are *their* explanations of an event or action, but as the researcher wishes to find people's own definition of reality, these reports are valid data. Researchers cannot always rely on the participants' accounts (Dey, 1993) but are able to take their words and actions as reflections of underlying meanings. The qualitative approach requires 'empathetic understanding', that is, the investigators must try to examine the situations, events and actions from the participants' – the social actors' – point of view and not impose their own perspective.

Of course, researchers can still theorise or infer from observed behaviour or participants' words. The researcher's view is the *etic perspective* – the outsider's view (Harris, 1976). The meanings of participants are interpreted or a phenomenon identified and described. Researchers have access to their world through experience and observation. This type of research is thought to empower participants, because they do not merely react to the questions of the researchers but have a voice and guide the study. For this reason, the people studied are generally called participants or informants rather than subjects. It is necessary that the relationship between researcher and informant is one of trust; this close relationship and the researcher's in-depth knowledge of the informant's situation make deceit unlikely (though not impossible).

Thick description

Immersion in the setting will help researchers use *thick description* (Geertz, 1973). It involves detailed portrayals of the participants' experiences, going beyond a report of surface phenomena to their interpretations, uncovering feelings and the meanings of their actions. Thick description develops from the data and the context. The task involves describing the location and the people within it, giving visual pictures of setting, events and situations as well as verbatim narratives of individuals' accounts of their perceptions and ideas in context.

The description of the situation or discussion should be thorough; this means that writers describe everything in vivid detail. Indeed Denzin (1989a: 83) defines thick description as: 'deep, dense, detailed accounts of problematic experiences ... It presents detail, context, emotion and the webs of social relationship that join persons to one another.' Thick description is not merely factual, but includes theoretical and analytic description. Janesick (1994: 216) declared that description is the 'cornerstone of qualitative research'. Thick description is related to the term 'exhaustive description' in phenomenological research

(Colaizzi, 1978). Strauss and Corbin (1994) go further by explaining that the emphasis in one of the approaches – grounded theory – is on conceptualisation rather than description.

Thick description helps readers of a research study to develop an active role in the research because the researchers share their knowledge with the readers of the study. Through clear description of the culture, the context and the process of the research, the reader can follow the pathway of the researcher, and the two share the construction of reality coming to similar conclusions in the analysis of research (Erlandson *et al.*, 1993). This shows readers of the story what they themselves would experience were they in the same situation as the participants, and therefore it should generate empathetic and experiential understanding.

Qualitative researchers are storytellers. Although the data collection and analysis are systematic and develop logically, writers present the findings and discussion in the form of a story with a distinct storyline.

The research relationship

In order to gain access to the true thoughts and feelings of the participants, researchers adopt a non-judgemental stance towards the thoughts and words of the participants. This is particularly important in interviews. The listener becomes the learner in this situation, while the informant is the teacher who is also encouraged to be reflective. Rapport does not automatically imply an inti-mate relationship or deep friendship (Spradley, 1979), but it does lead to nego-tiation and sharing of ideas. It makes the research more interesting for the participants because they feel able to ask questions. Negotiation is not a once and for all event but a continuous process.

The researcher should answer questions about the nature of the project as honestly and openly as possible without creating bias in the study. It is interesting that research books and articles differ in their advice on the relationship of researcher and informant. Some (for instance Patton, 1990) suggest a certain distance between the two, while others, such as Wilde (1992) feel that this could be a mistake because involvement and self-disclosure of the researcher facilitate disclosure and sharing of experiences from the participants. It is important for participants to realise that researchers, too, have human experiences just as they do and can empathise with them. The main goal of the meeting between researcher and informants is to gain knowledge.

Conflicting or complementary perspectives?

Some social scientists believe that qualitative and quantitative approaches are merely different methods of research to be used pragmatically, dependent on the research question (Bryman, 2001). Others decide that they are incompatible and mutually exclusive on the basis of their different epistemologies (Leininger, 1992; Lincoln and Guba, 1985; Denzin and Lincoln, 2000). Researchers sometimes use one or the other, depending on their own epistemological stance. Silverman (2001) asserts that neither school is superior to the other, and that an emphasis on the polarities does not result in a useful debate, as both are valid approaches.

Many sociologists, psychologists and medical professionals work in the positivist tradition. In much health, education and social work, however, the qualitative perspective is in the ascendant. One might suggest that qualitative research is a coherent way of researching human thought, perception and behaviour (not new or uni-linear but developed to answer different questions from those of traditional approaches).

The positivist and the interpretive/descriptive perspective of social research have their roots in different assumptions about social reality. While early positivism is based on the belief that reality has existence outside and independent of individuals, those who adopt new approaches to research claim that *social* reality is constructed and does not have independence from the people creating it, although they might acknowledge that there is a reality 'out there'.

Oakley (2000) claims that qualitative researchers sometimes use the term 'positivism' as a form of abuse. She criticises this and those researchers who neglect experimental and other forms of quantitative research. She asserts that both qualitative and quantitative approaches have a place. In any case, the terms are not absolute, as numbers are often used in qualitative research, and quantitative inquiry includes measurements of quality. Also, research, whether quantitative or qualitative, can be presented in a positivist or non-positivist frame, aim or direction. Crotty (1998: 41) suggests '. . . it is a matter of positivism vs non-positivism, not a matter of qualitative vs quantitative'. Methodological debates often suffer from oversimplification.

Bryman (2001) argues that qualitative research became popular initially because of dissatisfaction with quantitative research. The latter could not, in the view of many researchers, answer the important questions in which they were interested. In qualitative nursing and midwifery research, the 'voices' of patients and clients are heard, and feelings and experiences can be grasped. There are, however, distinct differences between the major methodological approaches.

Some of the differences of qualitative and quantitative methodologies and procedures can be seen in Table 1.1.

Triangulation

Many researchers believe that qualitative and quantitative methods can be used together, and indeed, they often are. A long debate has arisen about the use of triangulation. Triangulation is the process by which several methods (data sources, theories or researchers) are used in the study of one phenomenon. The

Table 1.1 Differences between qualitative and quantitative research

	Qualitative	**Quantitative**
Aim	Exploration of participants' experiences and life world Understanding, generation of theory from data	Search for causal explanations Testing hypothesis, prediction, control
Approach	Broad focus Process oriented Context-bound, mostly natural setting Getting close to the data	Narrow focus Product oriented Context free, often in artificial or laboratory setting
Sample	Participants, informants Sampling units such as place, time and concepts Purposive and theoretical sampling Flexible sampling that develops during research	Respondents, participants (the term 'subjects' is now discouraged in the social sciences) Randomised sampling Sample frame fixed before research starts
Data collection	In-depth non-standardised interviews Participant observation/fieldwork Documents, photographs, videos	Questionnaire, standardised interviews Tightly structured observation Documents Randomised controlled trials
Analysis	Thematic, constant comparative analysis Grounded theory, ethnographic analysis etc.	Statistical analysis
Outcome	A story, an ethnography, a theory	Measurable results
Relationships	Direct involvement of researcher Research relationship close	Limited involvement of researcher Research relationship distant
Rigour	Trustworthiness, authenticity Typicality and transferability	Internal/external validity, reliability Generalisability

concept has its origin in ancient Greek mathematics; in modern times it is employed in topographic surveying as a checking system. Denzin (1989a) differentiates between four different types of triangulation: triangulation of *data*, *investigators*, *theories* and *methodologies*. The triangulation of methodologies is most often used.

In *data triangulation* researchers gain their data from different groups, locations and times. For example: in a study of hospitalisation, old and young patients' perspectives could be explored and people from different locations might be asked for their experience. The surgical and medical wards might be the locations for the research. An admission in the middle of the night might be compared with one during the day.

Investigator triangulation means that more than one researcher is involved in the research. In student projects, dissertations or theses this does not often happen, but some well-known researchers have used investigator triangulation, for instance, Strauss researched work in psychiatric hospitals with a number of other researchers (Strauss *et al.*, 1964).

Theory triangulation – the use of different theoretical perspectives in the study of one problem – is rare.

Usually researchers use *methodological triangulation* in its two main forms: Within-method (intra-method) triangulation and between-method (across-method or inter-method) triangulation. Within-method triangulation adopts different strategies but stays within a single paradigm; for instance, participant observation and open-ended interviews are often used together in one qualitative study. A good example of this is Becker's study (Becker *et al.*, 1961). He and his co-workers observed new doctors in the hospital setting and asked them about their work through in-depth interviews about actions, problems and incidents they found through observation.

Researchers use between-method triangulation to confirm the findings generated through one particular method by another. An example would be if a nurse constructed a questionnaire about a problem but would also employ unstructured interviews to confirm the validity of the former. It is sometimes believed that triangulation can improve validity and overcome the biases inherent in one perspective (see Chapter 16). Sarantakos (1998), however, claims that triangulation is not necessarily more valuable than single method and not suitable for every type of research. It does not automatically confer validity. Desirability of triangulation depends on the particular project and research question. We suggest that only nurses and midwives who are experienced researchers in both qualitative and quantitative methods use triangulation.

Data triangulation is different from mixing methods. In triangulation, the researchers approach the same problem in different ways or from different angles. When they mix methods, they look at different problems in the same research study using different approaches.

The debate about triangulation

Social scientists are not in accord about the use of triangulation and the mixing of methods. Hammersley (1992) denies the existence of two methodological models and claims that distinctions are dangerous. Although fundamental differences may exist in these approaches, researchers should also consider the implications of the methods for practice and operational use, where a clear distinction is not always helpful. Miles and Huberman (1994) state that one of the differences lies in the description in words in qualitative research and numbers in quantitative research, but there are, of course differences in sampling, analysis and outcomes. Qualitative and quantitative methods are often used together in one single study for practical purposes only or to satisfy members of grant-making bodies who believe that a research study can be strengthened through using both methods.

Those with purist views suggest that the two main research methodologies have no place in one piece of research. Indeed, Leininger (1992) – who recognises that research findings from different philosophical directions can complement each other – warns researchers against mixing the two methodologies because they differ in philosophy, traits and aims. She does suggest that researchers mix methods *within* a paradigm. Triangulation *across* methods, which Leininger describes as 'multi-angulation', violates the integrity of both methodologies in her view. Clarke (1995) advises against using multiple methodologies for more practical reasons. He states that this produces a 'diffused picture' because of the lack of consistency and adequacy in analysis.

The practical angle should be considered: in a small undergraduate project a single method approach is less time consuming and gives an opportunity for in-depth use of the method. Creswell (1994) recommends that studies be based on a single paradigm, not only because of the limitations of time and size of the research, but also because each methodology has its roots in a particular worldview. Qualitative methods and procedures are appropriate to research some situations and problems, quantitative methods for others. Researchers must choose the methodology and methods which best suit the research question or topic. Depending on a particular project – triangulation between methods may be appropriate.

Nurse and midwife researchers rarely adopt the purist stance but are more pragmatic. They do not necessarily see a conflict or follow an extremist view, a standpoint irrelevant in nursing research. Evaluators of qualitative or quantitative methods must remember to judge each piece of work on its own terms within the specific approach taken. This becomes particularly important advice for qualitative research that is often evaluated by the use of criteria appropriate for quantitative methods. Hutchinson and Webb (1991: 311) note that 'qualitative research is not a substitute for quantitative inquiry. The two modes of research are not in competition.' Each has to be consistent within itself and fit the research topic or problem.

Mixing methods

Sometimes researchers employ the two methodologies which have their roots in distinctively different views of the world, not for validating the results of one through the other, but for different reasons, for instance, to gain a variety of information, to illuminate a particular problem from different angles, or to look at different aspects of a phenomenon. DePoy and Gitlin (1993) describe the three basic techniques for mixing methods: The *nested*, the *sequential* and the *parallel* strategies.

(1) When using the nested strategy, researchers choose a main framework and methodology to develop their research and then add a technique from another methodology. For instance, a nurse might employ participant observation and then conduct a survey on a particular issue that arose during the data collection or in the findings.

(2) Sequential strategies can also be used. They are the most common approaches to mixing methods. Nurses, for example, often use qualitative techniques, such as unstructured interviewing, as a first step in research to explore an issue. On the basis of these interviews they develop a hypothesis and construct a questionnaire for a large survey. Sometimes, on the other hand, a study starts with a quantitative approach that examines facts, and a qualitative strategy is added to explore feelings and perceptions that have not been explored before in depth.

(3) The parallel approach makes use of the qualitative and the quantitative at the same time while valuing both equally so that the topic can be illuminated from all sides.

Method slurring

Qualitative research includes a variety of diverse approaches for the collection or analysis of data, based on different philosophical positions and rooted in various disciplines. Some are in fact philosophies rather than methods of data collection and/or analysis – for instance phenomenology – others present approaches to data collection, analysis and theorising such as grounded theory and ethnography. Yet others are textual analyses like discourse and conversation analysis. Even within a single method different schools compete with each other and their followers sometimes take a strong position.

Students cannot always differentiate between methods, and some expert researchers strongly argue against 'slurring' or 'muddling' them (Boyle *et al.*, 1991; Baker *et al.*, 1992). These writers point out that each approach in qualitative research has its own assumptions and procedures. Morse (1994) stresses that, among other factors, application and use differentiate methods and give each approach its unique character. A researcher using one of the methods should make sure that language, philosophy and strategies 'fit' the chosen approach. Commonalities do exist, of course. Most of these approaches focus on the experiences of human beings and the perspectives of the participants, interpreted by the researcher. They uncover meanings that people give to their experiences. Most of these types of research result ultimately in a coherent story with a strong storyline.

The reasons for qualitative nursing and midwifery research

Qualitative researchers adopt a person-centred and holistic perspective. The approach helps develop an understanding of human experiences, which is important for health professionals who focus on caring, communication and interaction. Through this perspective, nurse and midwife researchers gain knowledge and insight about human beings – be they patients, colleagues or other professionals. Researchers generate in-depth accounts that present a lively picture of the participants' reality. They focus on human beings within their social and cultural context, not just on specific clinical conditions or professional and educational tasks. Qualitative nursing and midwifery research is in tune with the nature of the phenomena examined; emotions, perceptions and actions are qualitative experiences.

One could claim that a 'fit' exists between nursing philosophy and qualitative research. The essence of modern nursing contains elements of commitment and patience, understanding and trust, give and take, flexibility and openness (Paterson, 1978). These traits mirror those of qualitative inquiry. Indeed, flexibility and openness are as essential in qualitative study as they are in the tasks of the health worker. In the clinical arena too, health professionals often have to backtrack, return to the situation and try something new, because the situation is constantly evolving.

Health professionals have long recognised that individuals are more than diagnostic cases (Leininger, 1985), and therefore research must focus on the whole person rather than merely on physical parts. The researcher, taking a holistic view, observes people in their natural environment, and the researcher– informant relationship is based on trust and openness. Both professional caring and qualitative research depend on knowledge of the social context. The settings in which individuals live or stay for a time, the social support they have, and the people with whom they interact, have a powerful effect on their lives as well as on health and illness.

Built-in ethical issues exist in both caring and qualitative research. Health professionals and qualitative researchers are ethically bound to act in the interest of clients or participants in the setting and to empower them to make autonomous decisions. This does not mean that conventional forms of inquiry have no ethical basis; however, the closer relationships forged in qualitative research enable researchers to be more focused on ethical values and achieve empathy with the participants (*not* subjects) in the research. These relationships also help nurses and midwives be more aware that their clients are human beings and not just body parts.

In their assessment, nurses and midwives use inductive thinking before coming to conclusions, piecing together the full picture of the patient's or client's condition from specific observations and individual pieces of information. Listening carefully and asking relevant questions without being judgemental enables them to gain insights into problems and deeper understanding of the people with whom they interact. Qualitative research too, proceeds from collecting specific data to more general conclusions.

What methodology in nursing and midwifery research?

Adopting approaches because researchers find them easy or more interesting is not an appropriate way of doing research. Methodology and procedures depend on

- The nature and type of the research question or problem
- The epistemological stance of the researcher
- The skills and training of the researcher
- The resources available for the research project

> The methodology nurse and midwife researchers choose should depend on their intentions and goals. The research question, the ideas and the skills of the researcher determine the research approach and the procedures adopted.

Researchers do have to think of the practicalities of the research such as their own competence and interest, the scope of the research and available funds and resources, all factors that influence the undertaking of a project. A qualitative methodology is generally applied in healthcare settings when the focus is on feelings, experience and thoughts, change and conflict.

The research methodology and the methods inherent in it are not the only consideration for researchers though. We believe that 'methodolatry', about which Janesick (2000: 390) warns us, is a danger in any research. Methodolatry means an obsession with method without reflection, an overemphasis on the method rather than substance of the research. This can lead to distancing from participants by valuing method over their thoughts and ideas.

Nurses and other health professionals do not use qualitative approaches without reflection and evaluation. To be of value to health care, a critical and rigorous stance is necessary. We support the tenets of Atkinson, Coffey and Delamont (2001: 5)

'As qualitative research methods achieve ever-wider currency ... we need to apply a critical and reflexive gaze. We cannot afford to let qualitative research become a set of taken for granted precepts and procedures. Equally, we should not be so seduced by our collective success or radical chic of new strategies of social research as to neglect the need for methodological rigour.'

References

Atkinson, P. (1995) Some perils of paradigms. *Qualitative Health Research*, 5 (1) 117–124.

Atkinson, P., Coffey, A. & Delamont, S. (2001) A debate about our canon. *Qualitative Research*, 1 (1) 5–21.

Baker, C., Wuest, J. & Stern, P.N. (1992) Method slurring: the grounded theory/phe-
nomenology example. *Journal of Advanced Nursing*, **17**, 1355–60.

Banister, P., Bruman, E., Parker, I., Taylor, M. & Tindall, C. (eds) (1994) *Qualitative
Methods in Psychology: A Research Guide*. Buckingham, Open University.

Becker, H.S., Geer, B., Hughes, E. & Strauss, A.L. (1961) *Boys in White*. New Brunswick,
University of Chicago Press.

Benner, P. (ed.) (1994) *Interpretive Phenomenology: Embodiment, Caring and Ethics in
Health and Illness*. Thousand Oaks, Sage.

Boyle, J.S., Morse, J.M., May, K.M. & Hutchinson, S.A. (1991) Dialogue. On muddling
methods. In *Qualitative Nursing Research: A Contemporary Dialogue* (ed. J.M. Morse),
p. 257. Newbury Park, Sage.

Bryman, A. (2001) *Social Research Methods*. Oxford, Oxford University Press.

Burgess, R. (1984) *In the Field: An Introduction to Field Research*. London, Unwin
Hyman.

Burgess, R.G. (1985) *Issues in Educational Research: Qualitative Methods*. Lewes, Falmer
Press.

Chalmers, A.F. (1999) *What is This Thing called Science?* 3rd edn. Milton Keynes, Open
University Press.

Clarke, L. (1995) Nursing research: science, vision and telling stories. *Journal of Advanced
Nursing*, **21**, 584–93.

Colaizzi, P.F. (1978) Psychological research as the phenomenologist views it. In *Existential
Phenomenological Alternatives for Psychology* (eds R.S. Vallé & M. King), pp. 48–71.
New York, Oxford University Press.

Crabtree, B.F. & Miller, W.L. (eds) (1992; 2nd edn 1999) *Doing Qualitative Research*.
Thousand Oaks, Sage.

Creswell, J.W. (1994) *Qualitative and Quantitative Methods*. Newbury Park, Sage.

Creswell, J.W. (1998) *Qualitative Inquiry and Research Design: Choosing Among Five
Traditions*. London, Sage.

Crotty, M. (1998) *The Foundations of Social Research: Meaning and Perspective in the
Research Process*. London, Sage.

Darbyshire, P. (1997) Qualitative research: is it becoming a new orthodoxy? *Nursing
Inquiry*, **4**, 1–2.

Delamont, S. (1976) *Interaction in the Classroom*. London, Methuen.

Delamont, S. (1992) *Fieldwork in Educational Settings: Methods, Pitfalls and Perspectives*. London, Falmer.

Delamont, S. & Atkinson, P. (1995) *Fighting Familiarity: Essays on Education and
Ethnography*. Cresskill NJ, Hampton Press.

Denzin, N.K. (1989a) *The Research Act: A Theoretical Introduction to Sociological
Methods* 3rd edn. Englewood Cliffs NJ, Prentice Hall.

Denzin, N.K. (1989b) *Interpretive Interactionism*. Newbury Park CA, Sage.

Denzin, N.K. & Lincoln, Y.S. (eds) (1994) *Handbook of Qualitative Research*. Thousand
Oaks, Sage.

Denzin, N.K. & Lincoln, Y.S. (eds) (2000) *Handbook of Qualitative Research*, 2nd edn.
Thousand Oaks, Sage.

DePoy, E. & Gitlin, L.N. (1993) *Introduction to Research: Multiple Strategies for Health
and Human Services*. St. Louis, Mosby.

Dey, I. (1993) *Qualitative Data Analysis: A User-Friendly Guide for Social Scientists*. London, Routledge.

Erlandson, D.A. *et al*. (1993) *Doing Naturalistic Research*. Newbury Park, Sage.

Feyerabend, P. (1993) *Against Method*, 3rd edn. London, Verso.

Field, P.A. & Morse, J.M. (1985) *Nursing Research: The Application of Qualitative Approaches*. London, Chapman & Hall.

Filstead, W.J. (ed.) (1970) *Qualitative Methodology: Firsthand Involvement with the Social World*. Chicago, Markham.

Fuller, S. (2000) *Thomas Kuhn: A Philosophical History for our Times*. Chicago, University of Chicago Press.

Geertz, C. (1973) *The Interpretation of Cultures*. New York, Basic Books.

Giorgi, A. (ed.) (1985) *Phenomenology and Psychological Research*. Pittsburgh, Duquesne University Press.

Glaser, B.G. & Strauss, A.L. (1967) *The Discovery of Grounded Theory: Strategies for Qualitative Research*. New York, Aldine De Gruyter.

Greenhalgh, T. & Hurwitz, B. (1998) *Narrative Based Medicine*. London, BMJ Books.

Hammersley, M. (1992) *What's Wrong with Ethnography*. London, Routledge.

Hammersley, M. & Atkinson, P. (1995) *Ethnography: Principles in Practice*, 2nd edn. London, Tavistock.

Harris, M. (1976) History and significance of the emic/etic distinction. *Annual Review of Anthropology*, **5**, 329–50.

Hudelson, P.M. (1994) *Qualitative Research for Health Programmes*. Geneva, World Health Organisation.

Hutchinson, S. & Webb, R. (1991) Teaching qualitative research: perennial problems and possible solutions. In *Qualitative Nursing Research: A Contemporary Dialogue* (ed. J.M. Morse), pp. 301–21. Newbury Park, Sage.

Janesick, V.A. (1994) The dance of qualitative research design. In *Handbook of Qualitative Research* (eds N.A. Denzin & Y.S. Lincoln), pp. 209–19. Thousand Oaks, Sage.

Janesick, V.A. (2000) The choreography of qualitative research design. In *Handbook of Qualitative Research* (eds N.A. Denzin & Y.S. Lincoln), 2nd edn, pp. 379–99. Thousand Oaks, Sage.

Kuhn, T.S. (1962; 2nd edn 1970) *The Structure of Scientific Revolutions*. Chicago, University of Chicago Press.

Leininger, M. (ed.) (1985) *Qualitative Research Methods in Nursing*. New York, Grune and Stratton.

Leininger, M. (1992) Current issues, problems, and trends to advance qualitative paradigmatic research methods for the future. *Qualitative Health Research*, **2**, 392–415.

Lincoln, Y.S. & Guba, E.G. (1985) *Naturalistic Inquiry*. Beverley Hills, Sage.

Lincoln, Y.S. & Guba, E.G. (eds) (1990) *The Paradigm Dialogue*. Newbury Park, Sage.

Malinowski, B. (1922) *Argonauts of the Western Pacific: An Account of Native Enterprise and Adventure in the Archipelagos of Melanesian New Guinea*. New York, Datton.

Mays, M. & Pope, C. (eds) (1996) *Qualitative Research in Health Care*. London, BMJ Publishing Group (rev. edn. 1999).

Mead, G.H. (1934) *Mind, Self and Society*. Chicago, University of Chicago Press.

Mead, M. (1935) *Sex and Temperament in Three Primitive Societies*. New York, Morrow.

Melia, K. (1987) *Learning and Working*. London, Tavistock.

Miles, M.B. & Huberman, A.M. (1994) *Qualitative Data Analysis*, 2nd edn. Thousand Oaks, Sage.

Morse, J.M. (ed.) (1991) *Qualitative Nursing Research: A Contemporary Dialogue*. Newbury Park, Sage.

Morse, J.M. (ed.) (1994) *Critical Issues in Qualitative Research*. Thousand Oaks, Sage.

Morse, J.M. & Field, P.A. (1996) *Nursing Research: The Application of Qualitative Approaches*. Basingstoke, Macmillan.

Murphy, E., Dingwall, R., Greatbach, D., Parker, S. & Watson, P. (1998) Qualitative research methods in health technology assessment: a review of the literature. *Health Technology Assessment*, **2** (16).

Murphy, E. & Dingwall, R. (2001) Qualitative methods in health technology assessment. In *The Advanced Handbook of Methods in Evidence Based Healthcare* (eds A. Stevens, K. Abrams, J. Brazier, R. Fitzpatrick, & R. Lilford), pp. 166–178. London, Sage.

Nicholson, P. (1991) Qualitative psychology: Report prepared for the Scientific Affairs Board of the BPS. Cited in *Handbook of Qualitative Research Methods in Psychology and the Social Sciences* (1996) (ed. J.T.E. Richardson). Leicester, BPS Books.

Oakley, A. (2000) *Experiments in Knowing: Gender and Method in the Social Sciences*. Cambridge, Polity Press.

Park, R. & Burgess, E. (1925) *The City*. Chicago, University of Chicago Press.

Paterson, J.A. (1978) cited in *Nursing Research; A Qualitative Perspective* (1986) (eds P.L. Munhall & C. Oiler). New York, Appleton Century Fox (later editions also exist).

Patton, M.Q. (1990) *Qualitative Evaluation and Research Methods*, 2nd edn. Newbury Park, Sage.

Platt, J. (1985) Weber's *Verstehen* and the history of qualitative research: The missing link. *British Journal of Sociology*, **36**, 448–66.

Pike, K.L. (1954) *Language in Relation to a Unified Theory of the Structure of Human Behaviour*. Glendale CA, Summer Institute of Linguistics (later editions of this book have been published).

Popper, K. (1959) *The Logic of Scientific Discovery*. London, Routledge & Kegan Paul.

Potter, J.T.A. (ed.) (1996) *Handbook of Qualitative Research Methods in Psychology and the Social Sciences*. Leicester, BPS Books.

Potter, J. & Wetherell, M. (1987) *Discourse and Social Psychology: Beyond Attitudes and Behaviour*. London, Sage.

Richardson, J.T.E. (ed.) (1996) *Handbook of Qualitative Research Methods for Psychology and the Social Sciences*. Leicester, BPS Books.

Sarantakos, S. (1998) *Social Research*, 2nd edn. Basingstoke, Macmillan.

Silverman, D. (2001) *Interpreting Qualitative Data*, 2nd edn. London, Sage.

Smith, J.A., Harré, R. & Van Langehove, I. (eds) (1995) *Rethinking Methods in Psychology*. London, Sage.

Smith, J.K. (1983) Quantitative versus qualitative research: An attempt to clarify the issue. *Educational Researcher*, **12** (3) 6–13.

Smith, P. (1992) *The Emotional Labour of Nursing*. London, Macmillan Education.

Spradley, J.P. (1979) *The Ethnographic Interview*. Fort Worth, Harcourt Brace Johanovich.

Spradley, J.P. (1980) *Participant Observation*. Fort Worth, Harcourt Brace Johanovich.

Stake, R.E. (1995) *The Art of Case Study Research*. Thousand Oaks, Sage.

Strauss, A. & Corbin, J. (1990) (2nd edition 1998 Thousand Oaks, Sage). *Basics of Qualitative Research: Grounded Theory Procedures and Techniques*. Newbury Park, Sage.

Strauss, A. & Corbin, J. (1994) Grounded theory methodology: an overview. In *The Handbook of Qualitative Research* (eds N.K. Denzin & Y.S. Lincoln), pp. 173–285. Thousand Oaks, Sage.

Strauss, A.L., Schatzman, L., Bucher, R., Ehrlich, D. & Sabshin, M. (1964) *Psychiatric Ideologies and Institutions*. New Brunswick, Transaction Books.

Streubert, H.J. & Carpenter, D.R. (1996; 2nd edn 1999) *Qualitative Research in Nursing: Advancing the Humanistic Imperative*. Philadelphia, JB Lippincott.

Tesch, R. (1991) Software for qualitative researchers. In *Using Computers in Qualitative Research* (eds N.G. Fielding & R.M. Lee), pp. 16–37. London, Sage.

Thompson, N. (1995) *Theory and Practice in Health and Social Care*. Milton Keynes, Open University Press.

Thorne, S.E., Kirkham, S.R. & Henderson, A. (1999) Ideological implications of the paradigm discourse. *Nursing Inquiry*, **4**, 1–2.

Travers, M. (2001) *Qualitative Research through Case Studies*. London, Sage.

Webb, C. (1984) Feminist methodology in nursing research. *Journal of Advanced Nursing*, **9**, 249–56.

Wilde, V. (1992) Controversial hypotheses on the relationship between researcher and informant in qualitative research. *Journal of Advanced Nursing*, **17**, 234–42.

CHAPTER 2

Initial Steps in the Research Process

At the beginning of their research, nurses and midwives go through the process of selecting the research topic and defining the research question. They must make sure that they have a sound design and that this design fits the chosen topic. Although the initial steps in different types of research are similar, qualitative researchers use a different terminology and adopt different principles. The initial phase of the research is important as it sets the scene for future phases.

Selecting and formulating the research question

The first step in the process is the selection of the research area, topic and question. Although the terms are often used interchangeably, Punch (2000) suggests these as a hierarchy of concepts with different levels of abstraction. The research area and topic are more general than the research question. A research question is a question about an issue that researchers examine to gain new information. It differs from data collection questions that are at the lowest level of abstraction. They are the steps to gather data in order to answer the research question.

Examples

An *area* of research may be 'the experience of asthma', or 'living with pain'. A *topic* would be a more specific aspect of the area, for instance 'children's experience of asthma and their coping strategies' or 'chronic back pain and changes in identity'. The research questions might be phrased: 'How do children experience and cope with asthma?' or 'What is the relationship between chronic back pain and self perception?'

A *data collection question* is an interview question such as: 'How did you feel when you had that asthma attack?' or 'Tell me how you coped with your pain?'

Nurses and midwives often notice problems in their work setting which, they feel, need investigation so that solutions or remedies for unsatisfactory situations or behaviour may be found. Sometimes the topic emerges from the literature linked to a particular area of professional work where gaps in knowledge can be identified. Nursing and midwifery research studies contribute to existing knowledge and enhance understanding of the area under investigation. Knowledge and understanding are not always enough; health professionals also seek solutions to problems in the clinical setting.

Personal observation and experience, as well as discussion with others, guide individuals towards the topic for research. Events and interactions often provide nurses and midwives with an interest or a puzzle and generate the wish to know more. The research question is a statement about what they want to find out and stems directly from a problem experienced in the clinical area or in their personal and professional lives. Holliday (2002: 45) confirms: 'research questions vary from the very specific and instrumental to the broad and exploratory. They may change and develop as the research proceeds.'

It is important that the problem is related to professional work; for instance if nurses are working in the field of paediatrics it would be inappropriate for them to undertake a project with old people, however much it might arouse their interest. A nurse who worked on a ward for confused elderly people and had worried about accidents and falls, might explore nurses' perspectives on the care of old people and the problems involved in caring for them. A midwife who notices the reluctance of some women to breastfeed might use this as an area of investigation.

Certain criteria should be considered when identifying a research problem:

- The question must be researchable
- The topic must be relevant
- The work must be feasible within the allocated time span and resources
- The research should be of interest to the researcher

The question must be researchable

Nurses are often confronted with an important ethical or philosophical dilemma that cannot be solved through research. A moral or philosophical question is not researchable; for instance, the question of whether nurses should become involved in euthanasia is answerable only in philosophical but not in research terms. Although the problem need not be a practical one, it must nevertheless result in findings and outcomes. Research could not answer the question whether health professionals 'should' use euthanasia, while the topic of nurses' perceptions of euthanasia would be researchable. 'Do' and 'should' questions are difficult to answer. 'Do new mothers have feelings of inadequacy?' would become 'What are the feelings of new mothers about coping with their babies?' to transform it into a research question.

> **Examples of researchable questions**
>
> How do fathers perceive the role of the midwife?
>
> What are consultants' perspectives on specialist nursing?
>
> How do people with diabetes cope with their condition?

The topic should be relevant

Relevance means that the research is linked to clinical practice or professional issues. The question might also be important for patients or clients, the health professions or for society in general, and the answer will advance theoretical nursing and midwifery knowledge. The results should be applicable to practice, education or management, legitimising existing practices or leading the way towards change.

The work must be feasible

Nurses are sometimes overambitious, especially if they are new to research. Rather than reflecting on the time the study may take, some of the detailed procedures and the complexity of analysis, they want to start the study straight away, before they have a thorough knowledge of methodology. Time can become a problem in qualitative research because it is eaten up by transcribing, coding and categorising data. A simple small-scale study using a well documented research strategy is far less time consuming than a complex piece of triangulation.

The research should be feasible in terms of resources and accessibility of participants, and researchers should identify whose resources will be used. The topic might be inappropriate because of major ethical and access problems which cannot be overcome, such as superiors not giving permission to do the research, or patients' vulnerability. The research should also be feasible in terms of participant numbers or availability. Last but not least, it must be within the researcher's knowledge and capability.

The research should be of interest to the researcher

If the topic is interesting, it can stimulate and motivate rather than generate boredom after the study has been pursued even for a short time. The storyline of the project is not merely controlled by the participants but it reflects the interest of the researcher. The selection of the focus takes time, reflection and discussion with others who have knowledge in the field of study. Students in particular should discuss the focus of their work with their tutors and supervisors. All too often, new researchers in qualitative research choose a question that is designed to deal with factual issues and needs a survey rather than a qualitative approach.

Example

A nurse decides to research the availability of counselling services in the area. He or she decides to ask questions from patients and nurses in the community about access to these services. A qualitative study would not be useful, as a questionnaire is more appropriate to elicit this detailed information about facts.

Quantitative researchers focus on a very specific area and plan every detail, while qualitative researchers initially formulate the question in more general terms and develop it during the research process. Punch (2000: 14) calls this 'pre-structured versus unfolding research'. Qualitative researchers generally begin with a broad question in the data collection and become more specific in the process of the research, responding to what they hear and find in the setting (progressive focusing). The research design is evolutionary rather than strictly pre-defined. This needs flexibility on the part of researchers.

Example

A community nurse might be interested in the perspectives of diabetic patients on their condition. As many of her clients are elderly patients with diabetes, she decides that the focus of the study should be their experience. However, on searching the literature on this topic, she might find that a large number of studies exist on the perspectives of older people with diabetes, but nobody has yet examined children's experiences or those of their parents. The final aim of the project then could be 'to explore the experience and management of diabetes by children and their parents'.

Practical issues

Beginners, such as preregistration students, might undertake a simple study suitable to show that they understand the research process and can produce a valid and useful project. We advise novice researchers not to carry out research involving patients except in exceptional circumstances, for instance if they have long nursing experience, special expertise in their field and expert supervision. For inexperienced researchers it is particularly important to be clear and straightforward. The clearer the question, the clearer is the outcome of the study.

The literature review

After identifying the research question, investigators review the literature consisting of all the information published and closely related to the area of the project, including both *primary* and *secondary* sources. Primary sources are produced by researchers who developed original work on a subject or researched this topic. Secondary information is merely a report, summary or reference to original work in work originating by a person other than the researcher.

Researchers review the literature for the following reasons:

- To find out what is already known about the subject and identify gaps in knowledge
- To describe how the study contributes to existing knowledge of a topic area
- To avoid duplicating other people's work

Punch (2000) points out the importance of three aspects:

(1) The identification of the literature relevant to the topic
(2) The relationship of the literature to the proposed study
(3) The use of the literature in the research

Through reading reports, researchers can identify what knowledge about the subject of their study already exists, the way in which it was generated and the methods that were adopted. They may find a large number of studies on the particular topic and decide to avoid it, not wishing to focus on issues that others have thoroughly examined at an earlier stage. There is little justification for researchers to keep to their original ideas if the topic has already been addressed exhaustively and adequately elsewhere. However, the literature sometimes points to problems within the subject area that have not yet been investigated.

Example

One of our students works in a community hospital and was particularly interested in how patients viewed these places. She found that patient perceptions relating to small local hospitals had been studied in the USA, but that there were no data from Britain. This was the gap she identified.

Undergraduate student experience

The use of literature in qualitative research

Currently there is a debate about the place of the literature in qualitative research. We know that in quantitative studies researchers read the literature about a topic area and give a detailed report in the literature review before they start the fieldwork. In the early days of qualitative investigations, researchers were encouraged to start without a literature review so that they would not be directed in their research as it was believed that a detailed review would invalidate the qualitative research study, indeed Glaser (1978, 1992) strongly advises against any type of literature review. However, Morse (1994a) warns us that it is folly to 're-invent the wheel' because an answer to the question may already exist. In any case, a researcher's mind is not a *tabula rasa* or blank sheet, especially not when reaching the thesis stage (Glaser and Strauss, 1967; Morse, 1994a). Although it is inappropriate to start with a fully developed theoretical model and an in-depth literature review, it is dangerous to start without any prior ideas of what has already been done in the field. The introductory literature review (or overview) should not be seen to lead to *a priori* assumptions or the researchers could be accused of contaminating the data or their own interpretation (Morse, 1994b).

Researchers do not enter the study with a 'fixed framework' (Minichiello *et al.*, 1990), nor have they identified hypotheses or fully developed theories for their research, as do many quantitative researchers. However, in qualitative research a conceptual framework is necessary too, as the study must be linked to other research and ideas about the topic. An overview of the literature often takes place prior to the study, but the literature search and review is ongoing. The literature becomes another source for data in the main body of the study where it is guided by the emerging categories (Strauss and Corbin, 1998). The researchers compare or contrast their own findings with those of other studies and engage in an active debate with results reported in the literature. This happens throughout the study.

Often, a category or construct that researchers discover and develop is reflected in other disciplines or areas of knowledge. Ideas about the emerging concept can then be followed up in the literature. A look at the nursing literature does not always suffice; psychological or sociological literature might also be useful.

Example

An investigator finds that 'returning to normal' is a major issue for people who have had a myocardial infarction. He or she then follows up the idea of 'becoming normal, being normal, normalisation' etc. in other fields of study. Research in other studies about people with a disability or another illness condition, and how they try to achieve normality, can then become part of the data in the study of MI patients.

Practicalities

Hart (1998) identifies the steps to be taken by researchers in a literature review:

- Collect background information
- Start mapping the topic
- Focus the topic
- Search the sources of literature
- Build up early bibliographies
- Search for critical evaluations of the literature

Many researchers summarise research studies from the literature and the major concepts involved on cards that they file alphabetically from the beginning of their research. This way they can access the ideas and topic areas more quickly when they want them at a later stage. Novice researchers often take an uncritical stance to the literature, but it is important to evaluate critically rather than merely describe it.

If strong factual claims are made in the introduction or literature review (for instance: 'Recent research has shown ...' or: 'Some nurse researchers suggest...') they must be substantiated with names and dates; evidence should be given.

Writing a research proposal

Sometimes this process is called the research protocol; the term proposal is generally used in an academic setting. Before starting the project, researchers write a proposal – a summary of what they will be examining, why they adopt the particular research focus, and how they will proceed. It also includes information about where and when the research will be carried out. It is useful to add intended outcomes and the potential benefits for patients and service.

The proposal justifies and clarifies the proposed study for submission to ethics committees, funding agencies, official gatekeepers such as managers and, for student work, to supervisors. The proposal is a detailed plan of action to convince the reader that the researcher knows enough to undertake the project.

Structure of a proposal

The proposal consists of the following main elements:

(1) Working title
(2) Abstract
(3) Introduction
    Problem statement and rationale (justification for the study)
    Context and setting
    The aim of the research
(4) Brief discussion of the relevant literature
    A discussion of other researchers' work demonstrating the need for this particular study
(5) Design and methodology
    Theoretical basis and justification of the methodology
    Limitations of the study
    Sample selection and sampling procedure
    Data collection and analysis
    Ethical and entry issues

(6) Timetable and costing
(7) Dissemination

Researchers generally proceed in this order though reviewers (supervisors, ethics committees or funding bodies) might have their own format for the proposal. There may be change and reformulation at a later stage during the process. Sandelowski *et al.* (1989) remind qualitative researchers that the proposal is the beginning of a developing design that cannot be fixed and rigid in qualitative inquiry. We advise inexperienced researchers, however, to follow clearly structured, conventional guidelines.

Working title

The working title can be changed as the research evolves, although permission for change might have to be sought from supervisors, research committees or funding bodies. (There is a discussion of titles in Chapter 17.)

Abstract

The abstract in the research proposal is a brief summary of the aim, methods and reasons why the research will be done.

Introduction

This section sets the scene for the research and must be clear and precise. Readers can only understand the proposal in context. In the introduction researchers demonstrate quality and feasibility of the study and the reasons for it.

The problem statement and rationale

This briefly describes the research focus, the way in which the researcher(s) became aware of the problem, and why they want to find out about it. They describe the context in which it takes place. It is important that the research problem is not trivial but has significance for nursing. The potential usefulness of the project for the profession might be explained. Researchers can address a new problem that occurred in the setting or adopt a new approach to a familiar problem. They demonstrate the significance of the work by explaining why the research is important, and/or how it could possibly help in improving nursing or midwifery practice. Research funded by the National Health Service or related funding agencies must identify potential benefits to the NHS.

The rationale gives the reasons for the research that might have emerged through observation of a problem in a particular situation or were stimulated by reading about an event, a crisis or question in the clinical or community setting.

At this stage researchers can mention some of the claims and suggestions that other writers make about the topic or area of study. The investigation of the problem should fill a gap in professional knowledge, however small that gap may be. Stern (1985) suggests that qualitative research is particularly appropriate when little is known about the area of research, because the researcher does not start with preconceived ideas.

The proposal is a starting point for the writing up stage; indeed, some sections can be taken over directly into the research report and then extended or modified appropriately.

Context and setting

The context includes the environment and the conditions in which the study takes place as well as the culture of the participants and location. The setting is the physical location of the research, for instance a ward in a hospital, a clinic or the community.

The aim of the research

The aim of the study – a statement of the researcher's intentions – is made explicit. A statement of the aim is sufficient; objectives might constrict the study by directing it from the outset rather than following the guidance from the ideas of participants. Specific steps to reach the aim will develop as the research proceeds. The overarching purpose of the study reflected in the stated aim is usually concerned with an understanding of participants' feelings, experiences and perceptions as they have developed in the setting and context.

Examples of aims

The aim of this study is to explore the interactions of surgical patients and the nurses who care for them.

The purpose of my study is to describe the perspectives of experienced and new nurses on their expanded role.

The study aims to examine people's perceptions of their visits to alternative practitioners.

Creswell (1994) advises qualitative researchers to keep the aim non-directional, not to describe cause and effect but to give a general sense of the main idea using terms such as 'explore', 'develop', or 'describe'. Generally the statement of the study's aim should not exceed 25 words.

The literature

This is sometimes called the 'initial literature review' in qualitative research. The literature demonstrates the amount and level of knowledge that exists in the area of study. On the basis of an initial scan of relevant studies done by others, the researcher can decide whether to proceed with the work. It is important to mention seminal, classic studies on the subject – those which Hart (1998) calls 'landmark studies', but also to include the most recent writing.

In a qualitative literature overview the discussion of the literature tends to be more limited than in other types of research. As the data have primacy, qualitative researchers tend to avoid taking too much direction from the literature, and in consequence they only discuss a few major research studies. We would like to remind students, however, that the literature will become integrated at a later stage.

As data collection and analysis proceed at the same time, there is an ongoing process of searching the literature that is linked to the findings in the data. Researchers specify the use of resources and other costs to demonstrate that the research can be adequately funded. Resourcing and costs are of major importance in proposals for grant-giving bodies and must be detailed. These include clerical costs, paper, computer, letters and mailing as well as the researcher's time.

The research design and methodology

Theoretical bases and justification of the methodology

The research design is the overall plan and includes strategies and procedures. Researchers must also show how the conceptual framework will be developed during the research process. As stated before, methodology is concerned with the ideas and principles on which procedures are based. Methods consist of the procedures and strategies rooted in a methodology. Students must identify, describe and justify the methodology they adopt and the strategies and procedures involved. It is, of course important that the methods fit the research question. It must be remembered that some of the details of a qualitative research project cannot be prespecified as they arise during the research process.

Limitations of the study

Researchers should list the constraints and limitations of the study, and how they would overcome them. Locke *et al.* (2000) call limitations 'restrictive weaknesses' in the research. By stating these, researchers show their careful preparation for the study. For example, one of the limitations of qualitative research is the lack of generalisability of findings that must be acknowledged. When stating the limitations, researchers can sometimes suggest ways to overcome them. It may be explained, for instance, how the lack of generalisability need not be a problem by describing attempts to achieve typicality or specificity, or how theoretical ideas might be generalisable.

Example

A midwife might plan a study researching women's experience of labour and childbirth in water. She intends to do this in her workplace through in-depth interviewing of women. She then realises that the outcome of the study would only be related to her own setting and cannot be generalised. To achieve typicality, she studies three other settings in different areas of the country. Important similarities in the different settings might be found. When this study is finished, it might well show that the results show typicality, meaning that they are typical not only for one, but across similar settings.

Sample selection and procedure

The access to the participants and the initial sample size must be explained as well as other sampling procedures. An explanation of purposive and theoretical sampling is required.

Data collection and analysis

This section describes the way in which the data will be collected. These may include interviews, observations, diaries or other forms of data collection. The specifics of data analysis will also have to be discussed – for instance constant comparative or thematic data analysis.

Ethical and entry issues

Researchers will give an indication as to how they will deal with these issues, where and how will they recruit their sample, for instance. They will also demonstrate how they will protect the participants from risk and safeguard them from disclosure of identity and lack of confidentiality. A statement about ethics committee approval should also be included. There is further discussion of ethical issues later in this chapter and in Chapter 3.

Timetable and costing

Reviewers wish to see a timetable for the research to become convinced of its feasibility. Therefore qualitative researchers submit a projected work schedule for the research even though they cannot always predict how long exactly each step is going to take. Each step is recorded on the time line. This time line can be written or drawn as a diagram. It must be remembered that the analysis of data in qualitative research takes a long time. The literature has to be searched after the identification of major categories and built into the findings and discussion. The write-up is revised until a storyline is clearly discernible. All this takes time.

Dissemination

Researchers identify the readership for which they write and explain the useful-ness of the study for the particular group they address. They can state how they will disseminate the results of the study, be it through journals, books or other media, such as conferences, video and audiotapes.

Example of time frame for an undergraduate student project

(This could be presented in diagrammatic form)

June/July
- Initial literature review/ formulation of research question
- Gaining approval from gatekeepers, ethics committee and participants
- Writing proposal

August/September
- Data collection (for instance, interviewing and participant observation)
- Start of analysis (coding and categorising)

September–January
- Further data collection and analysis
- Literature review related to emerging categories
- Final decision on categories and major themes

January–March
Writing up

It is a good idea to look at one's own proposal in the light of an evaluation checklist. We have added an example below.

Example evaluation of a qualitative research proposal

(1)   The aim
    (a)   Is the aim linked to the discovery of feelings, perceptions and concepts rather than facts?
    (b)   Is the aim clearly and precisely stated?

(2) Methodology and methods
    (a) Is the methodology justified?
    (b) Does the researcher show an understanding of qualitative inquiry?
    (c) Are the methods, techniques and strategies clearly described in detail (this includes the data collection and analysis)?
    (d) Are the methods appropriate for the problem or topic under study?

(3) The sample
    (a) Do the researchers show how they will gain access to the sample?
    (b) Is there an explanation of purposive and/or theoretical sampling?
    (c) Does the researcher describe the essential features of the sample?

(4) The literature
    (a) Has a gap in knowledge been identified through an initial literature review?
    (b) Does the researcher state that the literature will be integrated into the discussion and become part of the study?

(5) Ethical and legal aspects
    (a) Are the relevant ethical and legal interests of the participants respected and any conflict of interests (fidelity) from the researcher identified?
    (b) Does the research study conform to the standards set out in the Research Governance Framework for Health and Social Care (DoH 2001a)?
    (c) Has permission been sought from the participants and the relevant gatekeepers including local research ethics committees?
    (d) Will the researcher guarantee anonymity to the participants and the right to withdraw at any time?

(6) Practical issues
    (a) Is the topic area researchable and feasible?
    (b) Does the researcher have enough time to undertake the study?
    (c) Are the resources sufficient for the proposed project?

(7) Application to nursing or midwifery
    (a) Are there any implications for clinical practice, education or management?
    (b) Will the outcome of the study have potential benefits for the participants?

Access and entry to the setting

Nursing and midwifery researchers, be they experienced or students, must ask permission for entry to the setting and access to the participants. Gaining access means that they can observe the situation, talk to members in the setting, read the necessary documents and interview potential participants. Formal permission is important in any research and protects both researchers and participants. Access is sought in various ways. Some health professionals put up a notice on a public board in the hospital in which they work. Others ask permission from a self-help group, such as a group of carers, to talk to the members and find out whether they wish to participate. Price (1993) recruited her sample via diabetes newsletters that were distributed locally. There are a number of ways to access potential informants, but voluntary participation must be ensured.

The choice of setting

Researchers search for an appropriate setting. The location where the research takes place must be suitable. For this the researcher has to know the setting intimately, and for nurse and midwife researchers who research their own setting it is not difficult. There is, of course, a very important difference between knowledge of, say, a paediatric oncology setting in general and researching it on the particular unit in which the nurse works. The more is known about the setting, the easier it is to find out whether the study is feasible in its proposed form (Jorgensen, 1989). Some settings are inappropriate for the particular research question. There is no point in planning an ambitious study if access to the setting proves impossible.

Hitchcock and Hughes (1995) give guidelines on the entry process and advise researchers to:

- Establish points of contact
- Describe the aims and scope of the project
- Anticipate sensitive aspects of the research
- Be aware of and sensitive to the organisational hierarchy in the setting
- Be conscious of the effects of change through research

First then, the researcher needs to make contact with people in the setting who can give permission for access and with those whom they wish to observe and interview.

Second, the researcher explains early and clearly the type of project and its scope and aims. It must be remembered, however, that the explanation cannot be too detailed as the research might be prejudiced if all the issues are explained at this early stage, and participants would be guided too firmly towards certain issues rather than give their own ideas and perceptions to the researcher.

Third, sensitive areas for research and vulnerable people must be treated with thoughtfulness and care.

Fourth, the researcher must be aware of the hierarchy in the system and know that conflicts between the interests of those at the top and those at the bottom of the hierarchy may exist. All individual participants involved should, of course be asked for permission to undertake the study.

Fifth, the researcher might have an effect on the setting, This may not only be threatening to the people involved but could also skew the research. This threat can be diminished if the researcher gets to know the people in the setting and establishes a relationship of trust.

Access to gatekeepers

Researchers negotiate with the 'gatekeepers' – the people who have the power to grant or withhold access to the setting. There may be a number of these at different places in the hierarchy of the organisation. Researchers should not just ask the person directly in charge but also others who hold power to start and stop the research. This includes managers, clinicians, consultants, GPs or other personnel, whose patients or clients might be observed or interviewed. For instance, if a nurse wishes to observe interaction on a ward, he or she must not only ask the consent of the manager of the NHS Trust and the local research ethics committee (LREC) but also that of the ward manager, the people working on the ward, and, most importantly, the patients involved. All gatekeepers have power and control of access, but those at the top of the hierarchy are most powerful and should be asked first because they can restrict access even if everybody else agrees. If they cooperate, the path of the research can be smoothed, and their recommendations might make others more willing to collaborate.

There can also be problems with gatekeepers. They may make demands that the researchers cannot fulfil, trying to guide them in a particular direction or denying access to some individuals. Often their knowledge of research is based on familiarity with randomised controlled trials or surveys, hence the nature of qualitative research and the aims and objectives of the study must be explained. The topic might have to be negotiated to fit in with the social organisation, physical environment or timetable of the setting. Although researchers cannot start without permission and must take the wishes of the gatekeepers into account, it is important that participants do not see researchers as a tool of management because this would affect the data.

Usually gatekeepers do not interfere in the research process, though ethics committees can and do. In research carried out with financial and social support from superiors, there is sometimes a danger that gatekeepers have their own expectations and attempt to manipulate the research, intentionally or unintentionally. This can affect the researchers' direction or report of the work, and they might find that they are influenced by these expectations. As gatekeepers are in a position of power, resistance might be difficult.

Example

As part of an undergraduate study, an experienced nurse intended to interview patients with a serious condition about their need for counselling. His immediate superior not only encouraged the research but she also saw it as important because of the support that might be given to future patients with the same condition. The ethics committee had given its approval. However, one of the consultants on the ward disagreed with the form of the proposed research and refused permission for interviews of the patients in his care.

A series of complications and difficulties followed. On the one hand the research was seen as important by the researcher and his colleagues. On the other, to go ahead meant directly contravening the consultant's wishes and generating conflict between him and the researcher's superiors. Endless debates and discussions would waste precious time, and in the end the researcher decided to explore the perceptions of the nurses who cared for the patients instead of interviewing the patients themselves. Although the piece of research did not directly explore the feelings of patients, it produced results that helped in their care and avoided conflict on the ward.

The above example shows that powerful people within the setting can generate difficulties for the researcher who often has to compromise. Contract arrangements might lead to more constraints on researchers as institutional objectives might take precedence over individual research interest because of the prioritising of resources. Staff time costs money.

Researchers are denied access for a variety of reasons:

- The gatekeeper sees the researcher as unsuitable
- It is feared that an observer might disturb the setting
- There is suspicion and fear of criticism
- Sensitive issues are being investigated
- Potential participants in the research may be embarrassed or fearful

Powerful gatekeepers might see researchers as unsuitable because of gender, age or lack of trustworthiness. They must be convinced that the researcher is both able to cope with the study and trustworthy. Friends and acquaintances who are already involved in the researcher's chosen location can sometimes persuade those in power of the ability and trustworthiness of the researcher. If researchers are very young, the gatekeepers might feel that they lack credibility. Some female writers such as Gurney (1991) have felt that men in a position of power did not take them seriously. On the other hand, Gurney felt that occasionally females are seen as less threatening, especially in a male dominated environment.

Managers might deny access if they feel that the setting will be disturbed by the presence of researchers. A ward climate might change because everybody feels that the researchers are watching every task and movement that occurs; therefore it is important that observers and interviewers immerse themselves in the setting until they become part of it and do not create an 'observer effect'.

Local research ethics committees

Ethics committees must scrutinise any research project:

'The Department of Health requires that all research involving patients, service users, care professionals or volunteers, or their organs, tissue or data, is reviewed independently to ensure it meets ethical standards.'

(DoH, 2001a: para 2.2.2)

Research ethics committees have existed within the NHS since 1968, and guidelines for local research ethics committees (LRECs) were first formulated by the Department of Health in 1990 and for multi-centre research ethics committees (MRECs) in 1997. These guidelines have recently been replaced in response to a number of changes that have occurred in the research culture in England and the European Union (new standards were set by the European Directive 2001/20/ EC). The government has provided a new

'... standards framework for the process of review of the ethics of all proposals for research in the NHS and Social Care which is efficient, effective and timely, and which will command public confidence.'

(DoH, 2001b: 1, para 6)

The Department of Health (DoH, 2001b: para 6) recommends that this is read in conjunction with the Research Governance Framework for Health and Social Care (DoH, 2001a) (see also Chapter 3).

An ethics submission form is filled out when researching patients or clients. This includes the name, position and location of the researcher, the title and aim of the study, the sampling and research methods, the number of participants and the way in which they will be asked for consent. The form is sent to the ethics committee for approval. The process of an ethical review is clearly identified in the *Governance Arrangements for NHS Research Ethics Committees* (DoH, 2001b) and the research governance framework states 'Before giving a favourable opinion, the REC should be adequately reassured about the following issues, as applicable' (DoH, 2001a: paras 9.12–9.18). These issues are:

- Scientific design and conduct of the study
- Recruitment of research participants
- Care and protection of research participants
- Protection of research participants' confidentiality
- Informed consent process and community considerations

If the submission does not meet with approval it must be resubmitted until it has passed the committee, as the research cannot start without approval. For research with clients, it does not suffice to gain permission from immediate superiors, managers, consultants or GPs. Any piece of health research that deals with sensitive issues should have approval from the ethics committee, even if it is research with colleagues rather than clients. At present under the new government arrangements for research, the Central Office for Research Ethics Committees (COREC) has sent to all ethics committees a draft of a proposed new national application form. This is far more extensive than the existing form and consists of three parts:

- Part A: Details of Research Project
- Part B: Ethical Issues
- Part C: Locality Issues

The researcher must also complete a summary of an ethical review form.

Ramos (1989) claims that not all health professionals have had formal instructions in the ethics of qualitative research, and members of committees are not always aware of the complex issues and dilemmas in these methods, although this position has been changing rapidly since 2000. The Association of Research Ethics Committees (2000) devoted a whole study day to the particular methodology of qualitative research and the ethical scrutiny required. During this, a number of issues arose in relation to qualitative research and academic research and the needs required to review these appropriately in both local and multi-centre research ethics committees. The qualitative researcher should, however, present a detailed statement of methods and procedures to the committee. Sometimes the committee demands a 'questionnaire'. The qualitative researcher must then send an interview guide with the type of questions that might be asked. Ethics committees can call on researchers to explain and defend their research and will demand to see written permission from participants.

Access to participants

Researchers ask potential participants for permission to interview or observe, stating clearly the right of refusal or withdrawal and assuring confidentiality. The Department of Health points out:

> 'Informed consent is at the heart of ethical research. All studies must have appropriate arrangements for obtaining consent and the ethics review process must pay particular attention to those arrangements.'
>
> (DoH, 2001a: para 2.2.5)

In research with children, the consent of parents and of the children themselves must be obtained. If the potential participants do not know the researchers, the latter should introduce themselves by name and identify their institution. It is useful to carry a short letter of introduction from the institution.

Consent forms are given or sent to each participant for signature. A copy of the signed consent form should be placed in the patient's notes. The form gives the aim and outline of the research and describes briefly the implications for the informants. The consent form should not be too long and must be clearly expressed in plain English, not in technical terminology or jargon. An example consent form is shown in Fig. 2.1.

This subject is discussed in more detail in Chapter 3.

CONSENT FORM   Organisation:

Title of study:

Researcher's name and contact details:

Researcher's position (for instance, oncology nurse, community midwife, research student, nurse specialist):

Manager's name and contact details:

Aim of the study: (Give a broad description of the aim of the study)

With your consent you will be interviewed and tape recorded. Tapes will not be shared by anybody other than the supervisors of the study (and possibly the typist of the transcripts). In the final report excerpts of the interview will be given, but these and quotes will remain anonymous; you will not be recognised because a pseudonym will be used. You need not answer any specific questions if you do not wish to, and you may withdraw at any time from the interview or the study. Your treatment will not be affected in any way whether or not you take part in this research.
The researcher will erase the tapes on completion of the project.

Consent to the research

I (name) _____

agree to take part in the study. I understand that I may withdraw from the study at any time, and that I will not be identified in the research report. I have been told that my treatment and care will not be affected if I take part in this study.

Signature of participant: _____ Date:

Signature of researcher: _____ Date:

Fig. 2.1 Consent form

When the main steps have been taken, the research can begin, always taking into account appropriate timing, site and situation.

Summary

Here is a brief summary of the research process:

- The first step in the process is selection of the research topic and focus. This is often based on experience of a problem in the clinical area, occasionally on personal experience or the professional literature.
- After an initial short overview of previous research the researcher identifies the gaps in knowledge; the specific topic area and methodology should be appropriate for the topic.
- Following ethical guidelines, the researcher then writes a research proposal and seeks access to gatekeepers and participants.
- It is essential that research with patients and clients, or other sensitive research, is vetted by the LREC, or MREC for studies involving several sites. Other research, involving professionals for instance, is also generally vetted by ethics committees when it takes place in healthcare settings.
- The researcher must obtain written consent from participants.

References

Creswell, J.W. (1994) *Research Design: Qualitative and Quantitative Approaches.* Thousand Oaks, Sage.

Department of Health (1990) *Local Research Ethics Committees.* Issued by NHS Management Executive HSG (**91**) 5.

Department of Health (1997) *Ethics Committee Review of Multi-centre Research Establishment of Multi-centre Research Ethics Committees.* Issued by NHS Management Executive HSG (**97**) 23.

Department of Health (2001a) *Research Governance Framework for Health and Social Care.* www.doh.gov.uk/research/RD3/nhsrandd/researchgovernance.htm

Department of Health (2001b) *Governance Arrangements for NHS Research Ethics Committees.* Issued by the Central Office for Research Ethics Committees (COREC) July 2001. htpp://www.doh.gov.uk/research

Glaser, B.G. (1978) *Theoretical Sensitivity.* Mill Valley CA, Sociology Press.

Glaser, B.G. (1992) *Basics of Grounded Theory Analysis.* Mill Valley CA, Sociology Press.

Glaser, B.G. & Strauss, A.L. (1967) *The Discovery of Grounded Theory: Strategies for Qualitative Research.* New York, Aldine De Gruyter.

Gurney, J.N. (1991) Female researchers in male-dominated settings: implications for short-term versus long-term research. In *Experiencing Fieldwork: An Inside View of Qualitative Research* (eds W.B. Shaffir & R.A. Stebbins), pp. 53–61. Newbury Park, Sage.

Hart, C. (1998) *Doing a Literature Review: Releasing the Social Science Research Imagination*. London, Sage.

Hitchcock, G. & Hughes, D. (1995) *Research and the Teacher: A Qualitative Introduction to School-Based Research*, 2nd edn. London, Routledge.

Holliday, A. (2002) *Doing and Writing Qualitative Research*. London, Sage.

Jorgensen, D.L. (1989) *Participant Observation*. Newbury Park, Sage.

Locke, L., Spirduso, W.W. & Silverman, S.J. (2000) *Proposals that Work: A guide for planning dissertations and grant proposals*, 4th edn. Newbury Park, Sage.

Minichiello, V., Aroni, R., Timewell, E. & Alexander, L. (1990) *In-Depth Interviewing: Researching People*. Melbourne, Longman Cheshire.

Morse, J.M. (1994a) Editorial: Going in 'blind'. *Qualitative Health Research*, **4** (1) 3–5.

Morse, J.M. (1994b) Emerging from the data: the cognitive process of analysis in quantitative inquiry. In *Critical Issues in Qualitative Research Methods* (ed. J.M. Morse), pp. 23–43. Thousand Oaks, Sage.

Price, M. (1993) An experiential model of learning diabetes self-management. *Qualitative Health Research*, **3** (1) 29–54.

Punch, K.F. (2000) *Developing Effective Research Proposals*. London, Sage.

Ramos, M.C. (1989) Some ethical implications of qualitative research. *Research in Nursing and Health*, **12**, 57–63.

Sandelowski, M., Davis, D.H. & Harris, B.G. (1989) Artful design: writing a proposal in the natural paradigm. *Research in Nursing and Health*, **12**, 77–84.

Stern, P.N. (1985) Using grounded theory in nursing research. In *Qualitative Research Methods in Nursing* (ed. M. Leininger), pp. 149–160. Philadelphia, WB Saunders Co.

Strauss, A. & Corbin, J. (1998) *Basics of Qualitative Research: Techniques and Procedures for Developing Grounded Theory*, 2nd edn. Thousand Oaks, Sage.

The Association of Research Ethics Committees (2000) Qualitative Research study day, 7 July (Bristol) reported in *The Association of Research Ethics Committees Newsletter*, Issue 3, September 2000 www.arec.org.uk

CHAPTER 3

Ethical Issues in Qualitative Research

Legal rights and ethical aspects have to be considered in all research methods, be they quantitative or qualitative. Researchers in nursing apply the principles that protect participants in the research from harm or risk and follow professional and legal rules which are laid down in the code of conduct (UKCC, 1992), and research guidelines. Most recently, the Research Governance Framework for Health and Social Care of the Department of Health (2001a) sets out standards for all those involved in the conduct of research and is not restricted to any one professional group. The standards for research governance in health and social care are organised into five domains:

(1) *Ethics:* the dignity, right, safety and well being of participants
(2) *Science:* the quality and appropriateness of research
(3) *Information:* the requirements for free access to research information
(4) *Health, safety and employment:* the safety of participants and of research and other staff must be given priority at all times
(5) *Finance and intellectual property:* research activity must show financial probity and compliance with the law

(DoH, 2001a)

Nurses and midwives, as all health and social care researchers, have to justify the research not only to ethics and research committees but also to superiors, gatekeepers and research participants. They must recognise the right of informants to refuse participation in the project or to withdraw from it if they wish. As human rights and civil liberties progress, individuals and groups are more aware of their right to bodily integrity in health care and are more prepared to challenge any infringement. Garwood-Gowers and Tingle (2001: 6) argue that health care is of central concern to all people and that the Human Rights Act 1998 'will stimulate the creation of a consciousness about rights'.

Lessons are still to be learnt concerning informed consent from situations such as the high death rate among children having surgery at Bristol (*Learning from Bristol* (2001)) and the retention of organs at Alder Hay Children's Hospital (*The Royal Liverpool Children's Inquiry* (2001)). As a consequence of these developments, researchers and practitioners must consider both the ethical and legal aspects of research and care. A study protocol that considered ethical aspects without due regard to the law would potentially infringe human rights and would be flawed, therefore legal aspects of informed consent are examined first in this chapter.

Legal aspects of informed consent

Legally the right of self determination and bodily integrity is protected in common law through the rules governing consent. As Montgomery (1997: 228) points out, healthcare professionals who do not obtain consent can potentially commit the crime of battery and the tort of trespass to the person. He does, however, argue that actions for battery have had a limited role in English courts concerning healthcare law, although there has been criticism of this stance. Battery instead serves to emphasise the right of refusal of treatment from a competent adult and there is no right in English law for proxy consent on behalf of an adult (Montgomery, 1997: 229). For research purposes and treatment this poses particular concerns for vulnerable groups such as those with mental illness and confused elderly people. There are as well particular issues concerning research with children discussed below. Where consent is not obtained or in dispute the action would be based on negligence and heard in the civil courts.

For consent to be valid however, Montgomery (1997) states it must be 'real', that is, based on certain factors; a person must be competent to give consent, they need to know in broad terms what they are consenting to and consent should be voluntary and not coerced. In order to address these features the notion of 'informed consent' has become the primary aim before research or any clinical intervention can take place. This is not unproblematic however, particularly in relation to disclosure of information and therapeutic intervention.

Case law in this country (*Sidaway* v. *Governor of the Bethlem Royal Hospital* ([1985] 1 All ER 643; 1 BMLR 132), *Gold* v. *Haringey Health Authority* ([1987] 2 All ER 888) and *Blyth* v. *Bloomsbury Health Authority* ([1993] 4 Med. LR 151) rests on the *Bolam* test (the standard of care test), that is, the information given is deemed adequate if it accords with a responsible body of medical opinion. Yet as McHale *et al.* (1997: 340–67) point out this interpretation by the courts uses a professional standard rather than the prudent patient standard (the patient should be given information concerning risks that they would attach significance to in deciding whether or not to forgo the proposed therapy). The prudent patient test is enshrined in the *doctrine* of informed consent, developed in Canada and the USA and is far more patient orientated. In the UK however, since the early 1990s, there have been significant developments in the case law on consent and the Department of Health in their *Reference Guide to Consent for Examination or Treatment* (DoH, 2001b: 2) point out that all health professionals have a legal duty to keep themselves regularly informed.

For research the same legal principles apply concerning informed consent and because some research may not have direct benefit for the participants, particular care is needed to provide the fullest possible information about the study and time to decide (DoH, 2001b: 9). In fact these features are expected in all patient information sheets provided to research participants and reviewed by institutional, local and multi centre research ethics committees. Rights of self determination and not to be harmed are implicit in the European Convention on Human Rights which is now given further effect in the UK in the Human Rights Act (1998) which came into force in October 2000. The Department of Health (2001b) suggest these articles are most relevant to health care:

- Article 2 (protection of right to life)
- Article 3 (prohibition of torture, inhuman or degrading treatment or punishment)
- Article 5 (right to liberty and security)
- Article 8 (right to respect for private and family life)
- Article 9 (freedom of thought, conscience and religion)
- Article 12 (right to marry and found a family)
- Article 14 (prohibition of discrimination in enjoyment of Convention rights).

Naturally, researchers would need to consider these in their study proposals to safeguard the interests and wellbeing of the research participants. For example Fennell (2001) draws attention to the European Commission on Human Rights statement concerning Article 3, which warns against experimental medical treatment without patient consent, as this would be contrary to this article. Further, he considers Article 8 pointing out that privacy has been held to include confidentiality, also compulsory medical intervention must be considered as an interference of the right of privacy.

Informed consent for children and frail older people

The issue of children and capacity to consent has developed in case law in England but it is not unproblematic in both clinical intervention and research. English law deems a child a minor until the age of 18 years. On reaching the age of 16 however, section 8 (1–3) of the Family Law Reform Act 1969 validates a minor's consent to some forms of medical treatment (McHale *et al.*, 1997). Yet as Montgomery (2001) points out, this presumption of competence to consent to treatment does not include research. There is no statutory guidance for research with children and the test for competence is governed in case law in *Gillick* v. *West Norfolk Area Health Authority* ([1985] 3 All ER 402). In this case, which reached the House of Lords, it was held that minors could give valid consent to treatment provided they had achieved 'sufficient understanding and intelligence to enable them to understand fully what is proposed'.

Montgomery (2001: 178, 179) identifies that for research purposes, to be 'Gillick competent', a child

'...must have the ability to appreciate the nature of the procedures (what would be involved, including the fact that they might not receive active treatment in a placebo-controlled trial), and their purpose (that they are for research and something of the reason for carrying out the study). In the research context, some understanding of the risks involved would also be necessary, although no legal case has yet arisen in which this has had to be established.'

Yet whilst parental consent may not be necessary if a child satisfies this test for competence, as Montgomery (2001) points out the guidance from the Medical Research Council and Royal College of Physicians is more cautious, recommending parental assent.

When children lack capacity to consent to research, the Department of Health *Reference Guide to Consent for Examination or Treatment* (2001b: 19, para 15) suggests that parents may give consent for their child to be entered into a trial, if the trial therapy is at least as beneficial as the standard therapy. When a child refuses consent to medical treatment Bridgeman (1998) highlights the cases where the courts have been reluctant to accept these consequences and overridden the autonomous refusal. Montgomery (2001: 178) argues that: 'There is no clear indication that the parental power to override a child's refusal would exist in relationship to research'. He outlines the presumption against child research that involves three principles: children should not be included in studies when the data can be obtained from adults; as much information as possible should be obtained from adult studies and risks assessed before children are involved; if research is necessary older children who can consent (or refuse) should be approached for participation.

It is unlikely that qualitative researchers would be undertaking therapeutic research and clinical trials. They may however wish to interview children about participation in these or the process of making decisions concerning medical treatment. For example, Priscilla Alderson, a social researcher, has made a particular contribution in the field of children's choices in health care (1993, 1995; Alderson and Montgomery, 1996) and children's rights (2000). She discovered in her research concerning children's consent to surgery (1993) that young children are often competent in their understanding of the consequence of clinical procedures. One example given is of a seven-year old girl weighing up the risks and benefits of a combined heart–lung transplant and choosing to be placed on a transplant list knowing it may not happen in time or may be unsuccessful (Alderson, 1993: 162–3). Alderson (2000: 83) supports the use of qualitative research methods arguing that they take a 'rainbow approach' allowing for exploration of differences in each child and circumstances that can improve understanding and empathy.

There are also particular issues to be considered when carrying out research with frail older people (Harris and Dyson, 2001). It is difficult for some, though by no means all, members of this group to give fully informed consent as they might be prevented from doing so by ill health, chronic disease or fatigue. Even factors such as size of writing in the information sheet or consent form or the clarity of the researcher's voice are important, as is the potential participant's ability to understand the information and to concentrate on it. Older people are sometimes loath to commit themselves to being interviewed for research purposes and must therefore be recruited with care and diplomacy.

Harris and Dyson add among other suggestions:

- Researchers should not underestimate difficulties in recruiting vulnerable older people
- Researchers need to develop skills in recruiting members of this group while also protecting their rights to refuse to take part
- Researchers should attempt to obtain genuine consent in a study

The basic ethical framework for research

Historically, attempts at establishing international rules for ethical research stem from the time after the Second World War, as a result of the criminal trials in Germany. The Nuremberg Code contained guidelines for consent and discontinuation of studies and advised on the balance between risks and benefits. Most of these rules were concerned with experimental research. The World Medical Association's Declaration of Helsinki (1964, revised 1975, 1983, 1989, 1996 and 2000) replaces the Nuremberg Code and has 32 paragraphs arranged into three sections:

A   Introduction
B   Basic Principles for All Medical Research
C   Additional Principles for Medical Research Combined with Medical Care

Although the terminology used references medical research and human subjects the Declaration is for all research investigators and research participants. Indeed the latest revision (2000) strengthens aspects of informed consent (paras 21–6) and paragraph 20 states 'subjects must be volunteers and informed participants in the research project'.

To appreciate specific features of ethics in qualitative and other research it is important to understand the philosophical assumptions on which they are based. Ethics originates from the Greek word *ethos*, meaning character (Tschudin, 1992) and refers to both individual character and ways of behaving. It is a branch of philosophy concerning value and there are two approaches in ethics: the *normative* approach (what we should do) and the *descriptive* approach (what we actually do).

Nursing and midwifery ethics take primarily the normative approach that is concerned with guiding professionals to 'safeguard the interest and well-being of patients and clients' (UKCC 1992). In order to achieve this, researchers need sufficient background in professional studies that focus on ethical and legal aspects of the professional–client relationship. Therefore, more than information about ethical codes is required. The researcher needs to draw on ethical principles and rules and balance these in the research process. Key ethicists in this field are Beauchamp and Childress (2001) in their work *Principles of Biomedical Ethics*, now in its fifth edition. They view ethics as a generic term for both understanding and examining the moral life (Beauchamp and Childress, 2001: 1). Much of their early work has been popularised in the UK by Gillon (1985) in his classic work *Philosophical Medical Ethics* and, despite the references to medical ethics, both texts involve all healthcare practice and practitioners. Beauchamp and Childress have developed their model of ethical reasoning over the course of their publications and since the first edition of their book. In their latest edition (2001) they emphasise a framework of moral norms that encompass principles, rules, rights, virtues and moral ideals. They outline four basic principles as pivotal to this framework:

(1) The principle of respect for autonomy (a norm of respecting the decision making capacities of autonomous persons)
(2) The principle of nonmaleficence (a norm of avoiding the causation of harm)
(3) The principle of beneficence (a group of norms for providing benefits and balancing benefits against risks and costs)
(4) The principle of justice (a group of norms for distributing benefits, risks, and costs fairly)

Respect for autonomy (from the Greek *autos*, self; *nomos*, law) means that the participants in the research must be allowed to make a free, independent and informed choice without coercion. The counterpart in law of this principle is the right of self determination (as stated above) and it underpins the notion of informed consent and refusal. It is often placed first in an ethical framework to focus ethicists, practitioners and researchers on the primary concern of respecting an individual's self rule. Yet Beauchamp and Childress (2001) do not assert that the principle of respect for autonomy overrides all other ethical considerations. Their concept of respect for autonomy aims not to be 'excessive' in three areas:

(1) Individualistic (ignoring the social nature of individuals and the impact of their choices and behaviour on others)
(2) On reason (ignoring the emotions)
(3) Legalistic (focusing mainly on legal rights and neglecting social practices)

As research is conducted for the benefit of individuals, patients, users, care professionals and the public in general (DoH, 2001a: para 2.4.1) these are pertinent features in the extension of considerations of this principle. Yet as the

Department of Health makes clear, the primary consideration in any research study is preserving the dignity, rights, safety and well being of participants (DoH, 2001a: para 2.2.1). Further it states 'Informed consent is at the heart of ethical research. All studies must have appropriate arrangements for obtaining informed consent and the ethics review process must pay particular attention to those arrangements' (DoH, 2001a: para 2.2.3). The interface between human rights and medical research is examined by Sommerville (2001). She argues that research ethics and human rights coincide in emphasising the centrality of participation in research through informed consent. Yet Sommerville points out that researchers need to balance the health needs of the whole population, with individual rights and this is sometimes a 'fragile' balance.

The principles of beneficence and nonmaleficence for research means that the good derived must be weighed against the potential harm, and the benefits must outweigh the risks for the individual and the wider society. The Declaration of Helsinki (see WMA, 2000: para 16) states: 'Every medical research project involving human subjects should be preceded by careful assessment of predictable risks and burdens in comparison with foreseeable benefits to the subject or others'. The Department of Health (2001a: para 2.2.8) acknowledges that an element of risk may be present in some research but that this should be kept to a minimum and fully explained to participants and ethics committees.

The principle of justice implies that the research strategies and procedures are fair and just. Increasingly fairness in research includes a proper representation in research samples and in a multi-cultural society research should take account of this (DoH, 2001a). Further the researcher must respect the diversity (age, gender, disability and sexual orientation) in human culture (DoH, 2001a: para 2.2.7). Significantly Sommerville (2001) shows that there has been a shift from protecting people from research intervention to campaigns to include them, such as in HIV treatment studies in Africa and Asia. Inclusion for treatment benefit is an important aspect of the principle of justice in research. This needs far more exposure and explanation in research studies especially in terms of fairness and access, particularly between so-called 'developed' and 'underdeveloped' countries.

In their ethical framework, Beauchamp and Childress (2001) specify ethical rules, although there is a loose distinction between rules and principles in the operation of these. They argue that rules are more specific giving more precise action guides. These will be examined in relation to research as set out below:

- Veracity (truth-telling)
- Privacy
- Confidentiality
- Fidelity (faithfulness)

Veracity in health care involves an accurate flow of information that is comprehensive and takes account of the patient's understanding. These features are naturally important for gaining participation in research studies and informed consent. Linking this rule with the principle of respect for autonomy it can be shown that clearly, telling the truth is part of that respect. Lying would simply not respect the autonomy of the individual and would impede the decision-making process. Similarly questions of veracity are necessary in terms of disclosure and nondisclosure of information. An individual cannot make a fully informed decision about participation in research if some information is withheld. This can be problematic however with respect to the flexibility of qualitative research methods as shown below.

Privacy is also part of the principle of respect for autonomy. Drawing on the work of Allen (1997) Beauchamp and Childress (2001) highlight five forms of privacy:

(1) Informational (a main focus in health care)
(2) Physical (personal space)
(3) Decisional (personal choices)
(4) Proprietary (genetic interests, tissue samples)
(5) Relational or associational (family and other significant persons)

For research, informational privacy is important. Researchers must respect this and that is why it is closely linked with the rule of confidentiality. Yet the other forms of privacy may well be important considerations, depending on the particulars of the research study. Article 8 of the European Convention on Human Rights, as stated above, provides a right to respect for private and family life, which gives legal force via the 1998 Human Rights Act to this ethical rule. The Declaration of Helsinki (WMA, 2000) as well, at paragraph 21, states: 'Every precaution should be taken to respect the privacy of the subject, the confidentiality of the patient's information and to minimize the impact of the study on the subject's physical and mental integrity and on the personality of the subject'.

Confidentiality in health care generally is recognised as underpinning the patient–practitioner relationship. Without such implicit expectations that information is kept confidential there would be no basis for trust in these encounters. Beauchamp and Childress (2001) highlight that one way of examining confidentiality is as a branch of informational privacy. Information disclosed in the course of health care or research must be protected. This information can only be given to a third party with the consent of the patient or research participant. Historically the ethical rule of confidentiality goes back to the Hippocratic oath and continues in the World Medical Association's Declaration of Geneva and The World Medical Association's International Code of Medical Ethics. The United Kingdom Central Council's *Code of Professional Conduct* (1992) devotes clause 10 to confidentiality. In the *Research Governance Framework* (DoH, 2001a), paragraph 2.2.5 highlights that the protection of patient data is paramount. Further the responsibility of all those involved in research to be aware of their ethical and legal duties and to ensure that systems are in place to protect confidentiality (DoH, 2001a).

Finally the ethical rule of fidelity concerns notions of faithfulness or loyalty. Beauchamp and Childress (2001) examine this rule in terms of conflicts of loyalty or conflicts of interest. They argue that traditionally, professional loyalty concerns giving priority to the patient's interests but this position has shifted. Third party interests, institutional interests and the changing profession of nursing have led to conflicts of interests and weakened traditional rules of fidelity. Significantly Beauchamp and Childress (2001) examine this rule with particular regard to research. They specifically examine aspects of conflicts of fidelity in clinical trials (such as the use of placebo controls, the problem of clinical equipoise and justifying conditions for randomised controlled trials), and highlight that fidelity conflicts can occur in both therapeutic and non-therapeutic research. The Declaration of Helsinki (WMA, 2000, para 22), states that the research participant must be informed of any institutional affiliations or possible conflicts of interest of the researcher. Returning to the *Research Governance Framework* (DoH, 2001a: para 3.6.3) it is quite clear that the first responsibility of the principal investigator is to ensure that: 'The dignity, rights, safety and well-being of participants are given priority at all times by the research team'. These values are enshrined in the ethical principles and rules specified in the ethical framework (Beauchamp and Childress, 2001) and outlined above.

The involvement of the researcher

Robinson and Thorne (1988) outline the dilemma of ethics in relation to qualitative healthcare research. They suggest four major issues: *informed consent, influence, immersion* and *intervention*. Informed consent is recognised as problematic in qualitative research because data collection and analysis occur simultaneously, and whilst consent may be implied at one stage of the research, it cannot be assumed at another stage when the researcher's objectives change on the basis of the information provided.

Influence in research means a process of changing something whilst studying it. Researchers influence the research and its findings. Qualitative researchers recognise clearly that biases occur and attempt to make these explicit in the report. The researcher as the major data-gathering tool must uncover the thought processes that lead to the findings. The findings are then explained within the social and interactional context of the research process. Nurses and midwives must account for the influences of their professional perspectives in the process and outcome of the research.

The third issue mentioned by Robinson and Thorne (1988) refers to immersion. Qualitative research requires the researcher to become immersed in the data. This immersion generates familiarity with the setting, the process and the world of the participants. Through this involvement, a certain amount of subjectivity may occur. As data collection and analysis are taking place at the same time, a measure of objectivity – standing back from the data – is needed. Robinson and Thorne suggest that health professionals engaged in qualitative research have to develop strategies to balance the subjective and objective elements inherent in immersion. They advocate that researchers describe how the tension between these elements was managed.

Intervention is perhaps the most contentious dilemma in qualitative research. The issue concerns the reality of the health professionals' clinical roles. Most research has no immediate result and researchers cannot easily intervene, but the tension between professional and researcher roles still exists.

One of us experienced all these aspects in her research (Wheeler, 1992). The following are the issues that arose in the study. Following ethical approval of the research proposal, individual informed consent was obtained from participating practitioners who reflected on their involvement in some distressing cases of child abuse (identities were not disclosed) that at times caused them to reconsider their participation in the research.

The ethical problem of influence in this study was concerned with the researcher's particular interest and experience in child protection work. It was impossible to 'bracket' out this background entirely. Rather, the aim was to express this as part of the research and make these experiences explicit in the report.

Immersion of the researcher in the data naturally caused tensions between the lived experiences of the research informants (which could be interpreted subjectively) and the emergence of potential new ideas about communication breakdowns (which could be expressed objectively). To resolve these differing perspectives the researcher had to describe how these were managed in the research process.

Intervention (the term that Robinson and Thorne suggest) was a contentious issue in this study. The researcher had both a previous practice and management role. Some themes that emerged from the data had immediate implications for current child protection work. Yet ethically it was not appropriate to intervene in practice structures prior to a completion of the study and critical analysis of the findings by others.

The implications of these issues for qualitative research mean continuous involvement of both project supervisors and colleagues in the research. Robinson and Thorne suggest that there should be an ongoing assessment in data gathering with others monitoring field notes and transcriptions. In student projects this means involvement and advice of the supervisor at all stages of the research.

Ethical problems and considerations

The question of ethics in qualitative healthcare research is complex and problematic. Qualitative researchers have to consider a variety of issues.

(1) Researchers explore the inner feelings and thoughts of the participants who are clients, colleagues or other health professionals, and they have to act with sensitivity and diplomacy.
(2) Informed consent is problematic as participants cannot be fully informed at the very beginning because of the tentative and exploratory nature of qualitative research.
(3) The informants' anonymity might be threatened by the detailed description of the research process, the data and the sample.
(4) The vulnerable position of clients and their feelings of obligation might prevent them from refusing participation in the research, although they may not actually wish to participate.
(5) The researcher has conflicting role expectations as investigator and professional.
(6) Participants do not always comprehend the research role of health professionals and see them primarily as carers.
(7) Patients may become fearful and distressed during interviews.
(8) Over-involvement and empathy could create assumptions and inaccuracies in the research.
(9) Ethics committees do not always fully understand the character of qualitative research.

Issues with informed consent and voluntary participation

Informed, voluntary consent is an explicit agreement by the research participants, given without threat or inducement and based on information which any reasonable person would want to receive before consenting to participate (Sieber, 1992).

Qualitative researchers have inherent problems with informed consent. When the research begins, they have no specific objectives for the research, though they may have general aims or a focus. The nature of qualitative research is its flexibility, the use of unexpected ideas arising during data collection and the prompts that are allowed during interviews. Qualitative research focuses on the meanings and interpretation of the participants. The researcher develops ideas that are grounded in the data rather than testing previously constructed hypotheses. Therefore, the researcher is not able to inform research participants of the exact path of the research, and informed consent is not a once and forever permission but an ongoing process of informed participation (Ford and Reutter, 1990).

The process of informed consent is set firmly within the principle of respect for autonomy. This principle demands that participation is voluntary and that informants are aware not only of the benefits of the research but also of the risks they take. First-time researchers, in particular, should take care that there is no major risk involved, though all research involves some dangers. Participants must be informed throughout about the voluntary nature of participation in research and about the possibility of withdrawing at any stage. This should be shown in the consent form (Fig. 3.1; see also Chapter 2 for a less specific consent form).

It is useful to anticipate potential problems in the course of the research and consider their solutions. The researcher must be aware that the research might threaten participants, superiors or institutions, even if it is intended to have a positive effect. Sim (1991) identifies a major dilemma of researchers: they experience conflict between the recognition of the rights of human beings and the wish to advance professional knowledge.

The researcher should try to be as clear as possible in stating the demands on the time of the participants and about the direction of the research so that they can agree or refuse to take part on the basis of information about it. Sometimes this might be difficult as the status of a health professional could prevent patients or colleagues from giving honest, open and non-biased answers.

Patients are in a particularly vulnerable position as they are ill and because of the perceived imbalance of power in their relationship with health professionals. Midwives' clients, too, are in a situation in which they have limited power. Researchers have to weigh benefits and risks of the research. Health professionals assess benefits of the project that might help future patients and clients, and they consider the risks involved for research participants.

Example

Consider a nurse who wishes to interview patients with a serious illness about their feelings and the support they receive. The study will almost certainly help in the future because of extended knowledge and information that nurses have gained. Patients, however, may well feel distressed and disturbed by the nurse's probing into private thoughts and feelings at a time when they experience pain, distress and anxiety about their future.

It can be seen that timing is an important issue in qualitative research (Cowles, 1988). Bad timing can inhibit informants, especially when they have recently had a traumatic experience. They might feel threatened at this particular time and too emotionally involved to make rational decisions about taking part or continuing the research. Qualitative interviews in particular can provoke distressing memories, and the researcher should be prepared to allow the participant to work through this and not abruptly terminate the interview.

CONSENT FORM

Wessex University
Faculty of Health Studies

15 St. John's Rd, Williamstown
Telephone: 03344 123 4567

Whetstone Hospital
Pain Clinic
St. Mary's Rd
Williamstown
Tel. 03344 788 899

January 1 2002

Dear Mrs Smith,

Re: People's experiences of back pain

I am a nurse currently studying people's experiences of back pain for my research degree at Wessex University. I understand from the doctor in the pain clinic that you have experienced lower back pain for some time and wonder if you would mind sharing your experiences with me. You will have met me before as I have been working in the clinic.

I do not necessarily wish to know the full details of any problems you may have had, but I am interested to know your feelings and experiences since you have had the back problem. I do not have a specific list of questions to ask, but would like you to describe your experience of having back pain in your own words. I anticipate that this will take up to an hour, depending on how much you have to tell.

I would like to tape-record our conversation so that I do not miss important details. Everything that you say will be treated in the strictest confidence. Your name and details will not appear in the research report, the tapes will be destroyed after use, and no information will be passed to any other person or agency without your express consent. The interview may take place in your home, in the clinic or in an office at the university, whichever you prefer.

If you are willing to talk to me, please return the attached consent form giving your name, address and telephone number so that I can contact you to make an appointment. If you would like further information please contact me on the telephone number at the top of this page. Please do not feel any pressure to participate – I fully understand if you prefer not to and your decision will not in any way affect your future treatment or care.

Thank you for reading this letter. I look forward to meeting you in due course, should you decide to accept this invitation.

Yours sincerely,

Janet Doe
Nurse specialist and research student

My manager's name is Christina Rie
Whetstone Hospital
Address as above

Fig. 3.1 Consent form (*Continued on next page*)

CONSENT FORM

People's experiences of lower back pain

I am quite happy for Janet Doe to interview me about my experiences of back pain.

I understand that everything I say will be treated in the strictest confidence, that I am completely free to withdraw from the study at any time I choose without any need for explanation, and that such a decision will not affect any aspect of my future treatment or care.

NAME (please print):

SIGNATURE:

ADDRESS:

TELEPHONE NUMBER:

The best time to contact me is:

Fig. 3.1 (Continued)

Example

A researcher was conducting lengthy interviews in the participants' own homes to find out how they coped with chronic pain. Towards the end, one woman became very upset when she described how her religious faith did not seem strong enough to help her to come to terms with her pain and disability. The researcher, who had no religious affiliation of her own, spent the next three hours persuading the participant that God did not demand perfection. The participant gradually responded positively and was left in a positive frame of mind. Indeed, she later wrote a note of thanks to the researcher.

Walker, 1989

Informants are not always aware of their rights to refuse participation in the research, particularly if it lasts over a long period of time, and when unexpected elements arise. The researcher must understand the feeling of obligation that participants might have. Often they feel powerless to deny the researchers access to their world.

Platt (1981) states that in interview situations informants are often in a position of inequality. Colleagues and other health workers have more choice in accepting or rejecting participation because they are generally in a situation of power equal or similar to that of the researcher. When researchers interview and observe their peers, a more reciprocal relationship exists which makes it easier for participants to become equal partners in the research enterprise – the aim, of course, of most qualitative research. 'Researching one's peers' may mean, however, that researchers sometimes impose a framework, which is based on the assumption of shared perceptions and does not allow informants to develop their own ideas.

Anonymity and confidentiality

Qualitative healthcare research might be more intrusive than quantitative research; therefore, the researcher needs sensitivity and communication skills. Usually, anonymity is guaranteed, and a promise is given that identities will not be revealed. Qualitative researchers work with small samples, and it is not always easy to protect identities. Even a detailed job description or an unusual occupational title of an informant may destroy anonymity. Geertz (1973) uses the term *thick description* as one of the characteristics of this type of research, meaning that everything is described in great detail, which might uncover the identity of the informant; this is why researchers must take care in the process.

Example

The research of one of our students involved just one man; all other participants were women. She did not mention anything that could have identified him. Fortunately no gender issues arose which would have been important for the study, because the student could not have discussed these without disclosing the identity of the participant.

Mayo, 1993

Researchers sometimes change minor details so that informants cannot be recognised. For instance, researchers may change the age of all participants by two or three years when age is not an important factor in the research (Archbold, 1986).

Only the researcher should be able to match the real names and identities with the tapes, report or description, and participants are given numbers or pseudonyms. Tapes, notes and transcriptions – important tools for the qualitative researcher – must be kept secure, and names should be not be located near the tapes. If other people, superiors, supervisors or typists have access to the information – however limited this might be – names should not be disclosed, participants' identities must be disguised, and they should be asked for permission. Videotapes, too, must be kept safe as participants are recognisable.

The researcher's dilemma is to decide what information can be made public; if there is doubt or ambiguity, the decision depends upon the client's wishes. Some informants may allow details to be given about them which would identify them to some people, but this can create problems for the researcher; discussing these issues with the informants can therefore be useful. Patton (1990) suggests that tapes should be erased a year after the research has been finished, but some ethics committees demand that they be kept for ten years. We erased our tapes soon after the research was finished because that was the wish of the participants.

Confidentiality is a separate issue from anonymity but also very important. In research where words and ideas from participants are used, full confidentiality cannot be promised. In these studies, confidentiality means that they keep confidential that which the participant does not wish to disclose to others. Patients, in particular, sometimes disclose intimate details of their lives which the researcher cannot divulge, although the information could be useful for the research.

The dual role

Fowler (1989) focuses on role conflict in qualitative research. Nurses and midwives have a dual role and responsibility, that of professional and that of researcher, and they may experience problems of identity. On the one hand they are committed to the research as they wish to advance health knowledge for the good of their clients and recognise that nursing and midwifery can only be professions if they become research based. On the other hand, nurses and midwives are dedicated to the care and welfare of clients. Health professionals cannot close their eyes to distress and pain because their professional training guides them towards being carers and advocates for their clients. Fowler stresses that nurses have a duty to their patients first, as the profession mainly exists for its clients. If informants are threatened by the research or feel that they are, then the professional has to give up the researcher role.

Nurses and midwives must be clear not only about their own identity but also about that of the client which may pose a dilemma. In the professional role, they recognise the person as patient or client while in their researcher role they see the person as informant, as participant in the research. The different elements of the professional identity cannot always be reconciled. Clients, too, do not always understand this duality and dichotomy in the health worker's role. They expect care and help from the person whom they perceive as a nurse or midwife and who professes to be a researcher.

Smith (1992) and Wilde (1992) stress the researcher's role as one of investigation rather than one of counselling or educating. Adopting the counselling or therapeutic role might shift the power balance and destroy the essential character of qualitative research which is based on equality between researcher and informant. Clients must recognise that professional intervention by the researcher is not always possible. Nevertheless, health professionals cannot completely detach themselves from their informants, particularly in the close relationship of the qualitative research process. They respond to distress and need, especially in emergency situations, or call on colleagues who perform caring roles in the setting.

Example

One of our students, an experienced nurse who worked on a renal dialysis unit, interviewed a number of individuals about kidney transplant failures that had happened in the preceding year. Although the participants welcomed the interviews, as they wanted to share their experiences, they also occasionally became distressed, as the failure was an emotional event for them. Our student recognised this and followed the first principle of ethical research, never to leave a participant in distress.

Mayo, 1993

If nurses find strong distress, there is need for a mechanism for following up the participants. For instance, perhaps a form of counselling could be built into the study. Robinson and Thorne (1988) state that the rights of the informants are more important than the interests of the researcher. Any interventions, however, should be made explicit in the research report.

Qualitative researchers must consider additional issues, which are somewhat different from those of quantitative research. Power relationships might affect the research.

Example

Seibold et al. (1994) recount research experiences Seibold had when interviewing a group of women in midlife. She found that the participants revealed parts of their lives that were highly personal. The women themselves were surprised about these revelations, and the researcher had to be very sensitive about the interviews. This demonstrates that consent given before the interview cannot be taken for granted and must be confirmed afterwards without putting pressure on the participants.

Mander (1988) claims that patients are particularly vulnerable because they are 'a captive population'. While official documents focus on the rights of patients, research in nursing and midwifery often deals with people who have little real power in their situation. The power balance is perhaps more equal in the client's own setting than in the hospital situation.

Patients and clients rarely refuse when asked to take part in research, as they feel dependent on the goodwill of carers. Because of the power differential, Archbold (1986) suggests that health professionals do not do research with people directly in their care. Occasionally, however, this cannot be avoided as the research might have been generated by a problem in the professional's own setting. Students do not always have access to settings other than their own.

Patients, of course, are vulnerable. Children, people with learning difficulties and those who have a mental or terminal illness need particular protection. Researchers are obliged to ask parents or legal guardians for permission to research, as well as the participants. Experienced health professionals only should undertake research with these groups after careful consideration.

Empathy and research mindedness

A research study requires both empathy and distancing. These traits appear contradictory. On the one hand, the researchers are asked to be non-judgemental and must be aware of personal values that could influence the research. On the other, health carers often have empathy and feeling for their clients. However involved, the researcher cannot allow preconceived attitudes or over-involvement to influence the data. This can be problematic because of the close relationship between the researcher and the participants. Researchers must be able to put themselves into the informant's place; this helps to establish the rapport that is important in this type of approach. The researcher might therefore experience intense emotions. Qualitative research into sensitive topics generates these problems to a greater extent than any other type. Perhaps support for researchers is needed, for example they could co-counsel each other when doing this sort of research.

Interviews, in particular, may deeply affect participants who do not just reveal their experiences and thoughts to the researcher but also might become aware of hidden feelings themselves for the first time. The interview, in this case, can change the life of the informant, although the initial aim of the researcher is the collection of data, which may or may not bring about future change in the setting (Patton, 1990). Towards the end of the research project another problem arises: the continuous, intimate nature of the interviewer–informant relationship generates trust and sometimes friendship; therefore, it is difficult for both researcher and participant to extricate themselves from it. A sensitive researcher does not leave the patient anxious or worried. May (1991) suggests the 'debriefing' of informants and the provision of emotional support if this is needed. This can be important for the interviewer who might find these conversations distressing and stressful.

Research interviews can, of course, be therapeutic although therapy is not the purpose of the interview. Lofland and Lofland (1995) suggest that there is often a *quid pro quo* in research. The researcher gains knowledge from informants who, in turn, find patient listeners for their feelings and thoughts. This means that reciprocity exists. Walker (1989), in her study on pain, relates that patients welcomed an opportunity to talk and found it beneficial.

Ethical questions arise in observation, too. Covert observation is problematic and its ethics debatable. Sapsford and Abbot (1992) suggest that in this type of research participants are sometimes deceived and exploited. Researchers in the field of health care generally disclose their presence as observers and reveal the purpose of the observation. However, this may generate the observer effect – the change that observers may bring about in the setting through their presence. Patton (1990) suggests that the effect is overestimated, as participants often forget the presence of the researcher. In any case, clients and colleagues generally trust the health professional to behave ethically.

Sometimes, however, non-disclosure of certain facts minimises the researcher effect.

Example

A ward sister wanted to explore bedside handover on her own ward from the patients' point of view. She explained this to her colleagues.

She intended to interview patients who had experienced several handovers about their feelings regarding them, but felt that disclosure of her position in authority would bias the research. Patients might not be comfortable talking to a ward sister about matters that involved her colleagues and might feel obliged to give positive comments only.

Much debate about ethical issues took place between the researcher, her colleagues and her supervisor. In the end she asked patients' permission for interviews in her role as nurse researcher but did not disclose her ward sister role until the completion of individual interviews and gave patients the opportunity to opt out of the research. She did not lie about her position and would have disclosed it, had she been asked. The researcher felt that in this way she did not compromise the veracity of the research, which would be accurate and truthful.

Waltho, 1992

Not everybody agreed with the solution to the problem in the above example, but researchers must often make difficult decisions after balancing advantages and disadvantages of certain procedures. This form of initial deception is only justifiable because it produces accurate data without harming the informants. Sieber (1992: 64, 65) states: 'If it is to be acceptable at all, deception should not involve people in ways that members of the subject population would find unacceptable'. In the above example, all informants remained in the research.

The nurse or midwife researcher has conflicting roles, that of health professional and that of researcher. The search for rich and deep data may cause distress but informants should not be left worried or anxious because of their participation in the research. It can be seen that nurses and midwives who attempt qualitative projects in clinical settings have to construct a complex ethical framework for the research which is all the more important when dealing with patients and clients.

Summary

Researchers should always abide by the principles below.

- Apart from seeking access to the setting from gatekeepers and ethics committees, the researchers also, and most importantly, ask permission from participants.
- The principles of ethical conduct must be followed and the rights and wishes of participants must be respected throughout the research, particularly the right of informed consent or refusal to take part.
- Consent involves the legal right of self-determination in common law and further rights are given legal force in the Human Rights Act 1998.
- The principles and rules in the ethical framework are expressed as well in the Declaration of Helsinki and the *Research Governance Framework* and must be adhered to.
- The 'dignity, rights, safety and wellbeing of participants' are paramount. They apply to veracity, privacy, anonymity and confidentiality, and fidelity and must be respected by the researcher.
- Vulnerable individuals and groups such as children require particular legal and ethical considerations.
- Participation can only be voluntary and the informants should be able to withdraw from the research, if they so wish, at any time.

References

Alderson, P. (1993) *Children's Consent to Surgery*. Buckingham, Open University Press.

Alderson, P. (1995) *Listening to Children: Ethics and Social Research*. Barkingside, Barnardo's.

Alderson, P. (2000) *Young Children's Rights: Exploring Beliefs, Principles and Practice*. London, Jessica Kingsley Publishers.

Alderson, P. & Montgomery, J. (1996) *Health Care Choices: Making Decisions with Children*. London, Institute for Public Policy Research.

Allen, A.L. (1997) Genetic privacy: emerging concepts and values. In *Genetic Secrets: Protecting Privacy and Confidentiality in the Genetic Era* (ed. M.A. Rothstein), pp. 31–59. New Haven, Yale University Press.

Archbold, P. (1986) Ethical issues in qualitative research. In *From Practice to Grounded Theory: Qualitative Research in Nursing* (eds W.C. Cheritz & J.M. Swanson), pp. 155–63. Menlo Park, Addison-Wesley.

Beauchamp, T.L. & Childress, J.F. (2001) *Principles of Biomedical Ethics*. 5th edn. York, Oxford University Press.

Bridgeman, J. (1998) Because we care? The medical treatment of children. In *Feminist Perspectives on Health Care Law* (eds S. Sheldon & M. Thomson), pp. 97–114. London, Cavendish Publishing.

Cowles, K.V. (1988) Issues in qualitative research on sensitive topics. *Western Journal of Nursing Research*, **10** (2) 163–79.

Department of Health (2001a) *Research Governance Framework for Health and Social Care*. London, Department of Health. www.doh.gov.uk/research/RD3/nhsrandd/researchgovernance.htm

Department of Health (2001b) *Reference Guide to Consent for Examination or Treatment*. London, Department of Health. www.doh.gov.uk/consent

Fennell, P. (2001) Informed consent and clinical research in psychiatry. In *Informed Consent in Medical Research* (eds L. Doyal & S. Tobias), pp. 182–92. London, BMJ Books.

Ford, J.S. & Reutter, L.I. (1990) Ethical dilemmas associated with small samples. *Journal of Advanced Nursing*, **15**, 187–91.

Fowler, M.D.M. (1988) Ethical issues in nursing research: issues in qualitative research. *Western Journal of Nursing Research*, **10**, 109–11.

Garwood-Gowers, A. & Tingle, J. (2001) The Human Rights Act 1998: a potent tool for changing health care law and practice. In *Healthcare Law: The Impact of the Human Rights Act* (eds A.J. Garwood-Gowers Tingle & T. Lewis), pp. 1–12. London, Cavendish Publishing.

Geertz, C. (1973) *The Interpretation of Cultures*. New York, Basic Books.

Gillon, R. (1985) *Philosophical Medical Ethics*. Chichester, John Wiley & Sons.

Harris, R. & Dyson, E. (2001) Recruitment of frail older people to research: lessons learnt through experience. *Journal of Advanced Nursing*, **36** (5) 643–51.

Learning from Bristol (2001) The Report of the Public Inquiry into Children's Heart Surgery at the Bristol Royal Infirmary 1984–1995. The Stationery Office, Cm 5207, London.

Lofland, J. & Lofland, L. (1995) *Analysing Social Settings*, 3rd edn. Belmont CA, Wadsworth.

Mander, R. (1988) Encouraging students to be research minded. *Nurse Education Today*, **8**, 30–35.

May, K.A. (1991) Interview techniques in qualitative research: concerns and challenges. In *Qualitative Nursing Research: A Contemporary Dialogue*, Revised edn (ed. J.M. Morse), pp. 188–201. London, Sage.

Mayo, A. (1993) *The Meaning of Transplant Failure*. Unpublished BSc project, Bournemouth, Bournemouth University.

McHale, J. & Fox, M. with Murphy, J. (1997) *Health Care Law: Text with Materials*. London, Sweet and Maxwell.

Medical Research Council (1991) *Issues in Research with Children*. London, Medical Research Council.

Montgomery, J. (1997) *Healthcare Law*. Oxford, Oxford University Press.

Montgomery, J. (2001) Informed consent and clinical research with children. In *Informed Consent In Medical Research* (eds L. Doyal & S. Tobias), pp. 173–81. London, BMJ Books.

Patton, M.Q. (1990) *Qualitative Evaluation and Research Methods*, 2nd edn. London, Sage.

Platt, J. (1981) On interviewing one's peers. *British Journal of Sociology*, **32** (1) 75–91.

Robinson, C.A. & Thorne, S.E. (1988) Dilemmas of ethics and validity in qualitative nursing research. *The Canadian Journal of Nursing Research*, **20**, 65–76.

Royal College of Physicians (1996) *Guidelines on the practice of ethics committees in medical research involving human subjects*, 3rd edn. London, Royal College of Physicians.

Sapsford, R. & Abbot, P. (1992) *Research Methods for Nurses and the Caring Professions*. Buckingham, Open University Press.

Seibold, C., Richards, L. & Simon, D. (1994) Feminist method and qualitative research about midlife. *Journal of Advanced Nursing*, **19**, 394–402.

Sieber, J.E. (1992) *Planning Ethically Responsible Research*. London, Sage.

Sim, J. (1991) Nursing research: Is there an obligation to participate? *Journal of Advanced Nursing*, **16**, 1284–9.

Smith, L. (1992) Ethical issues in interviewing. *Journal of Advanced Nursing*, **17**, 98–103.

Sommerville, A. (2001) Informed consent and human rights in medical research. In *Informed Consent in Medical Research* (eds L. Doyal & S. Tobias), Chapter 24, pp. 249–56. London, BMJ Books.

The Human Rights Act 1998 http://www.hmso.gov.uk/acts/1998/19980042.htm

The Royal Liverpool Children's Inquiry: Summary and Recommendations (2001) http://www.rlcinquiry.org.uk

Tschudin, V. (1992) *Ethics in Nursing: The Caring Relationship*, 2nd edn. Oxford, Butterworth Heinemann.

United Kingdom Central Council for Nursing, Midwifery and Health Visiting (1992) *Code of Professional Conduct*, 3rd edn. June.

Walker, J. (1989) *The Management of Elderly Patients with Pain: A Community Nursing Perspective*. Unpublished PhD thesis, Bournemouth, Bournemouth University.

Waltho, B.J. (1992) *Perception of the Nurse–Patient Relationship: Patients' Perceptions of Bedside Handover*. BSc project, Bournemouth Polytechnic (now Bournemouth University), Bournemouth.

Wheeler, S.J. (1992) Perceptions of child abuse. *Health Visitor*, **65** (9) 316–19.

Wilde, V. (1992) Controversial hypotheses on the relationship between researcher and informant in qualitative research. *Journal of Advanced Nursing*, **17**, 234–42.

World Medical Association (2000) *Declaration of Helsinki: Ethical Principles for Medical Research Involving Human Subjects*, 52 WMA General Assembly. Edinburgh, Canary Publications.

CHAPTER 4

Supervision in Qualitative Research

The importance of the supervisor

The supervisor is the most important support and critic during the research process. Supervisors oversee the research project, dissertation or thesis and give advice on the research topic, methodology and other research issues as well as guiding and supporting students through the process and the rules of the university.

Although supervision may differ according to circumstances – that is, the type of research, the topic as well as the level of study and experience of students – the principles remain similar for different students and types of research. The experience and expertise of the supervisors and their relationships with students will affect the success of the study. Delamont *et al.* (1997) stress the importance of the relationship between supervisor and researcher.

Supervisors have some responsibility for the quality and completion of the research project, for ensuring that students define and achieve aims and objectives and an obligation to the student to support and advise.

> The ultimate responsibility lies with the students; they are in charge of their own research.

Sometimes students can choose their own supervisors, after deciding on the research topic, from a given list of potential tutors and containing their specific interest and expertise. Both student and supervisor should feel comfortable with the topic and the relationship. Sometimes a programme leader allocates supervisors according to their particular expertise in research methods and/or because of their knowledge of the field. Sometimes students are able to choose a tutor with whom they can work, who is seen as helpful and supportive or whom they respect as a knowledgeable professional. Perhaps this is the most useful criterion, as the students will eventually become expert in their own research.

For supervisors, too, the match between them and the student is important because of the close connections that they will develop over time. The style of supervision will develop throughout the research process. Some students, for example, like having a highly structured timetable and want to be directed or organised by their supervisors, others are self-directed and see supervisors as an informal sounding board. The style of supervision has to be negotiated during the stages of the research. The stage of the research, whether at the start or towards completion and also the level of research – undergraduate or postgraduate – make a difference. Undergraduates and researchers starting out obviously need more guidance.

The responsibilities of supervisor and student

Supervisors and students have a common aim: to achieve a study of high standard that will be completed on time. Both student and supervisor(s) should be committed to the contract of respectively carrying out and supporting the research. The supervisor generally guides and advises rather than directs, except in circumstances where the student acts contrary to ethical or research guidelines.

Supervisor and student will have to negotiate the relationship from the beginning of the study. The frequency of contact depends on the student's needs and the stage in the research process. This can be negotiated at the beginning of the research and revised at intervals. Generally the student needs most help and support at the start and then again at the stage of writing up. Nevertheless, it is necessary for students to be in touch regularly rather than erratically. Some people need to see the supervisor often, others enjoy working on their own, though they too need feedback and constructive criticism. There should be a systematic and structured programme of work that forms the basis for the student–supervisor work relationship, but the instigation for this programme should come from students themselves.

The responsibility for contacting supervisors rests largely with students; indeed Cryer (1996) suggests that legally the responsibility to inform the supervisor of problems and getting in touch with them is likely to be the student's. Telephone contact can be useful, especially when a student experiences an academic or even a personal problem that affects the smooth process of the research.

Sharp and Howard (1996) advise students to inform the supervisor about the questions and problems they have in advance of a meeting. This means that both student and supervisor are prepared for the meeting, saving precious time. Many students and supervisors keep written notes on the supervision meetings; this is useful as a basis for further appointments and makes meetings more systematic and methodical. The supervisor generally advises the student to come with questions and problems. Most supervisors become involved and interested in the students' research topics. Students have the right to expect this interest.

Students do not always want to start writing after the start of the data collection; they believe that much of the research is 'in their head'. In our experience this is a fallacy, and it is useful to start writing early. The supervisor often asks for chapters on background, literature review and methodology, depending on the type of research. This ensures that students both understand the process and produce ideas that generate fresh motivation and interest, even though sections of the writing might have to be changed at a later stage. This way, students immerse themselves in the methodology, and some of the problems and pitfalls of the research become obvious and can be resolved at an early stage.

Often students are so enthusiastic about the research that they start data collection and analysis before becoming acquainted with the research methods. This can lead to inadequate interviewing and observation because methodological considerations have been neglected. Students must make sure that they are fully aware of the strategies, techniques and problems of their chosen research method. Indeed, students sometimes need a break so they can reflect on methods and topic.

Students sometimes find the writing up at the end an insurmountable task. The advice to start writing early will lessen this problem. The introduction, research strategies and writing up of ethical issues, might give direction to later chapters, and can be written quite early. If written work is sent to supervisors before a meeting, they are then able to give feedback and encouragement more easily. Students can expect that their supervisors have read the written work when they come for their pre-arranged supervision sessions, and that it will be criticised constructively. Sometimes supervisors may send their comments in writing to students before the meeting. Phillips and Pugh (2000) see the script as a basis for discussion. It is inadvisable to leave writing to the last stage of the research for two reasons: interesting and stimulating ideas will be forgotten and students might run out of time and hence panic. Seeing a chunk of the report in writing will motivate the student to proceed. All through the process, researchers make fieldnotes and memos as often as possible. The usefulness of carrying a small writing pad (as well as a field diary) to jot down ideas that arise cannot be underestimated.

Supervisors are not always gentle and diplomatic in their criticism; some students are easily hurt by it. The advice is best taken without seeing it as a personal attack but as an academic argument. In any case the relationship between supervisor and student develops over time as they learn about each other's weaknesses, strengths and idiosyncrasies, and both sides negotiate the process. The best supervisors are able to provide a supportive environment for students, draw out their ideas and are flexible and approachable (Phillips and Pugh, 2000), but even if students lack this type of supervisor, they can still learn. As in everyday life sometimes it is necessary for students to work with individuals to whom they cannot relate on a personal level. This does not mean that the professional relationship has to be problematic. Students do have some responsibility to try adapting to a style of tutoring with which they might not be familiar.

Supervisors cannot always help their students because they do not have unlimited knowledge about all the facets of the research. Researchers often find other experts who can advise them, and on whose knowledge they can draw without offending the supervisor. Indeed, supervisors often know their own limitations and help students find other experts. It is advisable, however, that students inform their supervisors when they seek advice from persons outside the supervisory relationship.

Students build up relationships with their supervisors on a one-to-one basis. Eventually the student becomes an independent researcher and expert in the field of study, and the supervisor acts as an adviser who takes a critical stance to the work.

Practical aspects of supervision

There are some other practical points that must be remembered. Students should make an appointment before coming to see their supervisors, if this is at all possible. Of course, open access to supervision is sometimes necessary and always valuable, but supervisors are busy with many other commitments, and an appointment system helps to save time for all parties. Students (and supervisors) should be available and punctual for a pre-arranged meeting, but if appointments have to be cancelled, the cancellation should be made as early as possible. If no other time for necessary supervision can be found, an occasional telephone session might do in an emergency. The main stress should be on regular and quality time of contact.

This is a summary of the roles and tasks of supervisors and students (adapted from Holloway and Walker (2000):

The responsibilities of the supervisors:

- They support and advise students
- They ensure that students adhere to ethical principles
- They give feedback such as constructive criticism and motivating praise
- They produce progress reports (if required)
- They introduce students to other experts or advisers (if needed)
- They make students aware of problems relating to progress and quality of the project
- They encourage students throughout the research process

The responsibilities of the students:

- They negotiate the process and style of supervision with the supervisor
- They regularly submit written work to the supervisor (as negotiated), generally well before supervisory meetings
- They give progress reports if required

- They negotiate major changes and modifications in the research with the supervisor
- They inform the supervisor of any problems which might interfere with the research project
- They observe ethical principles (which include not plagiarising the work of others)

In addition to the above, postgraduates attend agreed research sessions or training programmes.

Single or joint supervision

Students have either one or two supervisors for their research studies. One supervisor could be an expert in research method, the other might have specialist knowledge in the field of study. Supervisors generally differ in their skills and knowledge but complement each other.

There are a number of arguments for joint supervision. For the student, continuity is ensured when one supervisor is absent or ill. The student's experience can be enhanced by the support of two supervisors. For the supervisors there is support from colleagues who can discuss the appropriateness of advice about which they are uncertain. New supervisors gain from the guidance of experienced colleagues.

Taught masters' degrees in nursing and midwifery proliferate and recruit large numbers of students. Most part-time students work in the clinical setting and wish to carry out research in this environment in order to examine a problem or a major issue relevant to their work. Therefore one person in the supervisory team should have experience and knowledge of clinical practice and, if possible, the researcher's specialism.

When examining an educational problem, a student needs at least one supervisor with expertise in the educational field. This is different for undergraduate students. As novices to the research process and relatively inexperienced in the clinical setting, they need guidance to the principles of research while the topic is of lesser importance, although it should reflect the student's interest and advance knowledge in a more limited subject area.

The case for single supervision is not as strong. The main argument relates to the clear guidance of students who do not risk receiving conflicting guidance from different people if there is just one adviser. In universities and colleges where staff members move frequently, students have less risk of disruption to their project with two supervisors. To avoid conflicting advice to students, it is, of course, important that joint supervisors have a common ideology about supervision, a similar view about the particular method and topic, and that they stay in contact with each other. Students must be aware of some of the pitfalls and problems in supervision, because ultimately the responsibility is theirs.

Students often propose an ambitious project in which they intend to use both qualitative and quantitative methods – between-method triangulation – while it might be better to follow Leininger's (1992) advice and triangulate within-method, for instance through the use of both qualitative (unstructured or semi-structured) interviews and participant observation. For short student projects that take less than a year, between-method triangulation is too time-consuming though occasionally a student will successfully complete a project using this form of triangulation.

Supervisors have the task of asking questions about the particular circumstances, settings and people the students want to take into account when investigating the topic. Often they have knowledge of specific methodologies and are able to advise students on relevant and useful method texts. Although students cannot be forced to listen to their supervisors, they will usually find it profitable to do so.

Researchers have a duty to their discipline and should report data truthfully, accurately and as completely as possible (Kane, 1985). Trust and honesty are very important in establishing a supervisory relationship. In this process truth-telling is essential. There is an obvious duty for both to recognise the need to share all aspects of the study phases, be they positive or negative.

Supervisors are able to help because they have inside knowledge of the research and often spot distortions. In general, supervisors have lengthy experience of a variety of student projects. This knowledge helps students to trust the advice given and be guided appropriately.

Problems with supervision

Students who carry out research may have problems with their supervisors. Some are due to their own actions or inactions, others are the responsibility of the supervisor or the interaction between student and supervisor. Occasionally there may be a personality clash. The problems are more easily resolved at the beginning of the study, and it is important not to leave them for too long. Fortunately, there is rarely a major problem between researcher and supervisor. If it does occur, researchers, and particularly students who do research, can obtain advice from other members of the department or seek help from a senior staff member (such as the departmental research director, the departmental research degrees committee for research students, or the course tutor in the case of undergraduates) who will advise on an appropriate course of action. In most cases, negotiation with the supervisor(s) is not only possible but also desirable, and it resolves small problems.

Academic problems

The following problems may arise from time to time:

(1) The supervisor is inaccessible or lacks time to see the student
(2) The supervisor gives too little guidance or is uncritical
(3) The supervisor is too directive or authoritarian
(4) The student cannot keep to the agreed timetable
(5) The supervisor leaves the university or is allocated a different role

Students' most common complaints concern inaccessibility of supervisors. Supervisors are busy people who do not always see the student and supervision as their priority. Students can avoid this problem by making an appointment well before the supervisory session or by deciding on a future date at each meeting. It is important to inform the supervisor of cancellations. Students might supply supervisors with their home and (for part-time students) work telephone numbers so that they can cancel well before the meeting if they cannot attend.

When students have little guidance, feedback or criticism, they feel uninformed and unsure about their progress or the standard of their work. Students should not be afraid to ask for help. Most supervisors are willing to assist students in any way they can and have their interests at heart.

Students sometimes complain about too much guidance and over-direction. They may feel that the supervisor never allows them to make their own decisions and guides the work in a direction they do not wish to go. If the researcher is a novice, it is generally advisable to listen to the advice of the supervisor, particularly in the early stages. At a later stage, supervisors are generally open to academic argument and do not object to changes in direction as long as the student can justify these.

A problem sometimes occurs in joint supervision when supervisors have conflicting ideologies and different ideas about the research. Sometimes this is the outcome of misinterpretation. The situation can usually be negotiated. It is important for both researcher and supervisors to keep notes on meetings. It is generally advisable for all parties to get together to discuss the research, but of course, this is not always possible.

One of the main problems is the timetable that has been negotiated with the supervisor and that the institution demands. Many students neglect this issue until it becomes urgent. It is most important to look at the date for completion at the very beginning and plan the research carefully so that the timetable can be kept. This means that students and supervisors have to be realistic (Delamont *et al.*, 1997). Qualitative research is particularly demanding during the analysis and writing stages, and takes more time than the student might have originally envisaged. Also, during this stage, students have to gain access to the literature connected with their themes or categories, and the articles often take much time to arrive at the library.

Quite often supervisors change their roles or move on during the student's time at the university. They might be promoted and have little time for the student. They may have a sabbatical or a serious illness. In this case, joint supervision is valuable, and the department can add another supervisor if necessary. Also, telephone and e-mail tutorials are possible, and we have used these successfully. They cannot, however, replace face-to-face contact.

For postgraduates the guidelines for codes of practice of the National Postgraduate Committee (2001) are useful. They are available on the NPC website at http://www.npc.org.uk/publications/guidelines/research.htm, which also contains the address of the General Secretary of the Committee. The responsibilities of supervisors and postgraduate research students are made explicit on this website.

Summary

Supervision may be summarised as follows.

- Student and supervisor(s) have responsibility for the research project, but the main responsibility for the research lies with the student.
- Supervisors are chosen because of their knowledge in the area of methodology and topic.
- Negotiation between students and supervisors takes place early in the research when the ground rules are established.
- It is essential that close and regular contact is maintained between the student and the supervisor(s), and that they share ideas throughout the research.

Many of the ideas in this chapter were developed in Holloway and Walker (2000).

References

Cryer, P. (1996) *The Research Student's Guide to Success*. Buckingham, Open University Press.

Delamont, S., Atkinson, P. & Parry, O. (1997) *Supervising the PhD: A Guide to Success*. Buckingham, SRHE and Open University Press.

Holloway, I. & Walker, J. (2000) *Getting a PhD in Health and Social Care*. Oxford, Blackwell Science.

Kane, E. (1985) *Doing Your own Research*. London, Marion Boyars.

Leininger, M. (1992) Current issues, problems, and trends to advance qualitative paradigmatic research methods for the future. *Qualitative Health Research*, **2** (4), 392–415.

National Postgraduate Committee (2001) *Guidelines for Codes of Practice for Postgraduate Research*. Updated 21 June (first written in 1992).

Phillips, E.M. & Pugh, D.S. (2000) *How to get a PhD*, 3rd edn. Milton Keynes, Open University.

Sharp, J. & Howard, J.A. (1996) *The Management of a Student Research Project*, 2nd edn. Aldershot, Gower.

PART TWO

Data Collection

CHAPTER 5

Interviewing

Interviews as sources of data

In the last decade, interviews have become the most common form of data collection in qualitative research. Atkinson and Silverman (1997) suggest that we live in an 'interview society' where this form of research is favoured. Many novice nurse and midwife researchers rely on interviews as their main form of data collection because they want to gain the inside view of a phenomenon or problem.

It is easily understandable why health professionals wish to interview clients and colleagues. In their professional lives, too, they have conversations with patients in order to obtain information from them. They counsel their clients and already possess many interviewing skills. Nursing or midwifery assessment, for instance, relies on skilful questions and includes interviewing to elicit information from patients or clients. It might therefore be assumed that research interviews are easy to carry out, but interviewing is a complex process and not as simple as it seems.

Health professionals also discuss patients' or clients' conditions and progress and compare their own experiences with those of their colleagues. This means that they are used to the process of listening and talking. Burgess (1984) uses the term 'conversation with a purpose' for the qualitative interview (quoting the expression used by Beatrice and Sidney Webb who carried out social research around the turn of the last century). Rubin and Rubin (1995) add that researcher and informant become 'conversational partners'. Research interviews, however, differ from ordinary conversations, as the rules of the interview process are more clearly defined. The one-to-one interview consisting of questions and answers is the most common form of research interview. Other types include focus group and narrative interviews (discussed more fully in Chapters 7 and 13).

Considering interviews as a form of data collection, researchers might agree with Weiss (1994) who believes that interview studies have contributed a great deal to the understanding of society and human beings. In health research, interviewing has been the basis both for exploring colleagues' perspectives as well as for the understanding of clients. Interviews have sometimes been criticised for 'anecdotalism' (Silverman, 2001). If the researcher applies high standards and rigour to the research, they go beyond anecdotes and present the reality of the participant.

The interview process

Unlike everyday conversations, research interviews are set up by the interviewer to elicit information from participants. However, Holstein and Gubrium (1997: 113) suggest that the interview is more than 'a pipeline for transmitting know-ledge from informant to interviewer'. The purpose of the interview is the discovery of informants' feelings, perceptions and thoughts. Marshall and Rossman (1999) advise that the interviews focus on the past, present and, in particular, the essential experience of participants. The interview can be formal or informal; often informal conversations or chats with participants also generate important ideas for the project. Depending on the response of participants, researchers formulate questions as the interview proceeds rather than asking pre-planned questions. This means that each interview differs from the next in sequence and wording, although distinct patterns common to all interviews in a specific study often emerge in the analysis. Indeed, for many research approaches it is necessary that researchers discover these patterns when analysing data.

One-to-one interviews are the most common form of data collection. Examples can be given from much nursing research: for instance, Melia (1987) interviewed student nurses about learning their roles in the clinical setting. She acquired her knowledge by talking to individuals. One interview, however, does not always suffice. In qualitative inquiry it is possible to re-examine the issues in the light of emerging ideas and interview for a second or third time. Seidman (1998) sees three interviews as the optimum number, but these require much planning in the short time span available to undergraduates for their project. Many novice researchers therefore use one-off interviews although postgraduates and often other more experienced researchers carry out more than one with each partici-pant.

Pilot studies are not always used in qualitative inquiry as the research is developmental, but novice researchers could try interviews with their friends and acquaintances to get used to this type of data collection. We found that we lacked confidence when we started, and a practice run proved very useful. In our experience students become more confident as interviews proceed.

Most qualitative research starts with relatively unstructured interviews in which researchers give minimal guidance to the participants. The outcome of initial interviews guides later stages of interviewing. As interviews proceed, they become more focused on the particular issues important to the participants and emerge throughout the data collection. Flexibility and consistency must be balanced in the research (May, 1991) so that health professionals can compare the accounts of individuals and find common patterns, without neglecting the unique stories of their experience.

Types of interview

Researchers have to decide on the amount of structure in the interview. There is a range of interview types on a continuum, from the unstructured to the structured interview. Qualitative researchers generally employ the unstructured or semi-structured interview.

The unstructured, non-standardised interview

Unstructured interviews start with a general question in the broad area of study. Even unstructured interviews are usually accompanied by an *aide mémoire*, an agenda or a list of topics that will be covered. There are, however, no pre-determined questions except at the very beginning of the interview.

Example

Tell me about your experience at the time of the accident . . .

Aide mémoire

Feelings in the accident and emergency ward

Interaction with different types of professionals

Coping with the condition and the associated pain

The process of being in hospital

Social support from other patients, relatives and friends

Practical support etc.

This type of unstructured interviewing allows flexibility and makes it possible for researchers to follow the interests and thoughts of the informants. Sarantakos (1998) advises that unstructured interviews should not follow rigid procedures. Interviewers freely ask questions from informants in any order or sequence depending on the responses to earlier questions, although warm-up and simple questions are generally asked first. If the interviewer leaves the essential questions till the end of the interview the participant may be tired and reluctant to discuss deeper issues.

Researchers also have their own agenda. To achieve the research aim, they keep in mind the particular issues which they wish to explore. However, direction and control of the interview by the researcher is minimal. Generally, the outcomes of these interviews differ for each informant, though usually certain patterns can be discerned. Informants are free to answer at length, and great depth and detail can be obtained. The unstructured interview generates the richest data, but it also has the highest 'dross rate' (the amount of material of no particular use for the researcher's study), particularly when the interviewer is inexperienced.

The semi-structured interview

Semi-structured or focused interviews are often used in qualitative research. The questions are contained in an interview guide (not schedule as in quantitative research) with a focus on the issues or topic areas to be covered and the lines of inquiry to be followed. The sequencing of questions is not the same for every participant as it depends on the process of the interview and the responses of each individual. The interview guide, however, ensures that the researcher collects similar types of data from all informants. In this way, the interviewer can save time. The dross rate is lower than in unstructured interviews. Researchers can develop questions and decide for themselves what issues to pursue.

Example

Tell me about the time when your condition was first diagnosed. (Depending on the language use and understanding of the participant, this has to be phrased differently. For instance: What did you think when the doctor first told you about your illness?)

What did you feel at that stage?

Tell me about your treatment.

What did the doctor or nurses say?

What happened after that?

How did your husband (wife, children) react?

What happened at work?

And so on.

The interview guide can be quite long and detailed although it need not be followed strictly. It focuses on particular aspects of the subject area to be examined, but it can be revised after several interviews because of the ideas that arise. Although interviewers aim to gain the informants' perspectives, they must remember that they need some control of the interview so that the purpose of the study can be achieved and the research topic explored. Ultimately, the researchers themselves must decide what interview techniques or types might be best for them and the interview participants. Burgess (1984) suggests that the longer the questions, the longer the answers. Our students and other researchers found good questions of medium length with the use of prompts more useful.

The structured or standardised interview

Qualitative researchers rarely use standardised interviews as they are contradictory to the aims of qualitative research. The interview schedule contains a number of pre-planned questions. Each informant in a research study is asked the same questions in the same order. This type of interview resembles a written survey questionnaire. Standardised interviews save time and limit the interviewer effect. The analysis of the data seems easier as answers can be found quickly. Generally, knowledge of statistics is important and useful for the analysis of this type of interview. However, this type of pre-planned interview directs the informants' responses and is therefore inappropriate in qualitative approaches. Structured interviews may contain open questions, but even then they cannot be called qualitative.

Qualitative researchers use structured questions only to elicit socio-demographic data i.e. about age, length of condition, length of experience, type of occupation, qualifications etc. Sometimes research or ethics committees ask for a predetermined interview schedule so that they can find out the exact path of the research. For the purpose of gaining permission, a semi-structured interview guide would be advisable for nursing researchers.

Types of questions

When asking questions, interviewers use a variety of techniques. Patton (1990) lists particular types of questions, for example *experience*, *feeling* and *knowledge* questions.

Examples

Experience questions
Could you tell me about your experience of caring for patients with arthritis?
Tell me about your experience of epilepsy

Feeling questions
How did you feel when the first patient in your care died?
What did you feel when the doctor told you that you suffer from . . .

Knowledge questions
What services are available for this group of patients?
How do you cope with this condition?

Spradley (1979) distinguishes between *grand-tour* and *mini-tour* questions. Grand-tour questions are broader, while *mini-tour* questions are more specific.

Examples

Grand-tour questions
Can you describe a typical day in the community? (To a community midwife)
How did you see your condition? (To a patient)

Mini-tour questions
Can you describe what happens when a colleague questions your decision? (To a nurse)
What were your expectations of the pain clinic? (To a patient)

The sequencing of questions is also important.

Practical considerations

In qualitative studies questions are as non-directive as possible but still guide towards the topics of interest to the researcher. Researchers should phrase questions clearly and aim at the various participants' levels of understanding. Ambiguous questions lead to ambiguous answers. Double questions are best avoided; for instance it would be inappropriate to ask: How many colleagues do you have, and what are their ideas about this?

The researcher must be aware of practical difficulties in the data collection phase, particularly when interviewing in hospital. The routine of the hospital is disrupted by the presence of the nurse or midwife researcher whose activities might be viewed with suspicion by colleagues. A quiet place for interviews cannot always be found, and therefore the privacy of patients may be threatened. The ward might be full of noise and activity, and the researcher does not always find a convenient slot for interviewing without being interrupted by nursing activity, consultant round, cleaners, meals and so on. In the community, interviews are often interrupted by children or spouses and by the visits of friends or relatives.

Probing, prompting and summarising

During the interviews researchers can use prompts or probing questions. These help to reduce anxiety for researcher and research informant. The purpose of probes is a search for elaboration, meaning or reasons. Seidman (1998) prefers the term 'explore' and dislikes the word 'probe' as it stresses the interviewer's position of power and is the name for a surgical instrument used in medical or dental investigations.

Exploratory questions might be, for instance: What was that experience like for you? How did you feel about that? Can you tell me more about that? That's interesting, why did you do that? Questions can follow up on certain points that participants make or words they use. The researcher could also summarise the last statements of the participant and encourage more talk through this technique.

> **Example**
>
> You told me earlier that you were very happy with the care you received in hospital. Could you tell me a bit more about that?

Merkle Sorrell and Redmond (1995) suggest that both recapitulation and silence are effective techniques for eliciting information. Participants often become fluent talkers when asked to tell a story, reconstructing their experiences, for instance a day, an incident, the feeling about an illness. Unfortunately the data from interviews are sometimes better when the participants are articulate, and occasionally researchers may choose those who have language and interaction skills. This may create bias in the interviews.

> **Example**
>
> A number of years ago one of our students – an experienced midwife with good verbal and interactive skills – intended to interview clients about the nil-by-mouth policy of the maternity ward in which she wished to carry out research for her research diploma. She found that certain individuals only answered in very short sentences, could not be prompted and were generally in awe of the situation and the researcher. Also the policy was not an issue of interest to them – their concern focused only on the birth of their baby – but only for the midwives involved. The researcher had to abandon the topic area because she had not enough material for a long research study and also felt that there would be bias against less articulate and less confident clients.

The social skills of the researcher often, but not always, make a difference to the outcome of the interview.

Non-verbal prompts are also useful. The stance of the researcher, eye contact or leaning forward encourages reflection. In fact, listening skills, which some nurses and midwives already possess from the counselling of patients, will elicit further ideas. Patients often give monosyllabic answers until they have become used to the interviewer, because they are reluctant to uncover their feelings or fear that judgements might be made about them.

Length and timing of interviews

The length of time for an interview depends on the participants, the topic of the interview and the methodological approach. Of course, the researcher must suggest an approximate amount of time – perhaps an hour and a half – so that participants can plan their day, but many are willing or wish to go beyond this, some as much as three or four hours. Others, particularly elderly people or physically weak informants may need to break off after a short while, say 20 or 30 minutes. Children cannot concentrate for long periods of time. Nurses and midwives have to use their own judgement, follow the wishes of the informant and take the length of time required for the topic. One of our colleagues suggests that three hours should be the absolute maximum because concentration fails even experienced researchers or willing participants.

Phenomenological interviews focus on one phenomenon or a limited number of very specific phenomena. Because of the reflective character of the interviews, the participants may become tired as they uncover their feelings; hence the researcher may not be able to continue the research for long. Also, as the questions concentrate on the specific phenomenon, extraneous matters are not significant for the study, in contrast to ethnographic research for instance.

Stating an approximate time for the interview can ensure escape for the researcher who is pressed for time, although it is advisable to leave plenty of time for interviewing. For hard-pressed professionals this type of data collection is very time-consuming, however useful and therapeutic it may be for the informant. As stated before, researchers can, of course, re-interview one or more times.

Recording interview data

A number of techniques and practical points must be considered so that the data are recorded and stored appropriately.

Interview data are recorded in three ways

(1)   Tape-recording the interview
(2)   Note taking during the interview
(3)   Note taking after the interview

Tape-recording

Before analysing the data, researchers must preserve the participants' words as accurately as possible. The best form of recording interview data is tape-recording. As we said before, researchers must ask for permission before taping. Because tapes contain the exact words of the interview, inclusive of questions, researchers do not forget important answers and words and can have eye contact and pay attention to what participants say. Occasionally informants change their

minds about tape-recording, and their wishes should be paramount. The principle of respect for autonomy includes choice and free decision and must be
considered first in terms of consent. This allows for the participants' right to
refuse participation in research. This right can be exercised at any stage of the
research process.

Initially the informants may be hesitant, but they will get used to the tape-
recorder; a small recorder is easier to forget than a large one, but a larger recorder
can be placed further away so it is not necessarily always visible or disturbing. By
asking factual questions first, researchers allow the informants to relax and make
them feel more secure. Some interviewees have soft and quiet voices, particularly
if they feel vulnerable. Interviewers therefore place the tape-recorder near
enough, but not so prominently that it intimidates the hesitant person. Lapel
microphones allow a better quality of sound. A room away from noise and
disturbances enhances not only the quality of the tape but also the interview itself
as participants feel free to talk without interruption.

We have experienced some problems with tape-recorders. They sometimes
break down, and it is advisable to try them out at the beginning of the interview
and after it has been recorded. Researchers should remember to pack some extra
batteries and tapes. A good recording device is available – a portable mini
compact disc player made by Sony, but this is expensive. Each disc records 70
minutes and does not need to be turned over. Auto-reverse on tape-recorders is
useful, standard cassettes need not be turned over (the quality of non-standard
tape – for instance 120 minute tape – is not always very good). It is much better to
use tape-recorders with conference facility, although we know that students often
find them too expensive and have no access to them. The university often can
supply tape-recorders to staff and students for the duration of the data collection.

The tape is dated and labelled. Only pseudonyms should appear on the tape or
its transcription, and participants' names must be stored in a different place from
the tapes. The transcription of data will be discussed in Chapter 15.

Note taking

Note taking is important but might disturb the participant during the interview.
Contextual notes can be made before the interview, others immediately after-
wards when events and thoughts are still clearly in the mind of the researcher.
Note taking is further discussed in Chapter 15.

The interviewer–participant relationship

The relationship between researcher and participant is based on mutual respect
and a position of equality as human beings. The fallacy exists, however, that the
interviewer and the person interviewed work together in a relationship of com-

plete equality. Nurse and midwife researchers, by virtue of their professional expertise and skill in interviewing are in a position of some power, however much they attempt to achieve a relationship of equality with the participant. Researchers can empower patients and colleagues by listening to their perspective and giving voice to their concerns. The interviewer also respects the way in which participants develop and phrase their answers (Marshall and Rossman, 1999), they are, after all, not passive respondents but active participants in an important social encounter. Trust is built up through involvement and interest in the perspectives of the patient. It must also be remembered, however, that the interviewer is not a blank screen (*tabula rasa*) but also an active participant in the interview and thus takes part in co-constructing meaning.

Indeed, Wengraf (2001) reminds researchers that intersubjectivity is an important issue in interviews. Interviewer and participant inhabit a shared world and often a common culture. They have similar, though not the same, understandings of it and base interview questions and answers on shared meanings, but subjective ideas of both parties also must be taken into account.

Peer interviews

Many health professionals have an interest in the views and ideas of their colleagues. There are advantages and disadvantages in interviewing one's peers. Shared language and norms can be advantageous or problematic. A researcher who is involved in the culture of the participants more easily understands cultural concepts. Although there is less room for misinterpretation, misunderstandings can arise from the assumptions of common values and beliefs. Researchers do not always question ideas that are uncovered or constructs that arise from interviews with colleagues. This can be overcome by acting as 'cultural stranger', or 'naïve' interviewer, asking participants about their meaning and clarification of their ideas.

In many peer interviews, researcher and informant are in a position of equality (Platt, 1981), and the researcher is not distant or anonymous. The close relationship has the advantage that the participants will 'open up' and trust researchers, but there is the danger of over-involvement and identification with colleagues. In some cases it may be possible for the researcher to overcome this involvement with peers by eliciting responses from research informants outside the shared frame of reference (Hudson, 1986).

Example

SW investigated health visitors' and social workers' perceptions of child abuse. She was anxious to avoid over-identification with the members of her own profession, health visiting, with whom she shared the 'frame of reference'. This, she thought, might prejudice the information. As part of the background to her study, she visited Dr Dingwall then at Wolfson College, Oxford who had done academic work in the field of child abuse. He suggested interviewing the social workers first and using some of the information from the transcripts to interview the health visitors. She then presented the perceptions of the social workers to the health visitors for comment. There was a shift of focus, so that her own background did not interfere.

Wheeler, 1989

Students, however, sometimes interview friends and acquaintances for pragmatic and opportunistic reasons. Although this is useful to overcome the hurdles of getting to know informants and forming relationships, the selection from this group might create unease or embarrassment if the topic is a sensitive one. Informants and interviewers might hold assumptions about each other, which might prejudice the information. Therefore we suggest that students take great care in their choice of informants.

Interviewing through electronic media

E-mail and other online research as well as telephone interviews have become more popular in all research in recent years. Computer-mediated research entails the direct use of computers in research. So far, not many nursing research studies exist which have used this form of inquiry, although telephone interviews are quite popular.

Online research and e-mail interviews

The use of computers for research, however, is increasing. It is important to know about the possibilities of qualitative interviewing online and through e-mail correspondence where the researcher and the participant do not meet each other face to face. As in conventional one-to-one or focus group interviews, researchers seek special interest groups, or individuals with similar experiences or conditions, such as for instance a group of people in pain, supervisors of postgraduate students or patients with epilepsy etc. Chat rooms and newsgroups can also be observed and their contents analysed. Denzin (1999), for instance, obtained access to a newsgroup of people recovering from alcoholism to examine the 'gendered narratives of self'.

There are two types of online interviews: synchronous or asynchronous (Mann and Stewart, 2000). The synchronous interview takes place in real time and can be carried out with one participant or a group at the same time. This type of interview can proceed when researcher and participants read and write messages at the same time, using computers with software such as Internet Relay Chat (IRC). Morton Robinson (2001) suggests chat rooms as a source of data as dialogues and multiple conversations can take place. As more than one con-versation often proceeds at the same time, chat rooms can be confusing. Bulletin boards are also useful as messages and replies are posted there, and they stay in place for a time.

The researcher can ask questions and will receive an immediate response. The organisation of synchronous interviews is difficult because of differences in the time zones of various countries. It also limits the sample to those who own computers and use technology confidently, and without fear. Ethically access to chat rooms and bulletin boards is problematic unless the messages are completely public. It is more ethical in every case that the researcher uncovers his or her research identity to those who write the messages. The researcher also has to be careful about the trustworthiness of the data, as they are often provided anonymously.

Asynchronous or non-real time interviews are e-mail conversations. Data generation by e-mail correspondence entails asking a purposive sample of people with similar experiences to get in touch by e-mail and share these experiences with the researcher. These interviews enable correspondents to choose the best time for their writing. It means that they can be in touch when they wish to communicate in an 'ongoing dynamic process' (Kralik *et al.*, 2000: 18). This technique is less intrusive than face-to-face interviews, but the researcher can still obtain the same rich data. Because correspondents never meet the researcher, they can be more open and honest about their condition or experiences. Status issues and hierarchical positions have less influence in this type of interview because the contact is not face to face. The procedure will only work fully, however, if the research is a process of ongoing dialogue over a period of time, sometimes as short as three months, sometimes as long as a year.

Example

Kralik conducted a PhD study in which she aimed to find out about the effect of chronic illness on middle-aged women. Her sample consisted of 80 women who corresponded with her over the period of a year or so. The data were generated through e-mail correspondence. 13 women joined the research in the next year for further correspondence.

Kralik *et al.*, 2000

The advantage for the researcher is the instant availability of typed text that can be accessed at any time after the interview. Researchers can respond to questions or seek more answers when they find time and have considered the correspondents' narratives. Participants are able to enter the correspondence from an environment of their choice, often their homes. Bodily presence is not essential for a 'good' interview. Mann and Stewart (2000) give the example of

Picardie (1998) who described the use of e-mail and felt that it is useful for expressing emotions and being reflective about one's writing. Researcher and participant are able to get to know each other quite well over a period of time. These types of interview save travel, time and money. The e-mail interviewer can also avoid lengthy transcriptions as the message can be printed out immediately. In a geographical sense, the e-mail interview can widen the access to participants.

Example

Seymour (2001) discussed computer-aided methods when examining how individuals with disabilities use computer technology. In her article she states some of the advantages of this type of interview and exposes the limitations of traditional methods. Access to the participants was one of the main advantages.

Seymour (2001) lists several elements as important features of online research. She claims that 'the release of the interview from its imprisonment in time and space' makes it deeper, because the sites are open for longer periods of time and the response need not be immediate. Researchers can gain access to the participants in an ongoing process and clarify issues that are unclear, while participants too have the time to ask questions throughout the research process. The ongoing interaction, suggests Seymour, makes the position of the participants more egalitarian. There are also practical implications: the interviews need not be transcribed but are instantly available with little cost involved. Both researcher and participants have time to reflect on their answers.

One of the points relates to the lack of assumptions that researchers have about the participants. As the latter are not visible and cannot be identified as members of particular groups with specific group membership, personality or outside appearance, they cannot be instantly labelled.

These interviews are not, of course, as spontaneous as face-to-face or even telephone interviews but they give the participants time to reflect on the questions. It must be remembered though, that researchers who use this form of inquiry automatically exclude those who have no access to computers. These may well be members of a socio-economic or ethnic group of particular interest to the researcher (Graham and Marvin, 1996).

At the time of writing, e-mail interviews are possibly the most common form of research on the internet.

Telephone interviews

Telephone interviews are another effective way of interviewing. The telephone interview is immediate, and researchers and participants are able to respond spontaneously to each other.

Examples

In a multi-method study, which included a survey and qualitative research, Eloise Carr interviewed 29 patients who had volunteered to speak about their experiences of pain in hospital. She gained access to the individuals through asking every fourth respondent in the initial survey to take part in the telephone interviews.

Carr, 1999

Farnaz Heidari interviewed by telephone health professionals who were involved in the care and treatment of disabled children as part of a research project. The study aimed to gain access to the perspectives of health professionals – doctors, nurses and physiotherapists – on the use and effectiveness of complementary therapies.

Heidari et al., 2001

The telephone interviews in the above examples were more convenient for the health professionals with little time for interviews but also saved travel time for the researcher who had travelled long distances to interview parents and children.

The advantages of telephone interviews are obvious. They include the immediacy of response, anonymity of participants and the effective use of time. Researchers need not travel to the participants' home or work location. The disadvantage is the lack of deeper interaction, as the interviewer does not get to know the participants. A telephone talk must be more structured, and this is in contrast to the tenets of qualitative research which is designed to elicit rich and deep data. It is, however, a useful way of obtaining data when other types of interview are not possible.

Ethical issues

Ethical rules and principles that are considered in conventional forms of inquiry must also be considered in e-mail and other electronic research, for instance informed consent, confidentiality, the right not to be harmed or identified and the possibility of withdrawal at any time. Ethical issues are, however, particularly problematic in spite of the data protection law, as outsiders can gain access to the correspondence more easily than to tape-recorded interviews. It is therefore necessary that researchers inform the participants about the potential lack of security, and it is advisable to obtain written permission by post. Using e-mail, other online research and telephone interviewing means that the interviewer's words need to be more carefully considered and phrased, as they cannot be modified or accompanied by gestures and facial expressions like face-to-face conversations. Those obtaining access to a group site do not always ask for permission to 'listen in' or to use observations for research purposes, but we would suggest that nurse researchers inform the participants about the research and ask for this permission. In short, researchers must consider ethical issues most carefully and keep to ethical principles and procedures in electronic forms of inquiry.

Strengths and weaknesses of interviewing

There is an ever-increasing use of interviewing as data collection. Atkinson and Silverman (1997) speak of 'the rhetoric of interviewing' where the assumption exists that researchers gain full access to inner feelings and thoughts, uncovering the private self. These writers question the overuse of the interview and claim that it is often seen naïvely or uncritically by researchers who take the words of the informants at face value and do not reflect or take an analytical stance. Silverman (1998) also points out that gaps exist between words and actions – the old dilemma of 'what they say and what they do'. Therefore researchers need to observe situations and behaviour, so that they can collect data about social action and interaction. Observation is not only complementary to interviewing but is also a form of within-method triangulation. There are a number of critical comments about interviews listed by Kvale (1996: 292), which we will summarise. He suggests that much interview research:

- Centres on individuals and does not take social interactions into account
- Neglects the social and material context
- Does not take account of emotions
- Takes place in a vacuum and not in the real world
- Takes account of thoughts and experiences, not actions and focuses on verbal interaction
- Is atheoretical, trivial and ignores linguistic approaches to language

Researchers who interview will have to be aware of these issues to avoid the pitfalls in interviewing.

Advantages and limitations

One of the main features of qualitative interviewing is its flexibility. Researchers have the freedom to prompt for more information, and participants are able to explore their own thoughts as well as exert more control over the interview as their ideas have priority. This also includes opportunities for participants to react spontaneously and honestly to questions or to articulate their ideas slowly and reflect on them. Researchers can follow up and clarify the meanings of words and phrases immediately, but they can also take time so that trust can develop.

On the other hand, the collection and especially the analysis of interview data is time-consuming and labour intensive. Students who are very enthusiastic during the early data gathering process only realise when they are involved in transcribing and analysing how much time they need for the work.

The interviewer effect and reactivity

Participants sometimes react to the researcher and modify their answers to please or to appear in a positive light, consciously or unconsciously. For these reasons a monitoring process is necessary so that researchers recognise the interviewer effect and minimise it (Hammersley and Atkinson, 1995). This means spending time with the participant so that trust can develop. The interviewers too react to the words they hear. Within the framework of the research the researcher has different priorities from the participant. This has to be recognised so that both the insider's and the researcher's perspective can be made explicit in the research report. After all, health professionals are experts in care, informed about many health and illness issues and have their own perception of the phenomenon under study. Creswell (1998) also warns researchers of the possibility of misinterpreting the words of the participant. The interviewer effect is less noticeable in online interviews.

Summary

The in-depth interview is the most common form of data collection.

- Interviews can be face-to-face, online or by telephone.
- The qualitative research interview is relatively non-directive and depends largely on the participants whose ideas, thoughts and feelings researchers try to explore.
- The interviewer's agenda, the aim of the research and the research relationship influence the interview process.
- The advantage of the interview is obtaining the insiders' perspectives directly; its disadvantages are the problematic relationships between words and deeds and the change of participants' thinking over time.

References

Atkinson, P. & Silverman, D. (1997) Kundera's immortality: The interview society and the invention of the self. *Qualitative Inquiry*, **3** (3) 304–25.

Burgess, R.G. (1984) *In the Field: An Introduction to Field Research*. London, Unwin Hyman.

Carr, E.C.J. (1999) Talking on the telephone with people who have experienced pain in hospital: clinical audit or research? *Journal of Advanced Nursing*, **29** (1) 194–200.

Creswell, J.W. (1998) *Qualitative Inquiry and Research Design: Choosing Among Five Traditions*. London, Sage.

Denzin, N.K. (1999) Cybertalk and the method of instances. In *Doing Internet Research* (ed. S. Jones). Thousand Oaks, Sage.

Graham, S. and Marvin, S. (1996) *Telecommunications and the City: Electronic Spaces, Urban Places*. London, Routledge.

Hammersley, M. & Atkinson, P.A. (1995) *Ethnography: Principles in Practice*, 2nd edn. London, Tavistock.

Heidari, F., Dumbrell, A., Galvin, K. & Holloway, I. (2001) Brain injury: The use of complementary therapies. *Complementary Therapies in Nursing and Midwifery*, 7, 66–71.

Holstein, J.A. & Gubrium, J.F. (1997) Active interviewing. In *Qualitative Research: Theory, Method and Practice* (ed. D. Silverman), pp. 113–19. London, Sage.

Hudson, B. (1986) Lessons from the Jasmine Beckford Inquiry. *Midwife, Health Visitor and Community Nurse*, 22, 162–3.

Kralik, D., Koch, T. & Brady, B.M. (2000) Pen pals: correspondence as a method of data generation in qualitative research. *Journal of Advanced Nursing*, 31 (4) 909–17.

Kvale, S. (1996) *InterViews: An Introduction to Qualitative Research*. Thousand Oaks, Sage.

Mann, C. & Stewart, F. (2000) *Internet Communication and Qualitative Research: A Handbook for Researching Online*. London, Sage.

Marshall, C. & Rossman, G.R. (1999) *Designing Qualitative Research*, 3rd edn. Thousand Oaks, Sage.

May, K.A. (1991) Interview techniques in qualitative research. In *Qualitative Nursing Research: A Contemporary Dialogue* (ed. J.M. Morse), pp. 188–209. Newbury Park, Sage.

Melia, K. (1987) *Learning and Working*. London, Tavistock.

Merkle Sorrell, J. & Redmond, G.M. (1995) Interviews in qualitative nursing research: Differing approaches for ethnographic and phenomenological studies. *Journal of Advanced Nursing*, 21, 1117–22.

Morton Robinson, K. (2001) Unsolicited narratives from the internet: a rich source of data. *Qualitative Health Research*, 11 (5) 706–14.

Patton, M. (1990) *Qualitative Evaluation and Research Methods*, 2nd edn. Newbury Park, Sage.

Picardie, R. (1998) *Before I Say Goodbye*. Harmondsworth, Penguin.

Platt, J. (1981) On interviewing one's peers. *British Journal of Sociology*, 32 (1) 75–91.

Rubin, H.J. & Rubin, I.S. (1995) *Qualitative Interviewing: The Art of Hearing Data*. Thousand Oaks, Sage.

Sarantakos, S. (1998) *Social Research*, 2nd edn. Basingstoke, Sage.

Seidman, I.E. (1998) *Interviewing as Qualitative Research*, 2nd edn. New York, Teachers College of Columbia University.

Seymour, W.S. (2001) In the flesh or online? Exploring qualitative research methodologies. *Qualitative Research*, 1 (2) 147–68.

Silverman, D. (1998) The quality of qualitative health research: The open-ended interview and its alternatives. *Social Sciences in Health*, 4 (2) 104–18.

Silverman, D. (2001) *Interpreting Qualitative Data: Methods for Analysing Talk, Text and Interaction*, 2nd edn. London, Sage.

Spradley, J.P. (1979) *The Ethnographic Interview*. Fort Worth, Harcourt Brace Johanovich College Publishers.

Weiss, R.S. (1994) *Learning from Strangers: The Art and Method of Qualitative Interview Studies*. New York, The Free Press.

Wengraf, T. (2001) *Qualitative Research Interviewing: Biographic Narrative and Semi-Structured Methods*. London, Sage.

Wheeler, S.J. (1989) *Health Visitors' and Social Workers' Perceptions of Child Abuse*. Bournemouth, Bournemouth University. Unpublished BSc dissertation.

CHAPTER 6

Participant Observation and Documents as Sources of Data

Observation

Observation is a data collection procedure and, in particular, an essential element of ethnography. Although interviewing is a more popular strategy for those undertaking qualitative inquiry, participant observation contains the most typical features of this type of research. Indeed, Strauss and Corbin (1998) see it as qualitative research *'par excellence'*. It provides access not only to the social context, but also to the ways in which people act and interact. In any case, for nurses and midwives it is important to observe patients. There are many opportunities to do so: perhaps on a ward, in a reception area, in the emergency department, a clinic or any other relevant location inside the hospital or the community.

Savage (2000) sees parallels between observation and clinical practice:

(1) *Reliance on physical involvement:* The researcher is present in the setting. This means that health professionals need to be familiar with the location and learn about the behaviour and activities of the participants.

(2) *Claims to experiential knowledge:* Whether they act as researchers or as professionals in clinical practice, health professionals experience the situation in similar ways although they interpret the situation differently when carrying out research or when performing their professional activities.

(3) *Sharing of theoretical assumptions:* Similar underlying theoretical assumptions are shared both in research and clinical practice.

(4) *Reciprocity of perspectives:* In both roles, health professionals attempt to empathise with patients and put themselves in their shoes. This is perhaps easier for the researcher than for the busy professional in clinical practice carrying out routine business. The relationship between observer and observed in a health setting is strong, and many meanings (though not all) are shared.

When researchers decide to observe, they do not set up artificial situations but look at people in their natural settings. Qualitative researchers generally use the term 'participant observation', a phrase originally coined by Lindeman (cited in Bogdewic, 1999), which he described as the exploration of a culture from the inside. As Jorgenson (1989: 15) states: 'Participant observation provides direct experiential and observational access to the insiders' world of meaning.' The social reality of the people observed is examined. The researchers will become an integral part of the setting they enter and, to some extent, a member of the group they observe.

There has been a debate about the nature of participant observation, which we will not pursue in detail (see Savage, 2000 for some detail). Some see it as a research approach or methodology, others merely as a procedure or strategy for collecting qualitative data. Here it is being treated as a method within particular approaches to qualitative research such as ethnography, grounded theory or action research.

The origins of participant observation

Participant observation has its origins in anthropology and sociology. However, early travellers in ancient times wrote down their observation of cultures they visited, often as participants in those cultures, making it probably the earliest of all forms of data collection. From the early days of fieldwork, anthropologists and sociologists became part of the culture they studied and examined the actions and interactions of people in their social context, 'in the field'. Famous studies in anthropology are those of Malinowski (1922) and Mead (1935) on other cultures; in sociology the participant observations of Strauss and his colleagues on psychiatric hospitals (Strauss et al., 1964) and Spradley's work (1970) with tramps in the 1960s, typify some of the early well known studies. Atkinson (1995) observed the processes of interaction between doctors and examined the way they worked and talked while performing their occupational roles. In nursing, the study by Lawler (1991) describes observational procedures and interviewing in a study of nurses' work in relation to the management of the patient's body and its various functions and the process of patient recovery. She also observed the style of discourse within the ward.

Immersion in a setting can take a long time, often years of living in a culture. Participant observation goes on over a period of time, sometimes over one or several years (Atkinson, 1995; Roth, 1963), although some observation does not take as long. Health professionals, of course, are already members of and familiar with the culture they examine. For these reasons they may not need a long introduction to the setting; they may, however, miss significant events or behaviours in the locale because of familiarity. This also means that they should suspend prior assumptions, so as not to miss important aspects or misinterpret the situation.

Prolonged observation generates more in-depth knowledge of a group or subculture, and researchers can avoid disturbances and potential biases caused by an occasional visit from an unknown stranger. Observation is less disruptive and more unobtrusive than interviewing. However, participant observation does not just involve observing the situation, but also listening to the people under study.

Focus and setting

The focus of observation

The dimensions of social settings, according to Spradley (1980) focus on the features shown in Fig. 6.1 which catalogues some ideas about the focus of observation, although this focus also depends on the particular research question. Nurses and midwives centre particularly on the interaction of patients and professionals as well as the actions and activities of both groups.

Space:	the *location*
Actor:	the *members* or *participants* in the setting
Activity:	the *behaviour* and *actions* of people
Object:	the *things* that are located in the setting
Act:	*single actions* of people
Events:	what is *happening*
Time:	the *time frame* and *sequencing* of activities
Goal:	what people are *aiming* to do
Feeling:	the *emotions* that people have

Fig. 6.1 Dimensions of social settings (adapted from Spradley (1980: 78))

Setting of observation

Any appropriate setting can become the focus of the study. Participant observation varies on a continuum from open to closed settings. Open settings are public and highly visible such as street scenes, corridors and reception areas. In closed settings, access is more difficult and has to be carefully negotiated; personal offices or meetings and wards can be considered closed settings. It is useful to examine how people in the setting go about their routine and everyday business, how they act and interact with each other and how they relate to the space and the environment in which they are located. Hidden rituals and those activities that give a group special identities can also be discovered (Bogdewic, 1999), for instance through the use of language and laughter.

Researchers might observe critical incidents, dramatic events and examine language use, depending on location or topic, but they can also observe in detail exits and entrances of group members, body language, facial expressions and even choice of words (Abrams, 2000).

Observation provides a holistic perspective on the setting. Nurse and midwife researchers can observe as insiders and ask questions, which an outside spectator could not do. If they become deeply engaged and stay for a considerable time, participants will become used to them, and the observer effect will be minimal. The problems and unexpressed needs of the participants also can be observed. Although participants describe their experiences in interviews and reflect on events and actions, nurses and midwives will not have to rely only on participants' memories; they will be able to distinguish between words and actions, 'what they say and what they do', which is not always the same. Observation, however useful and appropriate, is time consuming; hence it is not generally used in undergraduate research, while postgraduates often include it.

Types of observation

Participant observers enter the setting without wishing to limit the observation to particular processes or people, and they adopt an unstructured approach. Occasionally certain foci crystallise early in the study, but usually observation progresses from the unstructured to the more focused until eventually specific actions and events become the main interest of the researcher.

Gold (1958) identified four types of observer involvement in the field:

(1) The complete participant
(2) The participant as observer
(3) The observer as participant
(4) The complete observer

The complete participant

The complete participant is part of the setting and takes an insider role that involves covert observation. Roth (1963), Rosenhan (1973) and Lawler (1991) attempted this (but only Lawler is a health professional).

Examples

Roth (1963), an American sociologist, was a patient in a tuberculosis hospital. While being part of the setting, he observed the interaction of patients with the health personnel, focusing on negotiation concerning time spent in and out of hospital.

The best known study of covert observation is that of Rosenhan (1973) who wanted to discover whether 'sane' and 'insane' individuals could be distinguished by health professionals. Eight pseudo patients were sent to psychiatric hospitals where they exhibited 'normal' behaviour apart from an initial statement that they could hear voices. (All except one were labelled by health professionals as schizophrenic with schizophrenia in remission, while other patients recognised their 'sanity'.)

Rosenhan (1973) wished to show that notions of normality and abnormality are not as clear and unambiguous as is sometimes believed. Lawler (1991), in her research on interactions of nurses and patients, also makes a case for covert observation. In spite of the value of these particular studies, complete participation generates a number of problems. First of all, one would have to question seriously whether covert observation in care settings, without knowledge or permission of the people observed, is ethical. After all, this is not a public, open situation such as a street corner or rally, where individuals can't be identified. In the public domain observation is permissible and may produce valuable data. For health professionals who advocate caring and ethical behaviour, covert observation in closed settings would be inadvisable. We would not advocate this type of observation, and undergraduates or novice researchers should never attempt it.

The participant as observer

Here, researchers have negotiated their way into the setting, and as participant observers they are part of the work group under study. This seems a good way of doing research, as they are already involved in the work situation. They might want to examine aspects of their own hospital or ward, for instance. The first stage is to ask permission from the relevant gatekeepers and participants and explain the observer role to them. The advantage of this type of observation is the ease with which researcher–participant relationships can be forged or extended. Nurses can move around in the location as they wish, and thus observe in more detail and depth. For new researchers, observation is more difficult than interviewing because of the ethical issues involved and the time needed for 'prolonged engagement'.

The observer as participant

An observer who participates only by being in the location rather than working there, is only marginally involved in the situation. In this case, researchers might observe a particular unit but not directly work as part of the work force; for instance they might observe a location where they have not been previously. They must, however, announce their interest and their public role and go through the process of gaining entry and asking permission from patients, gatekeepers and colleagues. The advantages of this type of observation are the possibility of asking questions and being accepted as a colleague and researcher but not called upon as a member of the work force. On the other hand, observers are prevented from playing a 'real' role in the setting. Restraint from involvement is not easy, particularly in a busy situation where professionals must be protected from intrusion when working.

The complete observer

Complete observers do not take part in the setting and use a 'fly on the wall' approach. Being a complete observer when the observer is not a participant is only possible when the researchers observe through a two-way mirror where they are not noticed and have no impact on the situation or when they use static video cameras fixed on the ceiling. Again, permission from participants should be requested in healthcare settings.

Access and permission to observe is more difficult to achieve than in other forms of data collection. All within the setting are included in gaining this permission and also those who have power to withhold and gain access, such as managers. When researchers have achieved the initial contact it is important to establish rapport with the group or cultural members. Researchers must make quite clear that they are not 'spies' for management in any of these situations.

There is no clear distinction however between the two latter types of observation; they overlap.

Progression and process

Progression

Spradley (1980) claims that observers progress in three steps; they use *descriptive*, *focused* and finally *selective* observation. Descriptive observation proceeds on the basis of general questions that the observer has in mind. Everything that goes on in the setting provides data and is recorded, including colours, smells and appearances of people. Description involves all five senses. As time goes by, certain important areas or aspects of the setting become more obvious, and the researcher focuses on these because they contribute to the achievement of the research aim. Eventually observation becomes highly selective, centring on very specific issues only.

LeCompte and Preissle (1997) give guidelines for observation, which we will summarise here.

The 'who' questions

Who and how many people are present in the setting or take part in the activities? What are their characteristics and roles?

Nurse and midwife researchers observe the situation and specifically focus on the many role performances and interactions.

The 'what' questions

What is happening in the setting, what are the actions and rules of behaviour? What are the variations in the behaviour observed?

Health professionals focus on the activities and behaviour of those involved.

The 'where' questions

Where do interactions take place? Where are people located in the physical space?

For health professionals this means looking at the ward, the clinic, the GP's surgery or meeting. Even discussions at the bedside or handovers are of importance.

The 'when' questions

When do conversations and interactions take place? What is the timing of activities?

Events, discussions and interactions take place at different times. Health professionals must ask whether there is any significance in the timing of these.

The 'why' questions

Why do people in the setting act the way they do? Why are there variations in behaviour?

The why questions are self-explanatory. Researchers examine the reasons for the activities, behaviour or critical incidents. This does of course, often include interviewing participants.

Process

Mini-tour observation leads to detailed descriptions of smaller and more intimate units, while *grand-tour observations* are more appropriate for larger settings. After the initial stages, certain dimensions and features of observation become interesting to the researcher who then proceeds to observe these dimensions specifically. 'Progressive focusing', which was discussed earlier, is not just a feature of interviewing but also of observation.

The study becomes more focused as time progresses, because the observer notices important behaviours or interactions. Focused observations are the outcome of specific questions. From broader observations researchers might proceed to observing a small unit. They could look for similarities and differences among groups and individuals. For this type of observation narrow focus and specificity are useful and necessary.

Marshall and Rossman (1995: 79) state: 'observation entails the systematic noting and recording of events, behaviours and artefacts (objects) in the social setting chosen for study.' The situation can then be analysed. Researchers observe social processes as they happen and develop. Although they are able to examine events, processes and behaviour, they cannot explore past events and thoughts of participants except in interviews. Often, interviewing is seen as part of participant observation. The study by Becker and his colleagues (1961) shows this clearly. The participants, namely medical students, were observed in their interaction with patients, colleagues and teachers, and the researchers then asked questions about what they saw and heard. Hammersley and Atkinson (1995), in fact, propose that one might see all social research as participant observation to the extent that the researcher actively participates in the situation.

Researchers may be reluctant to carry out formal participant observation because of time and access problems; for instance, it is easier to interview colleagues or clients than to observe them. Observation might change the situation, as people act differently in the presence of observers, although they often forget being observed in long-term research. The latter, however, takes more time than is available in student projects and therefore it is more often used by postgraduates and experienced researchers who have a longer time span for their research.

When observations are successful, they can uncover interesting patterns and developments, which have their basis in the real world of the participants' daily lives, and the task of exploration and discovery is, after all the aim of qualitative research.

Technical procedures and practical hints

Researchers might use cameras and video equipment to catch movements and expressions of participants more accurately, although video cameras could intimidate or disturb the participants and change their behaviour. If tape is used, it can be viewed over and over again so 'nothing is lost' (Abrams, 2000: 58). This also means, of course, that the tapes must be kept secure and confidential, and they cannot be shown to colleagues or friends, only to supervisors with permission of the participants.

A most important task is to take fieldnotes. Observations are translated into written records which researchers take while observing or immediately afterwards. These are detailed descriptions of the setting and the behaviour of participants. The researchers' own reflections on the situation and their feelings about it are also recorded in fieldnotes (see Chapter 9).

Nurses and midwives who are actively involved in patient care may not be able to observe as well as take notes at the same time. It is important to record impressions as soon as possible after the observation. Diagrams and charts also help in recording how people act and interact in the setting under observation.

The analysis of observation will be discussed in Part Four of the book. Once health professionals have collected the initial observational data, they start analysing them so that the collection and analysis of data interact and go in parallel. This way the observation can become progressively focused on emerging and interesting themes that are important to the research. Drawing maps of the location or indicating interaction through diagrams can be useful devices to help observation.

Documentary sources of data

The third kind of datum consists of documents and written records. Hammersley and Atkinson (1995) suggest that researchers use these because they give information for situations that cannot be investigated by direct observation or questioning. Also, documentary sources contain added knowledge about the group being studied. Typically they consist of autobiographies and biographies, official documents and reports, the latter ranging from informal documentary sources to formal and official reports such as newspapers or minutes of meetings. Timetables, case notes and reports can become the focus of nurses' investigation. The researcher treats them like transcriptions of interviews or detailed descriptions of observations; that is, they are coded and categorised. They act as sensitising devices and make researchers aware of important issues.

Example

Hawker (1991) examined the patterns of care in two Dorset parishes between the years 1700–1799. She investigated the records in the County Record Office to find out how medical and nursing care were administered to sick poor people in two parishes. As there were few diaries and letters she looked at the overseer reports and accounts (an overseer of the poor was appointed by the parishes), and from these she gleaned which people helped the poor and how they did so.

Many of these texts exist before researchers start their work, others are initiated and organised by the researchers themselves. Historical documents, archives and products of the media exist independently from researchers while personal diaries might be written through their intervention or instigation; for instance Hammersley and Atkinson (1995) cite a study of a midwife who used personal diaries in her research on student midwives.

Scott (1990) differentiates between types of document by referring to them as *closed, restricted, open-archival* and *open-published.* Access to closed documents is limited to a few people, namely their authors and those who commissioned them. As far as restricted documents are concerned, researchers can only gain access with permission of insiders under particular conditions.

Example

Nettleton and Harding (1994) examined all informal letters of complaint to a Family Health Service Authority in 1990. They analysed the complaints that did not proceed to a hearing. These letters showed that patients, their relatives and friends complained about practitioners' non-response to requests, their personal behaviour, and the health professionals' perceived mistakes.

Permission for access is asked from the living authors of diaries and keepers of other confidential documents. Open-archival documents are available to any person, subject to administrative conditions and opening hours of libraries. Published documents, of course, can be accessed by anybody at any time. Merriam (1988) stresses the non-reactivity of documentary data and claims that they are grounded in their context. This makes them useful and rich sources of information for researchers.

Qualitative researchers most often seek access to diaries – which are people's own accounts of their lives – and letters, but also to historical documents or the products of the media. Some researchers encourage participants to keep a diary for analysis. For instance, Seibold *et al.* (1994) relate that one of the researchers on whose research they report encouraged the participants to keep a diary for twelve months. Jones (2000) lists two different forms of diary: *solicited* and *unsolicited*. The former are accounts of conditions or treatments kept by patients at the behest of researchers. Unsolicited diaries are the personal and informal records patients keep about their stay in hospital, about their condition, illness or care. A researcher cannot easily access these documents.

Example

Jones (2000) describes the case of an elderly man who had kept diaries for many years. She learnt that in these he had kept a record of symptoms and events while dealing with the health service and health professionals. Jones felt very fortunate to have this personal account of events that happened while the man had treatment for his condition. She saw the document as both authentic and meaningful.

Through documents, researchers in the health professions acquire a perspective on history which gives them insiders' views on past lives and attitudes, or they can analyse contemporary documents – such as articles and comments in the press – and become aware of the significant features of issues or the dramatisation of particular events. Last, and most importantly, health professionals can trace the perspectives of diary or autobiography writers by collecting, reading and analysing these personal documents. Through this researchers can gain knowledge of the experiences of others in a particular context and at a particular time.

Researchers must be concerned about four major criteria that determine the quality of the documents: *authenticity*, *credibility*, *representativeness* and *meaning* (Scott, 1990). To demonstrate authenticity for historical documents, questions about their history as well as their writers' intentions and biases must be asked. Credibility involves some of these questions too. Accuracy might be affected by the writer's proximity in time and place to the events described and also the conditions under which the information was acquired at the time. Representativeness of documents is difficult to prove because researchers often have no information of the numbers or variety of documents about a particular event.

Scott (1990) claims that the most significant aim of the document collection and analysis is their meaning and interpretation. It is far easier to analyse a personal document written in the recent past where the researcher is familiar with language and context than to assess the representativeness or authenticity of a historical document whose context can only be assumed. Therefore, the researcher can only try to interpret the meaning of the text in context, study the situation and conditions in which it is written and try to establish the writer's intentions.

As in other types of data, the meaning is tentative and provisional only and may change when new data present a challenge and demand reappraisal. Hammersley and Atkinson (1995) warn that documents may generate biases as they are often written by and for élites or people in power. That in itself, however, might be useful because not many sources exist that give the ideas of these informants.

Images as sources of data

Prosser (1998) regrets the neglect of images as part of qualitative inquiry. This, he believes, is due to the status of films and other images as objects of mass consumption and entertainment. Audiences sit in front of television or cinema screens or in the theatre. There is another reason for the low position of image-based research: researchers who work with visual data do not form a coherent group; they have not had a serious impact on qualitative research.

Loizos (2000) declares that images are important records of social reality. Visual information generates primary data or can be used to supplement other data collection methods, although care must be taken in its use. Videos in particular, can enhance and expand the data derived from initial observation (the ethical issues inherent in filming are problematic, however). Still photographs are not as useful – they freeze the situation in time and do not demonstrate its processual character.

Loizos gives some practical advice in his chapter on images, such as videos, photos or films. He also points to some essential reading for the use of images. He suggests, for instance, that researchers:

(1)   Log film rolls, cassettes, photos and other images immediately with written details of locations, people and dates
(2)   Get permission from informants to reproduce their images
(3)   Make sure to get good quality sound
(4)   Do not forget that the technology is just a means to an end
(5)   Only use films and other images when they really enhance the research as they may be expensive and disturb the participants in the situation

As we have explained in Chapter 1, researchers sometimes triangulate within method. One such study is that of McClelland and Sands (1993) who collected their data through participant observation, interviewing and written and audio-visual record. This enhances the trustworthiness and authenticity of the study.

References

Abrams, W.L. (2000) *The Observational Handbook: Understanding how consumers live with your product*. Chicago, NTC Business Books.

Ashworth, P. (1995) The meaning of 'participation' in participant observation. *Qualitative Health Research*, 5 (3) 366–87.

Atkinson, P. (1995) *Medical Talk and Medical Work*. London, Sage.

Becker, H.S., Geer, B., Hughes, E. & Strauss, A.L. (1961) *Boys in White*. New Brunswick, University of Chicago Press.

Bogdewic, S.P. (1999) Participant observation. In *Doing Qualitative Research* (eds B.F. Crabtree & W.L. Miller), 2nd edn, pp. 47–69. Thousand Oaks, Sage.

Gold, R. (1958) Roles in sociological field observation. *Social Forces*, **36**, 217–23.

Hammersley, M. & Atkinson, P. (1995) *Ethnography: Principles in Practice*, 2nd edn. London, Tavistock.

Hawker, J. (1991) An investigation of care in two Dorset parishes. Unpublished research diploma; Bournemouth Polytechnic, now Bournemouth University, Bournemouth.

Jones, R.K. (2000) The unsolicited diary as a qualitative research tool for advanced capacity in the field of health and illness. *Qualitative Health Research*, **10** (4) 555–67.

Jorgensen, D.L. (1989) *Participant Observation*. Newbury Park, Sage.

Lawler, J. (1991) *Behind the Screens: Nursing, Somology and the Problem of the Body*. Melbourne, Churchill Livingstone.

LeCompte, M.D. & Preissle, J. with Tesch, R. (1997) *Ethnography and Qualitative Design in Educational Research*, 2nd edn. Chicago, Academic Press.

Loizos, P. (2000) Video, film and photographs as research documents. In *Qualitative Researching with Text, Image and Sound* (eds M. Bauer & G. Gaskell), pp. 93–107. London, Sage.

Malinowski, B. (1922) *Argonauts of the Western Pacific: An Account of Native Enterprise and Adventure in the Archipelagos of Melanesian New Guinea*. New York, Dutton.

Marshall, C. & Rossman, G.R. (1995) *Designing Qualitative Research*, 2nd edn. Thousand Oaks, Sage.

McClelland, M. & Sands, R.G. (1993) The missing voice in interdisciplinary communication. *Qualitative Health Research*, **3** (1) 74–90.

Mead, M. (1935) *Sex and Temperament in Three Primitive Societies*. New York, Morrow.

Merriam, S.J. (1988) *Case Study Research in Education*. San Francisco, Jossey Bass.

Nettleton, S. & Harding, G. (1994) Protesting patients: A study of complaints submitted to a Family Health Service Authority. *Sociology of Health and Illness*, **16** (1) 38–61.

Prosser, J. (1998) The status of image-based research. In *Image-based Research: A Sourcebook for Qualitative Researchers* (ed. J. Prosser), pp. 97–112. London, The Falmer Press.

Rosenhan, D.L. (1973) On being sane in insane places. *Science*, **1** (179) 250–58.

Roth, J.A. (1963) *Timetables*. Indianapolis, Bobbs Merril.

Sanger, J. (1996) *The Compleat Observer? A Field Research Guide to Observation*. London, The Falmer Press.

Savage, J. (2000) Participant observation: Standing in the shoes of others. *Qualitative Health Research*, **10** (3) 324–39.

Schensul, S.L., Schensul J.J. & LeCompte M.D. (1999) *Essential Ethnographic Methods: Observations, Interviews and Questionnaires*. Walnut Creek, Altmira Press.

Scott, J. (1990) *A Matter of Record: Documentary Sources in Social Research*. Cambridge, Polity Press.

Seibold, C., Richards, L. & Simon, D. (1994) Feminist method and qualitative research about midlife. *Journal of Advanced Nursing*, **19**, 394–402.

Spradley, J.P. (1970) *You Owe Yourself a Drunk: An Ethnography of Urban Nomads*. Boston, Little, Brown.

Spradley, J.P. (1980) *Participant Observation*. Fort Worth, Harcourt Brace Johanovich.

Strauss, A.L. and Corbin, J.M. (1998) *Basics of Qualitative Research: Techniques and Procedures of Developing Grounded Theory*, 2nd edn. Beverley Hills, Sage.

Strauss, A.L., Schatzman, L., Bucher, R., Ehrlich, D. & Sabshin, M. (1964) *Psychiatric Ideologies and Institutions*. London, Collier Macmillan.

CHAPTER 7

Focus Groups as Qualitative Research

What is a focus group?

A focus group in nursing research involves a number of people – often with common experiences or characteristics – who are interviewed by a researcher (or moderator) for the purpose of eliciting ideas, thoughts and perceptions about a specific topic or certain issues linked to an area of interest.

In the past researchers have employed these techniques in the area of marketing and business research, but recently they have become popular in social science and the caring professions. Indeed, in nursing and midwifery they are increasingly used as an alternative to one-to-one interviews for evaluation of services, interventions or programmes (Kingry *et al.*, 1990). The ideas generated are normally analysed by qualitative methods, although focus groups can result in quantitative or multi-method research; for instance, they may generate findings to be used in the construction of a questionnaire, or employed as a way to obtain in-depth data at the end of a survey. The type of group and the number of interviews are determined by the research question.

The origin and purpose of focus groups

The first literature on focus groups was written in 1946 by Merton and Kendall, as a result of working with groups during and shortly after the Second World War. In 1956 they expanded their knowledge into a book (Merton *et al.*, 1956). Business and market researchers had used this type of in-depth group interview since the 1920s. It became especially popular in market research in order to gather information about customers' thoughts and feelings about a product.

Today the focus group interview is used by a wide variety of researchers in the area of communications, policy, marketing and advertising. Focus groups in the social sciences and health professions have become fashionable since the growth of qualitative research methods in the 1980s. In nursing it is seen as a useful strategy for the evaluation of services, interventions or programmes (Kingry *et al.*,

1990). This approach does not rely merely on the ideas of the researcher and a single participant; instead, the members of the group generate new questions and answers. Through these group interviews, professionals are able to discover the needs and feelings of their clients, the perceptions and attitudes of their colleagues, and they can examine the thoughts of decision makers. The cultural values and beliefs of people can also be explored this way.

These interviews produce thoughts and opinions about a topic relevant to health care, treatment evaluation and illness experiences. Many examples are reported in nursing and social science journals (Morgan and Spanish, 1985; Reed and Payton, 1997; McNally *et al.*, 1998; Burrows, 1998; Robinson, 1999).

Example

Reed and Payton (1997), for instance, reported on a study carried out in 1996, which involved focus group interviews with older people moving to nursing and residential homes. The participants were interviewed in groups prior to and around six months after their move about their experiences. Reed and Payton also set up staff interviews in focus groups.

Focus groups are characterised by interaction between the participants from which researchers discover how people think and feel about particular issues. It is not the intention to examine a wide variety of issues in one study; interviews are set up 'to obtain accurate data on a limited range of specific issues within a social context where people consider their own views in relation to others' (Robinson, 1999).

Focus group members respond to the interviewer and to each other. The questions might start with eliciting knowledge about a specific condition, the use of a drug, a method of intervention or by putting the members at ease but should soon go on to a discussion of feelings or thoughts. Different reactions stimulate debate about the topic because group members respond to each other. Discussions in groups might help not only in the development of ideas about problems and questions which researchers have not thought about before but also by finding answers to some of these questions and solutions to problems.

The ultimate goal for the researcher is to understand the reality of the participants, not to make decisions about a specific issue or problem, although future actions may be based on the findings of the focus group interviews.

Focus group interviews differ from interviews with individuals in that they explore and stimulate ideas based on shared perceptions of the world rather than on individual ideas. Robinson (1999: 910) specifically suggests some areas for focus group research in nursing:

(1) As needs assessment with professionals and potential clients
(2) To identify advantages and flaws for potential improvement
(3) To collect information on outcomes of programmes
(4) To overcome time constraints when little time is available
(5) For mutual support of participants when the topic is sensitive

Sample size and composition

The sample is linked closely to the research topic. The people who are interviewed in a focus group usually have similar roles or experiences. They may be colleagues who share the same speciality, use the same technical equipment or nursing procedures. The purpose of the focus group generally determines its composition and size. Morgan (1998b) claims that a small group is better for controversial or complex topics, while larger groups tend to have lower levels of involvement with less highly intense topic areas.

Example

One of our colleagues conducted focus group interviews with nurses who had experience of caring for patients who controlled their own pain post-operatively through a device that administers a dose of analgesia intravenously (patient controlled analgesia or PCA). The aim of the study was an exploration of interaction between patient and nurse and their relationship in this situation. The researcher chose a homogeneous group of 15 registered nurses who were female and aged between 27 and 40 years. She conducted five focus groups consisting of three participants each over a period of two months.

Ratcliffe, 1994

Morgan (1998a) suggests that well defined criteria are needed for this selection. These might include demographic factors, gender, ethnic group membership and specific experiences or conditions. Patients in focus groups will have had common experiences, have the same condition or receive the same treatment. For instance, if a nurse wishes to interview a group of people with diabetes, she or he obviously involves individuals with this condition in the focus groups. A midwife might obtain the feelings and thoughts of pregnant women or new mothers by small focus groups. Colleagues who are interviewed generally share common interests, work in similar settings, or perform similar tasks. If the interviewer wants the thoughts of colleagues from a psychiatric setting, for example, then the sample has to be composed of nurses with psychiatric experience. Students too can be interviewed in focus groups about perspectives on their education. Health promotion often is a topic for research, particularly with client groups who are vulnerable or suffer from a specific condition.

Carey (1994: 229) states that the selection of participants generally proceeds 'on the basis of their common experience related to the research topic'. Although group members share experiences, this does not mean that they all have the same views about the topic area, or that they come from the same background or organisation. It might be useful to recruit members from naturally occurring groups such as antenatal classes or patient support groups. While they have similar experiences, they are nevertheless heterogeneous in other ways, and so could illuminate the topic from all sides.

The number of focus groups depends on the needs of the researcher and the demands of the topic area. For one research project the usual number is about three or four, but the actual number depends on the complexity of the research topic. The findings from the focus group interviews are often used as a basis for action.

Example

Robinson (1999) reports on a study by Kennedy *et al.* (1996). This project examined risk behaviour in young people. The researchers found that the young participants, although feeling positive about using condoms, did not behave accordingly. Relevant health and social care messages were designed based on research findings from young people, their parents and youth organisations.

Studies with large focus groups and many informants exist too. For instance Hart and Rotem (1990) used 15 groups, which included a total of 104 nurses from 44 wards. The normal group involved seven participants. Group sessions can last from one to three hours. We must stress, however, that three-hour interviews with patients would be far too long and demanding. In market research, participants are paid for their time and effort but not in nursing research, because this would coerce the informants and squander resources. Most new information emerges in the first groups (Kingry *et al.*, 1990); as in other qualitative research important themes emerge often at an early stage, although some serendipitous results might be found in a later phase.

Each group contains between four and twelve people, but six is probably the optimum number as it is large enough to provide a variety of perspectives and small enough not to become disorderly or fragmented. Indeed, one of our colleagues found that in her experience, a group of six was too large and that the optimum number of members in the group was three. Greenbaum (1998), a market researcher, however, claims that group dynamics work better if the group is not too small. The larger the group, the more difficult the transcription becomes. When several people start talking together and the group becomes lively, it can be difficult to distinguish voices.

There may well be a difference between groups who come together for market research purposes and those who gather for health research. The former will feel much less vulnerable because the area of discussion is rarely threatening or sensitive. The nature of the topic area is of importance: focus groups in which sensitive topics are discussed are more difficult to facilitate.

Members of the group, although sharing common experiences, do not have to know each other. In a group of immediate colleagues or friends, private thoughts or ideas might not be revealed, although occasionally the opposite could be true. One individual is more likely to dominate others and the past history of the group may inhibit or lead individuals in a particular direction. In nursing research, familiarity between participants, or participants and researchers could be useful because the 'warm-up' time – the time where informants get to know each other to facilitate interaction – is shorter, and the researcher can focus on the topic immediately. It is believed (Stewart and Shamdasani, 1990) that compatibility among group members is more productive than conflict or polarisation, although this too depends on the topic; sometimes conflict can generate new and different ideas.

Gender and age of the group members affect the quality and level of interaction and through this the data. For instance, evidence shows greater diversity of ideas in single sex groups than in those of mixed gender (Stewart and Shamdasani, 1990). The latter tend to be more conforming because of the social interaction between males and females; both groups sometimes tend to 'perform' for each other.

Conducting focus group interviews

Focus group interviews must be planned carefully. The informants are contacted well in advance of the interviews and reminded a few days before they start. As in other types of inquiry, ethical and access issues are considered. The environment for a focus group is important as the room must be big enough to contain the participants and the tape-recorder placed in an advantageous location, where they can all be heard and recorded. For focus group work, it is essential to have a top quality tape-recorder. Merton and King (1990) suggest a spatial arrangement of a circle or semi-circle, which seems the most successful seating arrangement.

The group interviews should have a clearly identified agenda otherwise they deteriorate into vague and chaotic discussions (Stewart and Shamdasani, 1990). Morgan (1997) believes in the importance of time management because both interviewer and informants have limited time. Time management is one of the tasks of the facilitator. Focus groups are more productive if the time for interchange is not too short. Usually focus group interviews last around $1\frac{1}{2}$ to 2 hours.

From the beginning the researcher establishes ground rules, so that all group members know how to proceed. Researchers plan initial questions and prompts. When the interviews start, the interviewer puts the group at ease and introduces the topic to be debated. Strategies such as showing a film or telling a story related to the topic sometimes stimulate interaction. Kitzinger and Barbour (1999) also suggest such stimulus material as vignettes or photographs. Researchers often adopt the strategy of asking stimulus questions and generally proceed from the more general to the specific, just as in other qualitative interviews. Involving all the participants, rather than letting a few individuals dominate the situation demands diplomacy and should be easier with a smaller group. Extreme views in a group of people are balanced out by the reactions of the majority when debating questions. As suggested before, focus groups can be combined with individual interviews, observation or other methods of data collection, though Morgan and Krueger (1993) maintain that it is not necessary to validate focus interviews by other methods.

In focus groups, as in all other research, ethical issues must be considered (see Chapter 3) Confidentiality, in particular, could be problematic in group interviews as members of the group might discuss the findings in other settings and situations. They should be reminded to keep the discussions confidential. Anonymity cannot be guaranteed, as members of the group might be able to identify other participants even when researchers only use first names. Participants may make remarks that are hurtful to others, or show prejudice, and the researcher has to find ways to deal with this.

The involvement of the interviewer

The interviewer becomes the facilitator or moderator in the group discussion although it could be useful to have another person who takes notes. In nursing or midwifery research, the health professional is usually the interviewer (while in market research focus groups professional moderators are employed). In health research generally a single interviewer facilitates the groups. The presence of a note-taker who can make fieldnotes, draw diagrams with the names of participants and generally help with practical matters, could be very useful. The researcher should have the particular qualities of the in-depth interviewer: flexibility, open-mindedness and skill in eliciting information. The creation of an open and non-threatening group climate is one of their initial important tasks.

Researchers must be able to stimulate discussion and have insight and interest in the ideas of the informants. The leadership role of the moderators demands abilities above that of the one-to-one interviewer. They must have the social and refereeing skills to guide the members towards effective interaction and sometimes be able to exert control over informants and topic without directing the debate or coercing the participants. If the group feels at ease with the interviewer, the interaction will be open and productive, and the participants will be comfortable about disclosing their perceptions and feelings. Researchers might experience difficulties with particular groups such as teenagers, while getting together groups of disabled people may present practical problems in the available space.

Morgan (1997) advises that the interviewers hold back on questioning if they want to examine the real feelings of participants; much of the discussion evolves from the dynamics of group interaction. This non-directive approach has particular importance in exploratory research where perceptions are examined. High involvement of the interviewer leads more quickly to the core of the topic, but special facilitation skills are needed if the focus groups are going to be successful. Biases of the interviewer should not be expressed in the focus groups. A special relationship with a specific individual, an affirmative nod at something of which the interviewer approves, or a lack of encouragement for unexpected or unwelcome answers may bias the interviews. Again, group behaviour is an important factor. Polarisation of views may generate a difficult group climate. Although conflicts of opinion can produce valuable data, the interviewer must defuse personal hostility between members, which demands good facilitating skills. Gestures and facial expressions have to be controlled to show members of the group that the interviewer is non-judgemental and values the views of all participants.

The analysis of interviews

Although there are a variety of different types of analysis for these interviews (Krueger, 1998), the principles of qualitative data analysis are similar to those of other non-structured or semi-structured interviews. Most often the interviews are recorded, and the researcher listens several times to each tape before making transcripts. Although this method has been used in market research, it is difficult to identify individuals' voices on a tape. The problem of identification might be overcome with videotaping, but Sim (1998) suggests that this might inhibit participants, particularly when they discuss a sensitive issue.

All tapes, fieldnotes and memos are dated and labelled. A wide margin is left on the transcript for coding and categorising. The transcription should include laughter, notes about pauses and emphasis, and the researcher makes fieldnotes on anything unusual, interesting or contradictory and writes memos about theoretical ideas while listening, transcribing and reading. It is important to be clear about who says what, because this can identify those individuals who try to dominate the discussion. The interviewer could note this while listening to the tape. At the listening stage, major themes and patterns can already be found. It is important, however, that researchers focus on the context of group interaction not just on the comments of individuals (Asbury, 1995).

Interviewers code paragraphs and sentences by extracting the essence of ideas within them and using labels which they put into the margin of the transcript. Through a reduction of these codes into larger categories, themes and ideas will be found. Krueger (1994) claims that not all data deserve equal importance, therefore the researcher must search for priorities and important themes from the vast amount of data. The method of analysis in focus groups is similar to those of other approaches; in fact, focus groups can be analysed by grounded theory analysis (see Chapter 10) or a simpler form of thematic analysis.

The analyst repeats the process with each focus group interview and compares the transcripts. The major themes arising from each interview are then connected with each other; topics in one interview will overlap with those of other focus groups. Once these themes have been formulated, the patterns described and their meaning interpreted, the literature connected with these ideas is discussed. The appropriate literature becomes part of the data as in other qualitative research. Researchers substantiate their work with relevant quotes from the participants, showing the data from which the patterns and constructs arise.

To write up the study, the interviewer develops a storyline, that is, he or she must produce an account that is readable and clear. The main concerns of the participants have to emerge from the report as the most important parts of the story.

Advantages and limitations of focus groups

In general the advantages and limitations in this approach are those of all qualitative interviews, but there are a number of strengths and weaknesses specific to focus groups (Stewart and Shamdasani, 1990; Sim 1998; Robinson, 1999). The main strength is the production of data through social interaction. The dynamic interaction stimulates the thoughts of participants and reminds them of their own feelings about the research topic. Informants build on the answers of others in the group. Second, on responding to each other's comments, informants might generate new and spontaneous ideas, which researchers had not thought of before or during the interview. Through interaction they remember forgotten feelings and thoughts. Third, all the participants, including the interviewer, have the opportunity to ask questions, and these will produce more ideas than individual interviews. Informants can build on the answers of others. Kitzinger (1994) maintains that group interaction gives courage to the informants to mention even sensitive topics. The interview might empower participants because as group members they often feel more able to express their views.

The interviewer has the opportunity for prompts and questions for clarification just like the other members of the group. These probes will produce more ideas than individual interviews, and the answers show the participants' feelings about a topic and the priorities in the situation under discussion. The researcher can clarify conflicts between participants and ask about the reasons for these differing views. Focus groups produce more data in the same space of time; this could make them cheaper and quicker than individual interviews.

There are also some disadvantages. The researcher generally has more difficulty managing the debate and less control over the process than in one-to-one interviews. As group members interact throughout the interview, one or two individuals may dominate the discussion and influence the outcome or perhaps even introduce bias, as the other members may be merely compliant. The group effect may, as Carey and Smith (1994) suggest, lead to conformity or to convergent answers. They use the term 'censoring', by which they mean the critical stance of group members towards each other. The participants affect each other, while in individual interviews the 'real' feelings of the individual informant may be more readily revealed. A person who is unable to verbalise feelings and thoughts will not make a good informant in focus groups. Indeed, Merton and King (1990) stress the importance of educational homogeneity of the group. If group members have similar educational backgrounds, the chance for contribution from all members is greater. The status of a few well educated individuals would inhibit the rest of the members in the group and might even silence them, and therefore similarity of social background is useful. The group members might know each other before the meeting, and it is important to take this into account. This means that sampling procedures which determine the composition of the group, are of paramount importance.

The group climate can inhibit or fail to stimulate an individual or it can, of course, be stimulating and lively and generate more data. Where a researcher feels certain that confrontation and conflict is likely to occur between potential group members, she or he has to be sensitive to group feelings and reconcile their ideas. Conflict can be destructive but can also generate rich data. In any conflict situation, ethical issues must be carefully considered. Sim (1998) identifies some problems with focus groups.

(1) It cannot be assumed that there is conformity and consensus between the individual members of the group, although it might seem so.
(2) Although some inferences may be drawn about the absence or presence of certain perspectives or feelings, the strength of the individual's emotions cannot be measured or assumed.
(3) Focus group findings based on empirical data cannot be generalised, though theoretical generalisation is feasible.

Krueger (1994) suggests that researchers experience greater difficulty getting groups together at a certain time and location while finding it easy to make appointments with individuals. Transcription can be much more difficult because peoples' voices vary, and the distance they sit from the microphone influences the clarity of individuals' contributions. As there are certain dangers of group effect and group member control, it is useful to analyse the interviews both at group level and at the level of the individual participants. The researcher must remember that the data must be seen within the context of the group setting (Carey and Smith, 1994). Fieldnotes should be made immediately after the session.

Critical comments on focus group interviews in nursing

There is some criticism about the use of focus groups in nursing. We would suggest that sometimes these interviews are used because researchers feel this is a new and easy way of gaining access to a larger sample. The complexities of setting up and facilitating focus groups are often forgotten. In a search through the Cumulative Index of Nursing and Allied Health Literature (CINAHL), Webb and Kevern (2001) found rather unsophisticated and uncritical uses of focus group research in the years 1990–1999. Few articles contained empirical research, and furthermore, some of the discussions were superficial and non-analytical. The writers suggest that researchers discuss the theoretical and methodological assumptions in their work and become more rigorous in their use of methodology. Webb and Kevern claim that the input from other disciplines, the social sciences in particular, would enhance and develop nursing knowledge.

Summary

A focus group consists of a small number of people with common experiences or areas of interest.

- Several focus groups with a small number of individuals are involved in each study.
- Whilst the interviews are carefully planned, the interviewer must at the same time be flexible and non-judgemental.
- The dynamic of the group situation is intended to stimulate ideas and elicit feelings about the focus of the study.
- It is important that an open climate exists so that group members feel comfortable about sharing their thoughts and feelings.
- The data can be analysed by any qualitative analysis method as long as researchers have adhered to the principles of the particular approach.

References

Asbury, J. (1995) Overview of focus group research. *Qualitative Health Research*, 5 (4) 414–20.

Burrows, D. (1998) Using focus groups in nursing research: a personal reflection. *Social Sciences in Health*, 4, 3–14.

Carey, M.A. (1994) The group effect in focus groups: planning, implementing and interpreting focus group research. In *Critical Issues in Qualitative Research Method* (ed. J.M. Morse), pp. 225–41. Thousand Oaks, Sage.

Carey, M.A. & Smith, M.W. (1994) Capturing the group effect in focus groups. *Qualitative Health Research*, 4 (1) 123–7.

Greenbaum, T.L. (1998) *The Handbook for Focus Group Research*, 2nd edn. Lexington, Lexington Books/DC Heath and Co.

Hart, G. & Rotem, A. (1990) Using focus groups to identify clinical learning opportunities for registered nurses. *Australian Journal of Advanced Nursing*, **8** (1) 16–21.

Kennedy, M.G., Rosenbaum, J., Doucette-Gate, A., Flynn, N., Miller, J. & Shepard, M. (1996) *Focus groups theme that will shape participating social marketing interventions in five cities*. Abstract 11, International Conference on AIDS, Vancouver.

Kingry, J.M., Tiedje, L.B. & Friedman, L.L. (1990) Focus groups: A research technique for nursing. *Nursing Research*, **39** (2) 124.

Kitzinger, J. (1994) The methodology of focus groups: the importance of interaction between research participants. *Sociology of Health & Illness*, **16** (1) 102–21.

Kitzinger, J. & Barbour, R.S. (1999) Introduction: the challenge and promise of focus groups. In *Developing Focus Groups Research: Politics, Theory and Practice* (eds R.S. Barbour & J. Kitzinger), pp. 1–20. London, Sage.

Krueger, R.A. (ed.) (1994) *Focus Groups: A Practical Guide for Applied Research*, 2nd edn. Thousand Oaks, Sage.

Krueger, R.A. (1998) Analysing and reporting focus groups. Vol. 6 of *The Focus Group Kit* (eds D.L. Morgan & R.A. Krueger). Thousand Oaks, Sage.

McNally, N.J., Phillips, D.R. & Williams, H.C. (1998) Focus groups in dermatology. *Clinical and Experimental Dermatology*, **23**, 195–200.

Merton, R.K., Fiske, M. & Kendall, P.L. (1956) *The Focused Interview*. New York, Columbia University Press.

Merton, R.K. & Kendall, P.L. (1946) The focused interview. *American Journal of Sociology*, **51**, 541–57.

Merton, R.K. & King, R. (1990) *The Focused Interview: A Manual of Problems and Procedures*. New York, Free Press.

Morgan, D.L. (1997) *Focus Groups as Qualitative Research*. Thousand Oaks, Sage.

Morgan, D.L. (1998a) The focus group guidebook. Vol. 1 of *The Focus Group Kit* (eds D.L. Morgan & R.A. Krueger). Thousand Oaks, Sage.

Morgan, D.L. (1998b) Planning focus groups. Vol. 2 of *The Focus Group Kit* (eds D.L. Morgan & R.A. Krueger). Thousand Oaks, Sage.

Morgan, D.L. & Krueger, R.A. (1993) When to use focus groups and why. In *Successful Focus Groups: Advancing the State of the Art* (ed. D.L. Morgan), pp. 3–19. Newbury Park, Sage.

Morgan, D.L. & Spanish, M.T. (1985) Social interaction and the cognitive organisation of health-relevant knowledge. *Sociology of Health and Illness*, **7** (3) 401–22.

Morgan, D.L. & Krueger, R.A. (eds) (1998) *The Focus Group Kit*. Thousand Oaks, Sage.

Ratcliffe, B. (1994) *Post-Operative Nurse–Patient Interaction During Patient Controlled Analgesia*. Unpublished MSc dissertation, Surrey University, Guildford.

Reed, J. & Payton, V.R. (1997) Focus groups: issues of analysis and interpretation. *Journal of Advanced Nursing*, **26**, 765–71.

Robinson, N. (1999) The use of focus group methodology – with selected examples from sexual health research. *Journal of Advanced Nursing*, **2**, 905–13.

Sim, J. (1998) Collecting and analysing qualitative data: issues raised by focus groups. *Journal of Advanced Nursing*, **28**, 345–52.

Stewart, D.W. & Shamdasani P.N. (1990) *Focus Groups: Theory and Practice*. Newbury Park, Sage.

Webb, C. & Kevern, J. (2001) Focus groups as a research method: a critique of some aspects of their use in nursing research. *Journal of Advanced Nursing*, **33** (6) 798–805.

CHAPTER 8

Sampling

Purposeful (or purposive) sampling

Patton (1990) states that the underlying principle of gaining rich, in-depth information guides the sampling strategies of the qualitative researcher. The selection of participants, settings or units of time are criterion-based, that is, certain criteria are applied, and the sample is chosen accordingly. Sampling units are selected for a specific purpose on which the researcher decides, therefore the term 'purposive' or 'purposeful' sampling is used. LeCompte and Preissle (1997) assert that 'criterion-based' is a better term for this type of sampling than 'purposive', because most sampling strategies, even random sampling, are highly purposive. However, *purposeful* is the term used by most qualitative researchers.

Researchers must ask two questions: *what* to sample and *how* to sample. People generally form the main sampling units. The useful informant is chosen by the researcher or may be self-selected. Sometimes researchers can easily identify individuals or groups with special knowledge of a topic, occasionally they advertise or ask for informants who have insight into a particular situation or are experts in an area of knowledge. Morse (1991b: 132) identifies the 'good' informant: 'Good informants must be willing and able to critically examine the experience and their response to the situation ... must be willing to share the experience with the interviewer'. Individuals are sampled for the information they can provide about a specific phenomenon, be it a condition, such as an illness, a treatment (for instance the use of counselling), a type of care, professional decision making, etc. They could be nurses who have cared for people undergoing treatment, patients who have had day surgery, or midwifery students who are interviewed about their clinical experience and so on. Identification of a particular population provides boundaries between those who are included in the study and those who stay outside it. The members of the sample share certain characteristics. The sample is thus chosen on the basis of personal knowledge about the phenomenon under study.

Useful informants would be people who have had experiences about which the researcher wants to gain information. For example, individuals who have diabetes might share experiences and the meanings that these have for them with the nurse researcher.

Informants with special knowledge or experience include newcomers, or those who are changing status in a setting. Individuals who are willing to talk about their experience and perceptions are often those persons who have a special approach to their work. Some have power or status; others are naïve, frustrated, hostile or attention seeking, although one must remember that the latter are not always the best informants because they may have a mainly negative perception of the organisation or institution under discussion. Ethically it is important that the persons in the sample are not jeopardised by uncovering their practices and ideologies.

Sampling types

There are various forms of sampling. We shall discuss only the most often used and important types. An overview of a whole range can be found in Patton (1990) and Kuzel (1999), although many sampling types overlap. The commonest methods are:

- Homogeneous sampling
- Heterogeneous sampling
- Total population sampling
- Chain referral sampling
- Convenience or opportunistic sampling
- Theoretical sampling

Homogeneous sampling

This involves individuals who belong to the same subculture or have similar characteristics. Nurses often use homogeneous sample units when they wish to observe or interview a particular group, for instance specialist nurses. Midwives may wish to examine the perspectives of community midwives on their role in the community. In these examples, a homogeneous group is being studied. The sample can be homogeneous with respect to a certain variable only – for instance, occupation, length of experience, type of experience, age or gender. The important variable would be established before the sampling starts.

Heterogeneous sampling

A heterogeneous sample contains individuals or groups of individuals who differ from each other in a major aspect. For instance, nurses may wish to explore the perceptions of nurses, social workers and doctors who care for patients with HIV. The three groups form a heterogeneous sample. Heterogeneous sampling is also called maximum variation sampling (Patton, 1990; Kuzel, 1999) because it involves a search for variations in settings and for individuals with widely differing experiences.

> **Example**
>
> A good example can be found in an ethnographic study by Tarasuk and Eakin (1995). These researchers investigated the link between work-related back injury and moral judgements that were made by others. The heterogeneous sample consisted of males and females, across a broad range of ages with different jobs and from a variety of different backgrounds. This was done to maximise contrasts between the participants.

May (1991) suggests that the initial sample might consist of a natural group, while later sampling is based on early findings with this group and cannot be determined prior to the study. For instance, a midwife could sample women who have just given birth to their first child and find that it would be interesting to select older and younger primiparae because they might have different ideas about childbirth. Sometimes married couples are chosen as samples or people who live together. Occasionally the sample consists of focus groups, for instance self-help groups, or groups with similar conditions or experiences.

Total population sampling

Morse (1991a) mentions a total population sample when all participants selected come from a particular group. For instance, all the nurses with specific knowledge or a skill, such as counselling, might be interviewed because the researcher focuses on this skill, and there might be few available with this skill. The researcher might interview all midwives in one midwifery unit because the specific setting in which they work or the special techniques they adopt are seen as important.

Chain referral sampling

A variation of a purposive sample is chain referral or *snowball* sampling (Biernacki and Waldorf, 1981). Morse (1991a) calls this type 'nominated sampling'. A previously chosen informant is asked to suggest other individuals with knowledge of a particular area or topic who participate and in turn nominate other individuals for the research. Researchers use snowball sampling in studies where they cannot identify useful informants, where informants are not easily accessible or where anonymity is desirable, for instance in studies about drug addiction or alcohol use.

Example

Three American researchers, Kearney and her colleagues (1994), interviewed women crack cocaine users about sexuality and reproductive issues. Instead of accessing these women directly, the researchers preferred chain referral sampling.

Convenience or opportunistic sampling

The terms *convenience or opportunistic* sampling are self-explanatory. The researcher uses opportunities to ask people who might be useful for the study. To some extent, of course, most sampling is opportunistic and arranged for the convenience of the researcher. Researchers usually adopt this strategy when recruiting people is difficult. The researcher always chooses individuals whose ideas or experiences will help achieve the aim of the research.

Example

One of our students put up posters in a day centre to obtain a sample of old people who lacked physical mobility, another advertised for students in a refectory. Sometimes a sample is chosen by an organisation although this can lead to problems.

Theoretical sampling

Glaser and Strauss (1967) advocate *theoretical sampling* in the process of collecting data. Theoretical sampling develops as the study proceeds, and it cannot be planned beforehand. Researchers select their sample on the basis of concepts and theoretical issues that arise during the research. The theoretical ideas control the collection of data; therefore researchers have to justify the inclusion of particular sampling units. At the point of data saturation, when no new ideas arise that are of value to the developing theory, sampling can stop. (For details of theoretical samples see Chapter 10.) Coyne (1997) discusses qualitative sampling in depth and differentiates between purposive and theoretical sampling (see Chapter 10), although she believes that theoretical sampling could be called 'analysis driven purposeful sampling'. Sandelowski (1995) also maintains that all sampling in qualitative research is purposeful; it is intended to achieve a specific aim. She claims that theoretical sampling is merely a variation of purposive sampling.

Other methods

LeCompte and Preissle (1997) identify other methods of purposeful or criterion-based sampling:

- Extreme-case selection
- Typical-case selection
- Unique-case selection

In *extreme-case selection*, the researcher identifies certain characteristics for the setting or population. Extremes of these characteristics are sought and arranged on a continuum. The cases that belong at the two ends of this continuum become the extreme cases. For instance, nurses may study a very large or a very small ward. These can be compared with cases that are the norm for the hospital population.

In *typical-case selection*, researchers create a profile of characteristics for an average case and find instances of this. They might exclude the very young or old, the almost healthy and the most vulnerable or any other participants at the end of a continuum.

When choosing *unique cases*, researchers study those that differ from others by a single characteristic or dimension such as people who share a particular condition but come from an unusual community, such as a sect or ethnic group.

Kuzel (1999) lists five important characteristics of sampling in qualitative research:

(1) Flexible sampling which develops during the study
(2) Sequential selection of sampling units
(3) Sampling guided by theoretical development which becomes progressively more focused
(4) Continuing sampling until no new relevant data arise
(5) Searching for negative or deviant cases

Sampling decisions

Early in a research project, and depending on the research question and focus, researchers have to make their sampling decisions. Qualitative approaches demand different sampling techniques from the randomly selected and probabilistic sampling used by quantitative researchers. It is, however, just as important for qualitative researchers to make their sampling decisions on a systematic basis and on rational grounds. A sample in qualitative research consists of sampling units of people, time or setting. Nurse and midwife researchers have to select the individuals or group members (*whom* to sample), the time and context (*what* to sample) and the place (*where* to sample), because they cannot investigate everything. It must be remembered that the people and places must be available and accessible.

The sampling strategies adopted can make a difference to the whole study. The rules of qualitative sampling are less rigid than those of quantitative methods where a strict sampling frame is established before the research starts. It is important, however, that the researchers describe how they gained access to the sample. Morse and Field (1996) advise that sampling be both appropriate and adequate. Appropriateness means that the method of sampling fits the aim of the study and helps the understanding of the research problem. A sampling strategy is adequate if it generates adequate and relevant information and sufficient quality data.

Sampling takes place after the research focus has been decided. Although qualitative researchers start selecting participants at this stage, they can continue the selection throughout the process if more are needed because of the changing focus or extension of ideas as the study progresses, especially in grounded theory and ethnography. It is not necessary to specify the overall sample and give an exact number of informants from the beginning of the study, although an initial sample should be stated. This sampling strategy differs from quantitative research where respondents are chosen before the project begins. A qualitative proposal could state, for instance, that the initial sample should consist of x (number of) informants. Grounded theory and ethnography favour this type of sampling while phenomenologists choose a sample and do not generally add to it at a later stage. Ethics committees do not always accommodate the idea of theoretical sampling and wish to know the exact number and clear description of the sample.

Sampling parameters

The investigators do not only decide on the participants in their study but also on the time and location of the research. Whatever the sample, the criteria for selecting it must be clearly identified. Some examples are shown in Fig. 8.1.

Hammersley and Atkinson (1995) suggest that the main dimensions on which sampling takes place are people, context and time. The people in the study are chosen for their experience and knowledge of the phenomenon under study.

Sampling parameters	Examples
People	Triage nurses Ward managers
Events and processes	Entry to hospital ward Interaction between nurse and patients
Activities	Giving injections, taking blood pressure
Time	Six months before and after visiting the pain clinic Morning and afternoon

Fig. 8.1 Examples of sampling parameters (adapted from Miles and Huberman, 1994)

Hammersley and Atkinson also claim that a particular context might be linked to specific kinds of action and interaction, and therefore researchers have to examine a range of contexts in which the phenomenon under study occurs. Different times of the day, year or stages in the process of care might also be a significant factor in the research.

Example 1: *Settings*

A midwife tutor has decided to examine the role of the clinical midwife teacher. She chooses three different hospitals in the South of England as the setting for her study.

Example 2: *Time*

A nurse researcher finds that patients are restless at a particular time of the morning. She might then focus on a specific time in the afternoon to see whether patients behave in a similar way at that time.

Sample size

The sample may be small or large, depending on the type of research question, material and time resources as well as on the number of researchers. Generally qualitative sampling consists of small sampling units studied in depth. Patton (1990) insists that no guidelines exist for sample size in qualitative research and sample size differs greatly in qualitative studies. Benner (1984), for instance, uses a very large heterogeneous sample (109 participants, but these are not all interviewed individually) in her study on nurses and their ideas about caring.

Although there are no rigid rules, research texts often mention that 6–8 data units are needed when the sample consists of a homogeneous group while 12–20 suffice for a heterogeneous sample (Kuzel, 1999). Most often, the sample consists of between 4 and 40 informants, though certain research projects contain as many as 200 participants. Qualitative studies that include a large sample do exist. Sample size, however, does not necessarily determine the importance of the study or the quality of the data.

Example

Field's (1983) sampling frame contained four informants, while Melia (1987) interviewed forty. Strong (1979) includes as many as 1000. Most studies comprise a small sample.

We do not see justification for a very large sample in qualitative research. Students or experienced researchers often use these to appease funding bodies, which are used to large samples, or research committees, which do not always know much about qualitative research. Wolcott (1994) asserts that the wish for a large sample size is rooted in quantitative research where there is a need to generalise. He maintains that a large sample in qualitative research does not enhance the research, indeed it can do harm as it might lack the depth and richness of a smaller sample. Banister *et al.* (1994) claim that when the sample size is too large, the specific response of the participants and their meanings might be lost or not respected. If the sample is too large, there is loss of the unique and idiographic.

What shall we call the people chosen for the sample?

It is difficult for researchers to know what term to use for the people they interview and observe, especially as this name makes explicit the stance of the researchers and their relationship to those being studied. We favour the terms 'participant' or 'informant'. In surveys, both by structured interviews and written questionnaires, the most frequent term has been 'respondents', and indeed, many qualitative researchers and research texts still use it (for instance Miles and Huberman, 1994), but it seems less frequent now in qualitative research texts and reports.

Morse (1991b) claims that 'respondent' implies a passive response to a stimulus – the researcher's question. It sounds mechanistic. Experimental researchers refer to 'subjects', again a word that expresses passivity of the people involved in a study. Interestingly this is still used in legal documents and ethical guidelines (see Chapter 3). Seidman (1998) argues that this term distinguishes between people as objects and subjects and can be positive, but it also demonstrates inequality between researchers and researched. In qualitative research it would be inappropriate. 'Interviewee' sounds clumsy and boring.

Anthropologists refer to 'informants', those members of a culture or group who voluntarily 'inform' the researcher about their world and play an active part in the research. Morse usually chooses this term, though she acknowledges the suggestion by some journal editors that it might be seen to have links to the word 'informant' as used by the police. Fetterman (1998) dislikes the term 'informant', as it reminds him of the language use of ethnographers during colonial times. Most ethnographers, however, still use the term and do not perceive it as negative. Most qualitative researchers prefer the term 'participant'; this expresses the collaboration between the researcher and the researched (DePoy and Gitlin, 1998) and the equality of their relationship, but the term could be misleading as the researcher, too, is a participant.

In the end, however, the nurses or midwives must choose for themselves which term suits their research. In Morse's words: 'Subjects, respondents, informants, participants – choose your own term, but choose a term that fits' (1991b: 406). We suggest that our students use the terms 'informant' or, better still, 'participant' but never the term 'subject'.

Summary

The important features of sampling are as follows.

- Sampling is purposeful, chosen specifically for the study and criterion-based.
- The sample of individuals in qualitative research is generally small.
- Sampling units can consist of people, time, setting, processes or concepts (the latter is called theoretical sampling).
- Sampling is not always wholly determined prior to the study but may proceed throughout.
- The individuals in the sample are usually called *participants* or *informants* rather than respondents (in qualitative research they are never subjects).

References

Banister, P., Burman, E., Parker, I., Taylor, M. & Tindall, C. (1994) *Qualitative Methods in Psychology: A Research Guide*. Buckingham, Open University Press.

Benner, P. (1984) *From Novice to Expert*. Menlo Park, Addison-Wesley Publishing.

Biernacki, P. & Waldorf, D. (1981) Snowball sampling: problems and techniques of chain referral sampling. *Sociological Methods and Research*, **10** (2) 141–63.

Coyne, I.T. (1997) Sampling in qualitative research: purposeful and theoretical sampling: merging or clear boundaries? *Journal of Advanced Nursing*, **26**, 623–30.

DePoy, E. & Gitlin, L.N. (1998) *Introduction to Research: Multiple Strategies for Health and Human Services*. St. Louis, CV Mosby.

Fetterman, D.M. (1998) *Ethnography: Step by Step*, 2nd edn. Thousand Oaks, Sage.

Field, P.A. (1983) An ethnography: four public health nurses' perspectives on nursing. *Journal of Advanced Nursing*, **8**, 3–12.

Glaser, B. & Strauss, A. (1967) *The Discovery of Grounded Theory*. Chicago, Aldine.

Hammersley, M. & Atkinson, P.A. (1995) *Ethnography: Principles in Practice*. 2nd edn. London, Tavistock.

Kearney, M.H., Murphy, S. & Rosenbaum, M. (1994) Learning by losing: sex and fertility on crack cocaine. *Qualitative Health Research*, **4** (2) 142–85.

Kuzel, A.J. (1999) Sampling in qualitative inquiry. In *Doing Qualitative Research* (eds B.F. Crabtree & W.L. Miller), 2nd edn, pp. 33–45. Thousand Oaks, Sage.

LeCompte, M.D. & Preissle, J. with Tesch, R. (1997) *Ethnography and Qualitative Design in Educational Research*, 2nd edn. Chicago, Academic Press.

May, K.A. (1991) Interview techniques in qualitative research: concerns and challenges. In *Qualitative Nursing Research: A Contemporary Dialogue* (ed. J. Morse), pp. 188–201. Newbury Park, Sage.

Melia, K. (1987) *Learning and Working*. London, Tavistock.

Miles, M.B. & Huberman, A.M. (1994) *Qualitative Data Analysis*, 2nd edn. Thousand Oaks, Sage.

Morse, J.M. (1991a) *Qualitative Nursing Research: A Contemporary Dialogue*, revised edn, pp. 127–45. Newbury Park, Sage.

Morse, J.M. (1991b) Subjects, respondents, informants and participants. Editorial in *Qualitative Health Research*, **1**, 403–406.

Morse, J.M. & Field, P.A. (1996) *Nursing Research: The Application of Qualitative Approaches*. Basingstoke, Macmillan.

Patton, M. (1990) *Qualitative Evaluation and Research Methods*. Newbury Park, Sage.

Sandelowski, M. (1995) Focus on qualitative methods: sample size in qualitative research. *Research in Nursing and Health*, **18**, 179–83.

Seidman, I.E. (1998) *Interviewing as Qualitative Research*. New York, Teachers College of Columbia University.

Strong, P.M. (1979) *The Ceremonial Order: Parents, Doctors and Medical Bureaucracies*. London, Routledge Kegan Paul.

Tarasuk, V. & Eakin, J.M. (1995) The problem of legitimacy in the experience of work-related back injury. *Qualitative Health Research*, **5** (2) 204–21.

Wolcott, H.F. (1994) *Transforming Qualitative Data: Description, Analysis, and Interpretation*. Thousand Oaks, Sage.

PART THREE

Approaches to Qualitative Research

CHAPTER 9

Ethnography

What is ethnography?

The meaning of the term ethnography is not unambiguous. Hammersley (1998) states that it lacks clear definition and is sometimes used as synonymous with qualitative research in general. In this chapter, however, we adopt the original meaning of the term, as a method within the anthropological tradition. Nurse and midwife ethnographers adopt mostly, though not always, qualitative procedures.

Ethnography is the direct description of a group, culture or community. As the oldest of the qualitative methods, it has been used since ancient times; for instance, in the descriptions of Greeks and Romans who wrote about the cultures they encountered in their travels and wars. Deriving from the Greek, the term ethnography means a description of the people, literally 'writing of culture' (Atkinson, 1992). Ethnographers use culture as a 'lens for interpretation' and therefore focus on cultural members, phenomena and problems (LeCompte and Schensul, 1999a). Ethnographic data collection takes place mainly through observations, interviews and examination of documents.

Ethnographers stress the importance of studying human behaviour in the context of a culture in order to gain understanding of cultural rules, norms and routines. Agar (1990) explains that the meaning of ethnography is ambiguous; it refers both to a process – the methods and strategies of research, and to a product – the written story as the outcome of the research. People 'do' ethnography: they study a culture, observe its members' behaviours and listen to them. They also produce an ethnography, a written text.

Applying ethnographic methods – especially observation – helps health professionals to contextualise the behaviour, beliefs and feelings of their clients or colleagues. Through ethnography, nurses and midwives become culturally sensitive and can identify the cultural influences on the individuals and groups they study. The goals of nurse ethnographers, however, differ from those of researchers in a subject discipline such as anthropology or sociology. Hammersley and Atkinson (1995) claim that ethnographers aim to produce knowledge rather than improve professional practice, but much ethnography in education, for instance, was intended to improve practice. Health professionals too, see the production of knowledge only as a first step; on the basis of this, they seek to improve their clinical practice.

The origins of ethnography

Modern ethnography has its roots in social anthropology and emerged in the 1920s and 1930s when famous anthropologists such as Malinowski (1922), Boas (1928) and Mead (1935), while searching for cultural patterns and rules, explored a variety of non-Western cultures and the life ways of the people within them. After the First and Second World Wars, when tribal groups were disappearing, researchers wished to preserve aspects of vanishing cultures by living with them and writing about them.

In the beginning these anthropologists explored only 'primitive' cultures (a term that demonstrates the patronising stance of many early anthropologists). When cultures became more linked with each other and Western anthropologists could not find homogeneous isolated cultures abroad, they turned to research their own cultures, acting as 'cultural strangers', that is, trying to see them from outside; everything is looked at with the eyes of an outsider. Sociologists, too, adopted ethnographic methods, immersing themselves in the culture or subculture in which they took an interest. Experienced ethnographers and sociologists who are researching their own society take a new perspective on that which is already familiar. This approach to a familiar culture helps ethnographers not to take assumptions about their own society or cultural group for granted.

The Chicago school of sociology, too, had an influence on later ethnographic methods because its members examined marginal cultural and 'socially strange' subcultures such as the slums, ghettos and gangs of the city. A good example is the study by Whyte (1943) who investigated the urban gang subculture in an American city. *Street Corner Society* became a classic, and other sociologists used this work as a model for their own writing.

The exploration of culture

Anthropology is concerned with culture, and ethnography differs from other approaches by its emphasis on culture. Culture can be defined as the way of life of a group – the learnt behaviour that is socially constructed and transmitted. The life experiences of members of a cultural group include a shared communication system. This consists of signs such as gestures, mime and language as well as cultural artefacts – all messages that the members of a culture recognise, and whose meaning they understand. Individuals in a culture or subculture hold common values and ideas acquired through learning from other members of the group. LeCompte and Preissle (1997) stress the researchers' responsibility to describe the unique and distinctive processes of the subculture or culture they study. Social anthropologists aim to observe and study the modes of life in a culture. This they do through the method of ethnography. They analyse, compare and examine groups and their rules of behaviour. The relationship of individuals to the group and to each other is also explored. The study of change, in particular, helps ethnographers understand cultures and subcultures. In areas where two cultures meet, they might focus on the conflict between groups if this is seen as important, for instance, in studies of interaction with doctors and other health professionals.

Sometimes nurses and midwives examine subcultures and situations with which they are familiar.

Examples

A nurse in the accident and emergency department (A&E) might wish to study the culture of the A&E setting in the local hospital. They will closely observe the events, critical incidents and behaviour of patients and professionals in this setting in order to improve the system.

A midwife explores the work of the local midwifery unit. She observes the situation and asks her colleagues about the routine actions they perform. She has also observed that some of the clients have problems with the way in which they are cared for and asks them about their feelings and perceptions.

Ethnographic methods

Sarantakos (1998) and Thomas (1993) distinguish between two types of ethnographic method:

- *Descriptive* or *conventional* ethnography
- *Critical* ethnography

Descriptive or conventional ethnography focuses on the description of cultures or groups and, through analysis, uncovers patterns, typologies and categories. Critical ethnography involves the study of macro-social factors such as power and examines common-sense assumptions and hidden agendas. It is therefore more political. Thomas (1993: 4) states the difference: 'Conventional ethnographers study culture for the purpose of describing it; critical ethnographers do so to change it'. Both kinds of ethnography use the same methods of analysis and will not be discussed separately in this chapter. Critical ethnography can be important for nurses and midwives because they are concerned with the empowerment of people.

Ethnography in nursing and midwifery

Ethnographic methods were first used in nursing and midwifery in the US. Some of the best known nursing ethnographers are Leininger (1978, 1985), and Morse (1991, 1994), who have written several well known texts. Leininger (1985) uses the term 'ethnonursing' for the use of ethnography in nursing. She developed this as a modification and extension of ethnography. Ethnonursing deals with studies of a culture like other ethnographic methods, but it is also about nursing care and specifically generates nursing knowledge, 'it is a specific research method focused primarily on documenting, describing and explaining nursing phenomena'. Muecke (1994) states that differences exist between studies in general anthropology and ethnography in nursing. She considers the goal of nursing ethnography to be more than the understanding of nursing or patient culture: it should lead to an advance in clinical practice. Nurse ethnographers differ from other anthropologists in that they only live with informants in their working day and spend their private lives away from the location where the research takes place. Nurses, of course, are familiar with the language used in the setting, while early anthropologists rarely knew the language of the culture they examined from the beginning of the research, and even modern anthropologists are not always familiar with the setting, the terminology and the people they study.

Ethnography in the healthcare arena is applied research. Chambers (2000) uses this term in approaches that are linked to making decisions in the interest of clients and in the area of decision making. In nursing and midwifery the method is used as a way of examining behaviours and perceptions in clinical settings, generally in order to improve care and clinical practice.

Example

Preston (1997) made a study of 'coronary families', studying health promotion in the weeks in which people had received preparation for and were recovering from coronary bypass surgery. Each family was seen as a small-scale group. Both observation and interviews were carried out. This had involved a structured programme for the prevention and management of heart disease.

Ethnographies in this field incorporate studies of healthcare processes, settings and systems. They are typified by observations of wards or investigations of patient perspectives or specific groups whose members have experienced a condition or illness. Socialisation studies are also important in the field of professional practice. They often examine the negotiation and interaction in the subculture of clinical practice or classroom settings.

Schensul *et al.* (1999) give useful advice that might be adopted by nurses and midwives. They can take a number of steps:

- They describe a problem in the group under study
- Through this, they understand the causes of the problem and may prevent it
- They help the cultural members to identify and report their needs
- They give information to affect change in clinical or professional practice

Nurse ethnographers do not always investigate their own cultural members. In modern Britain, nurses care for patients from a variety of ethnic groups and need to be knowledgeable about their cultures. Culture becomes part of all aspects of nursing because both nurses and patients are products of their group. DeSantis (1994) advises that nurses, in encounters with patients of different values and belief systems, temporarily suspend their own. She states that at least three cultures are involved in interaction with patients: the nurse's professional culture, the patient culture and the context in which the interaction takes place.

The main features of ethnography

The main features of ethnography are:

- Data collection from observation and interviews
- The use of 'thick' description
- Selection of key informants and settings
- The emic–etic dimension

Data collection through observation and interviews

Researchers collect data by standard methods mainly through observation and interviewing, but they also rely on documents such as letters, diaries and taped oral histories of people in a particular group or connected with it. Wolcott (1994) calls these strategies 'experiencing' (participant observation), 'enquiring' (interviewing), and 'examining' (studying documents).

As in other qualitative approaches, the researcher is the major research tool. Direct participant observation is the main way of collecting data from the culture under study, and observers try to become part of the culture, taking note of everything they see and hear as well as interviewing members of the culture to gain their interpretations.

Health researchers commonly observe behaviour in the clinical or educational setting. LeCompte and Preissle (1997) advise novices not to get lost in detail, as it is difficult to describe the social reality of a culture in all its complexity. The decisions about inclusion and exclusion depend on the research topic, the emerging data and the experiences of the researchers. The participants and their actions are observed as well as the ways in which they interact with each other. Special events and crises, the site itself and the use of space and time can also be examined. Observers study the rules of a culture or subculture and the change that occurs over time in the setting. Richardson (1990) warns us that the findings don't just consist of the interviews and fieldnotes; the participants' accounts must be formed into a story and a text that emerges from the data.

Observations become starting points for in-depth interviews. The researchers may not understand what they see, and ask the members of the group or culture to explain it to them. Participants share their interpretations of events, rules and roles with the interviewer. Some of the interviews are formal and structured, but often researchers ask questions on the spur of the moment and have informal conversations with members. Often they uncover discrepancies between words and actions – what people do and what they say – a problem discussed by Deutscher (1970) and, more recently, by LeCompte and Schensul (1999a). On the other hand there may be congruence between the spoken work and behaviour. Germain (1993) advises that these congruencies or discrepancies should be evaluated and explained.

Nurse and midwife ethnographers take part in the life of people; they listen to their informants' words and the interpretation of their actions. In essence, this involves a partnership between the investigator and the informants.

The use of 'thick description'

One of the major characteristics is *thick description*, a term used by the anthropologist Geertz (1973) who borrowed it from the philosopher Ryle. It is description that makes explicit the detailed patterns of cultural and social relationships and puts them in context. Ethnographic interpretation cannot be separated from time, place and events. It is based on the meaning that actions and events have for the members of a culture within the cultural context. Description and analysis have to be rooted in reality; researchers think and reflect about social events and conduct. Thick description must be theoretical and analytical in that researchers concern themselves with the abstract and general patterns and traits of social life in a culture. Denzin (1989) claims that thick description aims to give readers a sense of the emotions, thoughts and perceptions that research participants experience. It deals with the meaning and interpretations of people in a culture.

Thick description can be contrasted with thin description, which is superficial and does not explore the underlying meanings of cultural members. Any study where thin description prevails is not a good ethnography.

Selecting key informants and settings

As in other types of qualitative research, ethnographers generally use purposive sampling that is criterion-based and non-probabilistic (LeCompte and Preissle, 1997). This means ethnographers adopt certain criteria to choose a specific group and setting to be studied, be it a ward, a group of specialist nurses or patients with a specific condition. Some of our students have used samples taken from groups of recovering alcoholics, patients with myocardial infarction, children with asthma and many others. The criteria for sampling must be explicit and systematic (Hammersley and Atkinson, 1995). Researchers should choose key informants carefully to make sure that they are suitable and representative of the group under study. Key actors often participate by informally talking about the cultural conduct or customs of the group. They become active collaborators in the research rather than passive respondents.

The sample is taken from a particular cultural or subcultural group. Ethnographers have to search for individuals within a culture who can give them specific detailed information about the culture. Key informants own special and expert knowledge about the history and subculture of a group, about interaction processes in it and cultural rules, rituals and language. These key actors help the researcher to become accepted in the culture and subculture. Researchers can validate their own ideas or perceptions with those of key informants by going back to them at the end of the study and asking them to check the script and interpretation (member checking).

Example

One of our students examined the thoughts and perceptions of relatives who cared for old people. She chose as her key informants a group of individuals who were part of an informal carers' group. They allowed her to sit in on meetings and listen to their ideas and thoughts helping her to become acquainted with the subculture of care and also other carers. When she found something that seemed interesting or puzzling to her, she went to the key members of the group for information and eventually for confirmation of her interpretations.

Undergraduate experience

The bond between researcher and key informant strengthens when the two spend time with each other. Through informal conversations, researchers can learn about the customs and conduct of the group they study, because key informants have access to areas which researchers cannot reach in time and location. For instance, a midwife might wish to gain information about midwifery during the war, or a nurse to discover the problems of nursing abroad and have no access themselves to the past or the location. These researchers use informants who have this special knowledge, in these instances midwives who practised during the war or nurses who have worked extensively abroad. Key informants may be other health professionals or patients. DeSantis (1994) sees patients as the main cultural informants in nursing ethnography. They tell the nurses of their culture or subculture, and of the expectations and health beliefs that form part of it. Spradley (1979) advises ethnographers to elicit the 'tacit' knowledge of cultural members – the concepts and assumptions that they have but of which they are unaware.

Fetterman (1998) warns against prior assumptions which key informants might have. If they are highly knowledgeable they might impose their own ideas on the study and the researcher, therefore the latter must try to compare these tales with the observed reality. There might be the additional danger that key actors might only tell what researchers wish to hear. This danger is particularly strong in the health system. Clients are aware of labelling processes and often want to please those who care for them or deal with them in a professional relationship. However, the lengthy contact of interviewer and informants and 'prolonged engagement' in the setting help to overcome this.

The emic–etic dimension

Ethnographers use the constructs of the informants and also apply their own scientific conceptual framework, the so-called *emic* and *etic* perspectives (Harris, 1976). First, the researcher needs an understanding of the emic perspective, the insider's or native's perceptions. Insiders' accounts of reality help to uncover knowledge of the reasons why people act as they do. A researcher who uses the emic perspective gives explanations of events from the cultural member's point of view. This perspective is essential in a study, particularly in the beginning, as it prevents the imposition of the values and beliefs of researchers from their own culture to that of another. The outsider's perspective, the etic view, has been prevalent for too long in health care and health research. Outsiders, such as health professionals or professional researchers, used to identify the problems of patients and described them rather than listening to the member's own ideas. Now, those who experience an illness are allowed to speak for themselves as they are 'experts' not only on their condition but also on their own feelings and perceptions; as Harris (1976: 36) states: 'The way to get inside of people's heads is to talk with them, to ask questions about what they think and feel'.

The emic perspective corresponds to the reality and definition of informants. The researchers who are examining a culture or subculture gain knowledge of the existing rules and patterns from its members; the emic perspective is thus culturally specific. For nurses and midwives who explore their own culture and that of their patients, the 'native' view is not difficult to obtain because they are already closely involved in the culture. This prior involvement can be dangerous, because health professionals, by being part of the culture they examine, lose awareness of their role as researchers and sometimes rely on assumptions which do not necessarily have a basis in reality. Therefore reflection on prior assumptions is important.

Of course, the etic view is important too. Etic meanings stress the ideas of ethnographers themselves, their abstract and theoretical view when they distance

Example

One of our colleagues carried out research on the emotional experience of people in hospital. She assumed that fear would be the most predominant aspect of the hospital experience. However she found that embarrassment was also a strong emotion of many older people. This is a significant finding, because it suggests certain types of treatment and care which do not generate embarrassment.

Warren et al., 2000

themselves from the cultural setting and try to make sense of it. Harris (1976) explains that etics are scientific accounts by the researcher, based on that which is directly observable. The researchers place individuals' ideas within a framework and interpret it by adopting a social science perspective on the setting. Emic and etic perspectives provide a partnership between researchers and participants. Sometimes researchers – as outsiders – recognise patterns and ideas of which the informants are not themselves aware (Katz, 1997).

These ideas correspond directly to those of Denzin (1989) who speaks of first- and second-order concepts. First-order concepts are those used in the common-sense perspective on everyday life, while second-order concepts are more abstract and imposed by the researcher. For instance, individuals often mention the term 'learning the job' which could be called a first-order concept recognised by people in everyday life. A social scientist would call the same concept 'occupational socialisation', a second-order concept. The two terms show the difference between 'lay language' and 'academic language'. It must be kept in mind, however, that the emic view cannot be simply translated into an etic perspective. The meaning of the participants differs from scientific interpretations. Researchers move back and forth, from the reality of informants to scientific interpretation, but they must find a balance between involvement in the culture they study and scientific reflections and ideas about the beliefs and practices within that culture. This can be described as 'iteration', where researchers revise ideas and build upon previous stages (Fetterman 1998).

Fieldwork

The term fieldwork is used by ethnographers and other qualitative researchers to describe data collection outside laboratories. The major traits of ethnography have their basis in 'first-hand experience' of the group or community, and this usually, though not only, involves participant observation and interviewing (Atkinson *et al.*, 2001). Ethnographers gain most of their data through fieldwork. They become familiar with the community or group that they want to investigate. Fieldwork in qualitative research means working in the natural setting of the informants, observing them and talking to them over prolonged periods of time. This is necessary so that informants get used to the researcher and behave naturally rather than putting on a performance. The observation of a variety of contexts is important. Spradley (1980: 78) provides a list in order to guide researchers when they observe a situation, although these guidelines cannot be seen as complete or all inclusive (see Chapter 6).

The initial phase in the field consists of a time for exploration. Nurses and midwives learn about an area of study and become familiar with it. This is not difficult, because they are already part of the community and well aware of patient and professional cultures. Acceptance need not be earned because health professionals have been part of these cultures, while anthropologists in foreign cultures must achieve entry through learning the ways of the group from the beginning. Fieldwork aims to uncover patterns and regularities in a culture which the people living in that community can recognise. Germain (1993) identifies three stages in fieldwork. In the first stage the researchers gain an overview of the culture under study and write notes on their observations. In the second stage researchers start focusing on particular issues. They question the informants on the initial observations. In the third stage researchers realise that saturation has occurred, and they start the process of disengagement.

The best method of data collection in ethnographic research is participant observation, the most complete immersion in a culture. For instance, a nurse who intends to explore the work of a nursing development unit would either be a member of this unit or take part in it in order to observe the practices and reactions of the individuals within.

Micro- and macro-ethnographies

Micro-ethnographies focus on subcultures or settings such as a single ward or a group of specialist nurses. Fetterman (1998) claims that micro-studies consist of research in small units or focus on activities within small social settings. Ethnographers might select a setting such as a pain clinic, an operating theatre, a labour ward or a GP practice; two of our students, for instance, examined a mixed gender ward. Most students choose a micro-ethnographic study as it makes fewer demands on their time than macro-ethnography. It also seems more immediately relevant to the world of the nurse and the midwife.

There is a continuum between large- and small-scale studies, macro- and micro-ethnographies. A macro-ethnography examines a larger culture with its institutions, communities and value systems. In nursing and midwifery this might be a hospital, or the nursing culture. A large-scale study means a long period of time in the setting and is often the work of several researchers. Both types of ethnography demand a detailed picture of the community under study as well as similar strategies for data collection and analysis. The type of project depends, of course, on the focus of the investigation and the researcher's own interests.

Ethnographic research can be very useful during changes in a culture. In a changing healthcare system, health professionals sometimes study developments not only in larger settings such as hospitals or communities but also in the smaller world of wards and theatres. Change – the transition from one stage or one ideology to another – can provide a useful focus for nursing and midwifery research. In Britain, for instance, the document *Changing Childbirth* (DoH, 1993) might have made a significant impact on midwifery practice. Whether it has actually changed practices in a local midwifery unit could usefully be evaluated by an observation study. Small social units are the most appropriate setting for ethnography by health professionals (Boyle, 1994).

Example

Holland (1993) was very interested in ritual in nursing practice. She observed a group of nurses – a cultural group – in a surgical ward setting to find out whether ritual behaviour was prevalent. She established that rituals and cultural rules existed. They were an outcome of the common values of the group members and helped to create cohesion among them while not adversely affecting patients.

The ethnographic record: field and analytic notes

Researchers collect data by standard methods, mainly through observing and interviewing but also rely on documents such as letters, diaries and the oral history of people in the culture they study. From the beginning of their research, nurse and midwife ethnographers record what goes on 'in the field' – the setting and situation they are studying. This includes noting down fleeting impressions as well as accurate and detailed descriptions of events and behaviour in context. While writing notes and describing what occurs in the situation ethnographers become reflective and analytic.

Spradley (1979) lists four different types of fieldnotes in ethnography:

- The condensed account
- The expanded account
- The fieldwork journal
- Analysis and interpretation notes

Condensed accounts are short descriptions made in the field during data collection while expanded accounts extend the descriptions and fill in detail. Ethnographers extend the short account as soon as possible after observation or interview if they were unable to record during data collection. In the field journal ethnographers note their own biases, reactions and problems during fieldwork. Researchers use additional ways to record events and behaviour such as tapes, films or photos, flowcharts and diagrams.

Fieldwork proceeds in progressive stages. Initially researchers gain the broad picture of the group and the setting. They observe behaviour and listen to the language that is used in the community they study. For nurses and midwives in a clinical setting this is not difficult because patients, colleagues and other health professionals trust them to record accurately and honestly. After initial observation, researchers focus on particular issues that seem important to them. Finally, writing becomes detailed analysis and interpretation of the culture under study.

Doing and writing ethnography

Ethnographers start by 'experiencing', 'enquiring' and 'examining' (Wolcott, 1992). We have discussed these initial procedures. When writing up, researchers take all these into account, and they form part of an ethnography. As Wolcott states, an ethnography consists of description, analysis and interpretation. Ethnographers describe what they see and hear while studying a culture; they identify its main features and uncover relationships between them through analysis; they interpret the findings by asking for meaning and inferring it from the data. According to Stewart (1998) an ethnography is holistic in the sense that researchers create a portrait of the group under study. This also means that they take into account the social context in which the study takes place.

Description

'Description – in its everyday sense . . . – is at the heart of qualitative inquiry' says Wolcott (1994: 55). We must warn however, that it is never as simple as it seems. Writers select specific situations for observation, disregard some events and interactions in favour of others and focus on particular issues that they perceive as relevant and significant. Not everything observed or heard is described but only that which is relevant for the study at hand. This involves at least some analysis and interpretation.

Researchers describe by writing a story, which is a report of the actions, interactions and events within a cultural group. The reader should get a sense of the setting or a feel for it and understand what is going on there. The description is enhanced by the portrayal of critical events, rituals or roles. Wolcott demands that during description the writer follow an analytical structure that gives a framework to the account.

Analysis

Analysis entails working with the data. After processing them by coding, we transform them from the raw data by recognising patterns and themes and making linkages between ideas. Analysis cannot proceed without interpretation but is more scientific and systematic; it brings order to disorderly data, and the researchers must show how they arrived at the structures and linkages. At this stage other people's research connected with the emergent themes becomes part of the analytic process through comparison and integration in the study. It is important that the analysis accurately reflects the data. Whatever the analyst finds has to be related back to the data in order to see whether there is a fit between them and the analytic categories and themes.

Steps in the analysis

As in other qualitative research, data analysis takes place from the beginning of the observation and interviews. The focus becomes progressively clearer. In the data analysis the researcher revisits the aim and the initial research question. Analysis takes more time than data collection. Fielding (1993) claims, that in the analysis, description of behaviour and events does not suffice, and that the aim of ethnography is more than the description of a group or a culture. The process of analysis involves several steps:

(1) Ordering and organising the collected material
(2) Rereading the data
(3) Breaking the material into manageable pieces
(4) Building, comparing and contrasting categories
(5) Searching for relationships and grouping categories together
(6) Recognising and describing patterns, themes and typologies
(7) Interpreting and searching for meaning

Spradley (1979:92) claims that analysis involves the 'systematic examination of something to determine its parts, the relationship among parts, and their relationship to the whole'. Agar (1980) stresses the non-linear nature of the process: researchers collect data through which they learn about a culture, they try to make sense of what they saw and heard, and then they collect new data on the basis of their analysis and interpretation.

The data are scanned and organised from the very beginning of the study. If gaps and inadequacies occur, they can be filled by collecting more data or refocusing on the initial aims of the study. While this work goes on, researchers choose to focus on particular aspects which they examine more closely than others.

While rereading the data, thoughts and observations are being recorded, and a search for regularities can begin. The first interview – or the first detailed description of observation – is scanned and marked off into sections, which are then given codes. The second and third interview transcripts are then coded and compared with the first. Commonalities and similar codes are sorted and grouped together. This happens for each interview (or observation). Thematically, similar sets are placed together. The researcher then tries to find the ideas that link the categories, and describes and summarises them. From this stage onwards diagrams are helpful because they present the links and patterns graphically. The text by Miles and Huberman (1994) is the classic example of the use of diagrams in qualitative research.

The regularities and emerging themes are grouped into categories, which the researcher compares and reduces to major constructs. Broad patterns of thought and behaviour emerge. The patterns and regularities have their basis in the actual observations and interviews; they will be connected with the personal experiences of the researcher and the categories and themes drawn from the literature. LeCompte and Preissle (1997) advise occasional written summaries as useful organising devices (see Chapter 15).

Interpretation

Researchers take the last step, that of interpretation during and after the analysis, making inferences, providing meaning and giving explanations for the phenomena. While describing and analysing, they interpret the findings, that is, they gain insight and give meaning to them. Interpretation involves some speculation, theorising and explaining although it must be directly grounded in the data. It links the emerging ideas derived from the analysis to established theories through comparing and contrasting others' work with the researcher's own.

Eventually the story is put together from the descriptions, analyses and interpretations. LeCompte and Preissle (1997) compare this to assembling a jigsaw puzzle where a frame is quickly outlined and small puzzle pieces are collected together and placed in position within the frame. The difference is that one knows about the final picture of a jigsaw and has something to work towards, while in qualitative research one merely has an emerging picture whose outline one can only imagine, and which may change in the process of assembly.

Pitfalls and problems

There are a number of problems with ethnographic research in the nursing and midwifery culture. First, it is difficult to examine one's own group and become a 'cultural stranger' questioning the assumptions of the familiar culture whose rules and norms have been internalised. Vigilance and advice from outsiders are very important. Second, because health professionals often have a background in the natural sciences and are taught to adopt a systematic approach to their clinical work, they sometimes may find it difficult to suffer ambiguity. It is better, however, to admit to uncertainty than to make unwarranted claims about the research. It resembles nursing diagnosis: signs and symptoms are examined for meaning but should never become once-and-for-all interpretation. Findings can be re-interpreted at a later stage in the light of reflection or new evidence.

Our students often write up their research, making statements that seem to be applicable to a whole range of similar situations. An ethnography, like other qualitative research, cannot simply be generalised. Findings from one subculture, or one setting are not automatically applicable to other settings. However, Wolcott (1994) asserts that there is always a possibility for generalisation, and often the readers can themselves make that leap. The researcher can compare with other specific situations similar to the case studied and can achieve typicality.

Novice researchers are often too descriptive and present raw data without analysis and interpretation. Even the quotes in the study are not raw data but should have gone through the process of analysis. Nevertheless, at the start of a research career, it is advisable to give more descriptive detail, clear analysis and to be careful with interpretation. With experience the balance might change. It is interesting that on revisiting the work at a later stage, many researchers start reinterpreting the data.

Summary

The main features of ethnography as a research method are as follows.

- Ethnographers immerse themselves in the culture or subculture they study and try to see the world from the cultural members' point of view.
- Data are collected through work in the field through participant observation and interviews with key informants as well as through documents.
- Researchers observe the rules and rituals in the culture and try to understand the meaning and interpretation that informants give to them.
- They compare these with their own etic view and explore the differences between the two.
- Fieldnotes are written throughout the fieldwork about events and behaviour in the setting.
- Ethnographers describe, analyse and interpret the culture and the local, emic perspective of its members.
- The main evaluative criterion is the way in which the study presents the culture as experienced by its members.

References

Agar, M. (1980) *The Professional Stranger: An Informal Introduction to Ethnography*. Newbury Park, Sage.
Agar, M. (1990) Exploring the excluded middle. *Journal of Contemporary Ethnography*, **19** (1) April; Special Issue: The Presentation of Ethnographic Research, 73–88.
Atkinson, P. (1992) *Understanding Ethnographic Texts*. Newbury Park, Sage.

Atkinson, P., Coffey, A., Delamont, S., Lofland, J. & Lofland, L. (eds) (2001) Introduction to part one. In *Handbook of Ethnography*, pp. 9–10. London, Sage.

Boas, F. (1928) *Anthropology and Modern Life*. New York, Norton.

Boyle, J.S. (1994) Styles of ethnography. In *Critical Issues in Qualitative Research*, pp. 159–85. Thousand Oaks, Sage.

Chambers, E. (2000) Applied ethnography. In *Handbook of Qualitative Research* (eds N.K. Denzin & Y.S. Lincoln), 2nd edn, pp. 851–69. Thousand Oaks, Sage.

Denzin, N.K. (1989) *Interpretive Interactionism*. Newbury Park, Sage.

Department of Health (1993) *Report of the Expert Maternity Group (Changing Childbirth)*. London, HMSO.

DeSantis, L. (1994) Making anthropology clinically relevant to nursing care. *Journal of Advanced Nursing*, **20**, 707–15.

Deutscher, I. (1970) Words and deeds: social science and social policy. In *Qualitative Methodology: Firsthand Involvement with the Social World* (ed. W.J. Filstead), pp. 27–51. Chicago, Markham Publishing.

Emerson, R.M., Fretz, R.I. & Shaw, L.L. (2000) Participant observation and fieldnotes. In *Handbook of Ethnography* (eds P. Atkinson, A. Coffey, S. Delamont, J. Lofland & L. Lofland), pp. 352–367. London, Sage.

Fetterman, D.M. (1998) *Ethnography: Step by Step*, 2nd edn. Thousand Oaks, Sage.

Fielding, N. (1993) Ethnography. In *Researching Social Life* (ed. N. Gilbert), pp. 154–71. Newbury Park, Sage.

Geertz, C. (1973) *The Interpretation of Cultures*. New York, Basic Books.

Germain, C.P. (1993) Ethnography: the method. In *Nursing Research: A Qualitative Perspective* (eds P.L. Munhall & C. Oiler Boyd), 2nd edn, pp. 237–67. New York, National League for Nursing Press.

Goetz, J.P. & LeCompte, M.D. (1984) *Ethnography and Qualitative Design in Educational Research*. Orlando, Academic Press.

Hammersley, M. (1998) *Reading Ethnographic Research*, 2nd edn. London, Longman.

Hammersley, M. & Atkinson, P. (1995) *Ethnography: Principles in Practice*, 2nd edn. London, Tavistock.

Harris, M. (1976) History and significance of the emic/etic distinction. *Annual Review of Anthropology*, **5**, 329–50.

Holland, C.K. (1993) An ethnographic study of nursing culture as an exploration for determining the existence of a system of ritual. *Journal of Advanced Nursing*, **18**, 1461–70.

Katz, J. (1997) Ethnography's warrant. *Sociological Methods and Research*, **31**, 391–423.

LeCompte, M.D. & Schensul, J.J. (1999a) *Designing and Conducting Ethnographic Research*. Walnut Creek, CA, Altamira Press.

LeCompte, M.D. & Schensul, J.J. (1999b) *Analyzing & Interpreting Ethnographic Data*. Walnut Creek, CA, Altamira Press.

LeCompte, M.D. & Preissle, J. with Tesch, R. (1997) *Ethnography and Qualitative Design in Educational Research*, 2nd edn. Chicago, Academic Press.

Leininger, M. (1978) *Transcultural Nursing: Concepts, Theories and Practices*. New York, John Wiley & Sons.

Leininger, M. (ed) (1985) *Qualitative Research Methods in Nursing*. Philadelphia, WB Saunders Co.

Leininger, M. (1994) Evaluation criteria and critique of qualitative research studies. In *Critical Issues in Qualitative Research Methods* (ed. J.M. Morse), pp. 95–115. Thousand Oaks, Sage.

Malinowski, B. (1922) *Argonauts of the Western Pacific: An Account of Native Enterprise and Adventure in the Archipelagoes of Melanesian New Guinea*. New York, Dutton.

Mead, M. (1935) *Sex and Temperament in Three Primitive Societies*. New York, Morrow.

Miles, M.B. & Huberman, A.M. (1994) *Qualitative Data Analysis*, 2nd edn. Thousand Oaks, Sage.

Morse, J.M. (ed.) (1991) *Qualitative Nursing Research: A Contemporary Dialogue*, Rev. edn. Newbury Park, Sage.

Morse, J.M. (ed.) (1994) *Critical Issues in Qualitative Research Methods*. Thousand Oaks, Sage.

Muecke, M. (1994) On the evaluation of ethnographies. In *Critical Issues in Qualitative Research Method* (ed. J.M. Morse), pp. 187–209. Thousand Oaks, Sage.

Preston, R.M. (1997) Ethnography: studying the fate of health promotion in coronary families. *Journal of Advanced Nursing*, **25**, 554–61.

Richardson, L. (1990) Narrative and sociology. *Journal of Contemporary Ethnography*, **19** (1) 116–35.

Sarantakos, S. (1998) *Social Research*, 2nd edn. Basingstoke, The Macmillan Press.

Schensul, S.L., Schensul, J.J. & LeCompte, M.D. (1999) *Essential Ethnographic Methods: Observations, Interviews and Questionnaires*. Walnut Creek CA, Altamira Press.

Spradley, J.P. (1979) *The Ethnographic Interview*. Fort Worth, Harcourt Brace Johanovich College Publishers.

Spradley, J.P. (1980) *Participant Observation*. Fort Worth, Harcourt Brace Johanovich College Publishers.

Stewart, A. (1998) *The Ethnographer's Method*. Thousand Oaks, Sage.

Thomas, J. (1993) *Doing Critical Ethnography*. Newbury Park, Sage.

Warren, J., Holloway, I., Smith, P. (2000) Fitting in: maintaining a sense of self during hospitalisation. *International Journal of Nursing Studies*, **37**, 229–35.

Whyte, W.F. (1943) *Street Corner Society: The Social Structure of an Italian Slum*. Chicago, University of Chicago Press.

Wolcott, H. (1992) Posturing in Qualitative Enquiry. In *Handbook of Qualitative Research in Education* (eds M. LeCompte, W.L. Millroy & J. Preissle), pp. 121–52. San Diego, Academic Press.

Wolcott, H.F. (1994) *Transforming Qualitative Data: Description, Analysis, and Interpretation*. Thousand Oaks, Sage.

CHAPTER 10

Grounded Theory

The use of grounded theory

Grounded theory (GT) is an approach to data collection and analysis initially developed by Glaser and Strauss in the 1960s. It has its origins in sociology, particularly in symbolic interactionism. Grounded theory procedures, however, are not specific to a particular discipline or type of data collection. The way of analysing data (constant comparison) can be used in any field of study, be it nursing or health studies, psychology or sociology and for any type of material, such as interview transcripts, observations or documents. Grounded theory is a favoured approach in nursing, due to the systematic and structured way in which the data are collected and analysed. Wuest (1995) claims that GT is particularly appropriate in nursing because researchers take account of the findings and act on them after having identified the ground of informants' experiences. There is a case for grounded theory in situations where little is known about a particular topic or problem area, or where a new and exciting outlook is needed in familiar settings (Stern, 1980).

History and origin

Grounded theory was first used in the 1960s by Barney Glaser and Anselm Strauss, two sociologists who worked together on research about health professionals' interaction with dying patients. This generated two books (Glaser and Strauss, 1965; 1968), which have become exemplars of grounded theory. From research and teaching the classic text emerged, *The Discovery of Grounded Theory* (Glaser and Strauss, 1967). Four other books on grounded theory followed, *Field Research: Strategies for a Natural Sociology* (Schatzman & Strauss, 1973) *Theoretical Sensitivity* (Glaser, 1978), *Qualitative Analysis for Social Scientists* (Strauss, 1987), and *Basics of Qualitative Research* (Strauss and Corbin, 1990, 1998). The last – which Strauss (who died in 1996) co-authored with a nurse researcher – is by far the clearest and most practically useful book on grounded theory as it describes an approach which has been tried and developed. The book edited by Chenitz and Swanson (1986) discusses GT specifically in relation to nursing research. Strauss and Corbin (1997) also edited a book in which they show how researchers have applied GT in practice. In 1999 Ian Dey analysed the approach of GT and developed guidelines for it.

In nursing and health care the approach has been popular from its inception, starting with Benoliel's (1973) study on the interaction of nurses with dying patients. She (Benoliel, 1996: 419–21) lists the GT research studies that have been carried out in nursing between 1980 and 1994. Stern (1985), Charmaz (1991, 2000) and Hutchinson (1993) in the United States; Melia (1987) and Smith (1992) in Britain are some of the better known nurse researchers who have used this approach.

Symbolic interactionism

The theoretical framework for grounded theory is derived from the insights of symbolic interactionism, focusing on the processes of interaction between people exploring human behaviour and social roles. Symbolic interactionism explains how individuals attempt to fit their lines of action to those of others (Blumer, 1971), take account of each others' acts, interpret them and reorganise their own behaviour. Mead (1934) and Blumer contributed to GT the idea that human beings are active participants in their situation rather than passive respondents.

Mead, the main proponent of symbolic interactionism, sees the self as a social rather than a psychological phenomenon. Members of society affect the development of a person's social self by their expectations and influence. Initially, individuals model their roles on the important people in their lives, 'significant others'; they learn to act according to others' expectations, thereby shaping their own behaviour. The observation of these interacting roles is a source of data in grounded theory.

In symbolic interactionism the model of the person is active and creative rather than passive. Individuals plan, project, create actions and revise them. People share their attitudes and responses to particular situations with members of their group. Hence members of a culture or community analyse the language, appearance and gestures of others and act in accordance with their interpretations. On the basis of these perceptions, they justify their conduct, and this conduct can only be understood in context. Grounded theory therefore stresses the importance of the context in which people function.

Symbolic interactionism focuses on actions and perceptions of individuals and their ideas and intentions. The Thomas theorem states: 'If men [*sic*] define situations as real, they are real in their consequences' (Thomas, 1928: 584), thereby claiming that individual definitions of reality shape perceptions and actions. Participant observation and interviewing trace this process of 'definition of the situation'.

Denzin (1989) links symbolic interactionism to naturalistic, qualitative research methods by stating that researchers must enter the world of interactive human beings to understand them. By doing this, they see the situation from the perspective of the participants rather than their own. Qualitative methods suit the theoretical assumptions of symbolic interactionism. As human beings are seen as active and creative, they can be observed in the process of their work and their negotiations with others, particularly with 'significant others'. Researchers use grounded theory to investigate these interactions, behaviours and experiences as well as individuals' perceptions and thoughts about them. The intention of the research is 'the idiographic study of particular cases rather than the nomothetic study of mass data' (Alvesson and Sköldberg, 2000:13) (see Chapter 1).

The aims and features of grounded theory

The main aim of the grounded theory approach is the generation of theory from the data. Existing theories, too, can be modified or extended through GT. It emphasises the development of ideas from the data similar to other qualitative methods but goes further than these. Researchers start with an area of interest, collect the data and allow relevant ideas to develop, without preconceived theories and hypotheses to be tested for confirmation. Glaser and Strauss (1967) advised that rigid preconceived assumptions prevent development of the research; imposing a framework might block the awareness of major concepts emerging from the data.

Researchers are able to create their own theories as long as these are rooted in the real world and clearly understandable to the participants and professionals who are linked to the area of study. Wiener and Wysmans (1990: 12) claim that theory in this approach means: 'identifying the relationship between and among concepts, and presenting a systematic view of the phenomena being examined, in order to explain what is going on'. The theory must be applicable to a variety of similar settings and contexts.

Grounded theory researchers are able to adopt alternative perspectives rather than follow previously developed ideas. For this they need flexibility and open minds, qualities related to the processes involved in nursing.

Example

Orona (1990) examined the experience of care giving by relatives of people with Alzheimer's disease. The researcher had expected that carers go through a process of decision making before placing their relatives in an institution. However, she found that there was no such conscious process, and relatives did not focus on decision making but on the process of identity loss of their relative. Identity loss of the person with Alzheimer's became the core theme. For Orona, the analytic development was not linear or systematic and ordered. She needed flexibility to deal with the findings that arose directly from the data.

The grounded theory style of research uses constant comparison. The researcher compares each section of the data with every other throughout the study for similarities, differences and connections. Included in this process are the themes and categories identified in the literature. All the data are coded and categorised, and from this process major concepts and constructs are formed. The researcher takes up a search for major themes that link ideas to find a 'storyline' for the study.

Strauss (1987) sees the processes of induction, deduction and verification as essential in grounded theory. The approach is both inductive and deductive. Grounded theory does not start with a hypothesis though researchers might have 'hunches'. After collecting the initial data, however, relationships are established and provisional hypotheses conceived. These are verified by checking them out against further data. Corbin (1986) reminds the analyst that this process of grounded theory is very similar to the nursing process and should prove easy to use for nurses. Glaser (1992) however, questions the process of verification as discussed later in this chapter (p. 165–66).

Strauss and Corbin (1998) acknowledge that grounded theory has similarities with other qualitative methods in data sources and emphasis. Grounded theorists accept their role as interpreters of the data and do not stop at merely reporting them or describing the experiences of participants. Researchers search for relationships between concepts, while other forms of qualitative research often generate major themes but do not always uncover patterns and links between categories or develop theories.

Data collection

Data are collected through observations in the field, interviews of participants, diaries and other documents such as letters or even newspapers. Researchers use interviews and observations more often than other data sources, and they supplement these through literature searches. Indeed, the literature becomes part of the data that are analysed.

Everything, even researchers' experience, can become sources of data. Glaser and Strauss (1967) recognise that the researcher does not approach the study with an empty mind. In fact, most forms of inquiry are based on prior interest and problems that researchers have experienced and reflected on even when there is no hypothesis.

GT processes do not always follow in chronological order. For instance, data collection and analysis are linked from the beginning of the research, proceed in parallel and interact continuously. The analysis starts after the first few steps in the data collection have been taken; the emerging ideas guide the analysis. The gathering of data does not finish until the end of the research because ideas, concepts and new questions continually arise which guide the researcher to new data sources. Researchers collect data from initial interviews, observations or documents and take their cues from the first emerging ideas to develop further interviews and observations. This means that the collection of data becomes more focused and specific as the process develops.

While observing and interviewing, the investigator writes fieldnotes from the beginning of the data collection throughout the project. Certain occurrences in the setting or ideas from the participants that seem of vital interest are recorded either during or immediately after data collection. They remind the researcher of the events, actions and interactions and trigger thinking processes.

According to Glaser (1978) the following are necessary for grounded theory:

- Theoretical sensitivity
- Theoretical sampling
- Data analysis: coding and categorising
- Constant comparison
- The literature as a source of data
- Integration of theory
- Theoretical memos and field notes

Theoretical sensitivity

Researchers must be theoretically sensitive (Glaser, 1978). Theoretical sensitivity means that researchers can differentiate between significant and less important data and have insight into their meanings. There are a variety of sources for theoretical sensitivity. It is built up over time, from reading and experience which guides the researcher to examine the data from all sides rather than stay fixed on the obvious.

Professional experience can be one source of awareness, and personal experiences, too, can help make the researcher sensitive.

Example 1

An expert nurse explores patient experience in hospital. She knows from her long professional career that patients feel a number of emotions when they first come to hospital. This experience makes her sensitive to patients' feelings and perceptions which she then explores.

Example 2

A midwife was given little information about some aspects of childbirth when she had her first child. She therefore knows, from personal experience, about the problems of lack of information. When she observes or asks questions about the experience of childbirth, she might include questions on the feelings that lack of information can generate.

The literature sensitises in the sense that documents, research studies or autobiographies create awareness in the nurse of relevant and significant elements in the data.

Example

A health professional has read a study about nurses' role learning in an academic journal. He or she might follow up some of the aspects of role learning that are discussed in the article.

Strauss and Corbin (1998) believe that theoretical sensitivity increases when researchers interact with the data because they think about emerging ideas, ask further questions and see these ideas as provisional until they have been examined over time and are finally confirmed by the data.

Theoretical sampling

Sampling guided by ideas with significance for the emerging theory is called *theoretical sampling*. In theoretical sampling 'the emerging theory controls the research process throughout' (Alvesson and Sköldberg, 2000: 11). One of the main differences between this and other types of sampling is time and continuance. Unlike other sampling, which is planned beforehand, theoretical sampling in grounded theory continues throughout the study and is not planned before the study starts. Cutcliffe (2000) shows that the initial data collection and analysis guides the direction of further sampling.

At the start of the project nurses make initial sampling decisions. They decide on a setting and on particular individuals or groups of people able to give information on the topic under study. Once the research has started and initial data have been analysed and examined (one must remember that data collection and analysis interact) new concepts arise, and events and people are chosen who can further illuminate the problem.

Researchers then set out to sample different situations, individuals or a variety of settings, and focus on new ideas to extend the emerging theories. The selection of participants, settings, events or documents is a function of developing theories. Theoretical sampling continues until the point of saturation. Students do not always understand the meaning of the concept 'saturation'. They believe that saturation has taken place when a concept is mentioned frequently and is described in similar ways by a number of people, or when the same ideas arise over and over again. This does not necessarily mean that saturation has occurred, and it is difficult to establish when saturation has been achieved (Backman & Kyngäs, 1999). Morse (1995: 149) suggests that researchers can recognise when saturation has been achieved by the quality of the theory that has been developed.

Saturation occurs at a different stage in each research project and cannot be predicted at the outset.

Theoretical sampling, though originating in grounded theory, is occasionally used in other types of qualitative analysis (see Chapter 8).

Data analysis: coding and categorising

Coding and categorising goes on throughout the research. From the start of the study, analysts *code* the data. Coding in grounded theory is the process by which concepts or themes are identified and named during the analysis. Data are transformed and reduced to build *categories*. Through the emergence of these categories theory can be evolved and integrated. Researchers form clusters of interrelating concepts not merely descriptions of themes.

In this process, the first step is concerned with open coding which starts as soon as the researcher receives the data. Open coding is the process of breaking down and conceptualising the data. Hutchinson (1993) differentiates between level 1, 2, and 3 codes. Level 1 codes are relatively simple. For instance, a novice midwife might describe experiences in hospital: 'I was shocked when I observed the first birth I had ever seen on the ward'. The code for this might be 'initial shock'.

Sometimes these codes consist of words and phrases used by the participants themselves to describe a phenomenon. They are called *in vivo* codes (Strauss, 1987). A new recruit to nursing might declare in an interview: 'I was thrown in at the deep end'. The code might be 'thrown in at the deep end'. *In vivo* codes can give life and interest to the study and can be immediately recognised as reflecting the reality of the participants.

In grounded theory, all the data are coded. Initial codes tend to be provisional and are modified or transformed over the period of analysis. At the beginning of a project or a study, line-by-line analysis is important, although it may be a long drawn-out process for analysts. Codes are based directly on the data, and therefore the researcher avoids preconceived ideas. An example of an interview with a nurse tutor gives some idea of level 1 coding.

Example

Well I suppose most people get fed up with doing the same things year in, year out.	Getting bored
I really felt like a change.	Desire for change
Regular hours are important to me.	Wish for regularity
I hadn't been promoted to the level to which I could function.	Lack of promotion

The analyst groups concepts together and develops categories. At the start a great number of labels are used, and after initial coding analysts attempt to condense (or collapse) codes into groups of concepts with similar traits which are categories. Hutchinson (1993) calls these level 2 codes. These categories tend to be more abstract than initial codes and are generally formulated by the investigator. These are examples of level 2 codes.

Example

I had this fear that I was not going to survive.	Fear of dying
Nobody, but nobody was there to help me and I felt that I was completely alone.	Lack of support Feeling isolated
We all need somebody close to be with us when we're ill.	Need for significant other

---

The broken down data must be linked together again in a new form. The main features (properties) and dimensions of these categories are identified.

Level 3 constructs are major categories which, although generated from the data and based in them, are formulated by the analysts and rooted in their nursing and academic knowledge. These constructs contain developing theoretical ideas and themes and through building these constructs, analysts reassemble the data. Categories are linked to subcategories. This process of reassembling the data is called *axial coding*. There is no reason why researchers cannot use the categories that others have discovered. For instance Melia (1987) borrows the term 'awareness context' from Glaser and Strauss (1965), but usually nurses and midwives develop their own useful categories.

Although there is no initial hypothesis in grounded theory, during the course of the research working propositions or hypotheses are generated. These must be based in and indicated by the data. The process of testing and verification for the hypotheses which link the categories goes on throughout the research in the Straussian version of GT. Researchers also seek deviant or negative cases which do not support a particular working proposition. When these are found, the researcher must modify the proposition or find reasons why it is not applicable in this particular instance.

The process of coding and categorising only stops when:

- No new information on a category can be found in spite of the attempt to collect more data from a variety of sources
- The category has been described with all its properties, variations and processes
- Links between categories are firmly established

(Strauss and Corbin, 1990)

The core category

The researcher must discover the *core category*. In grounded theory, the major category which links all others is called the core category or core variable. Like a thread the category should be woven into the whole of the study and provide the story line. The linking of all categories around a core is called selective coding. This means that the researcher uncovers the essence of the study and integrates all the elements of the emergent theory. The core category is the basic social-psychological process involved in the research (BSP). The BSP is a process that occurs over time and explains changes in behaviour. It represents the ideas that are most significant to the participants.

Example

A project about the perceptions of young people with diabetes shows in essence that they want to be seen as normal by their peers. Thus, 'being normal' may be a core category. On the other hand the study might show that these young people, after discovering diabetes, want to be seen as they were before their illness and try to achieve this by a variety of means. 'Reclaiming a normal self' could be identified as a basic social-psychological process.

Strauss (1987) claims some major characteristics for the core category:

(1) It must be the central element of the research related to other categories and explain variations
(2) It must recur often in the data and develop as a pattern.
(3) It connects with other categories without a major effort by the researcher
(4) In the process of identifying, describing and conceptualising the core category develops
(5) The core category is usually fully developed only towards the end of the research

Constant comparison

Coding and categorising involves constant comparison. Initial interviews are analysed and codes and concepts developed. By comparing concepts and sub-categories, researchers are able to group them into major categories and label them. When they code and categorise incoming data, they compare new categories with those that have already been established. Thus, incoming data are checked for their 'fit' with existing categories. Each incident of a category is compared with every other incident for similarities and differences. The comparison involves the literature. Constant comparison is useful for finding the properties and dimensions of categories. It helps in looking at concepts critically as each concept is illuminated by the new, incoming data. Strauss and Corbin (1998: 4) stress that they do not offer prescriptions but 'essentially guidelines for suggested techniques'. However, it is useful if researchers are completely familiar with the main features of the GT approach.

The literature as a source of data

The literature becomes a source for data. When categories have been found, researchers trawl the literature for confirmation or refutation of these categories. Analysts try to discover what other researchers have found, and whether there are any links to existing theories.

Strauss and Corbin (1998) list a number of points about the use of the literature.

(1) Concepts from the literature can be compared with those deriving from the study.
(2) The literature can stimulate theoretical sensitivity. It can make analysts aware of existing ideas.
(3) The literature can generate questions and problems.
(4) Knowledge of existing theories can be useful in influencing the stance of the researcher.
(5) The literature can be used as an added source of data although these do not have priority over the researchers' own data.
(6) Researchers have to consider why the literature confirms or refutes their own ideas or data.
(7) Even before the study starts, initial questions can help develop conceptual areas.
(8) During the analysis process more questions can be generated, especially when the researchers' data and the findings of the literature show a discrepancy.
(9) The literature can guide theoretical sampling. It can help decide where to go next. Ideas might arise which increase the chance of developing further the emerging theory.
(10) The literature can be used to validate the researcher's categories. Concepts in the literature may confirm or refute the findings of the researcher.

Researchers can also use the literature to compare their own theories with those previously developed.

Integration of theory

To be credible the theory must have 'explanatory power', linkages between categories and specificity. In a good project, categories are connected with each other and tightly linked to the data. Researchers do not just describe static situations but take into account processes which occur. Glaser and Strauss (1967) state that two types of theory are produced: substantive and formal.

Substantive theory emerges from a study of just one particular context – such as a ward, or patients with myocardial infarction, or nurse education – hence this type of theory is very useful for nurses or midwives. This type of theory has specificity and applies to the setting and situation studied; this means that it is limited. Formal theory is generated from many different situations and settings, and it is conceptual. It might be a theory about vocational education, general experiences of suffering or being a mother. Layder (1993) demonstrates the links between substantive and formal theory. The 'career' of the dying patients in hospital, the stages through which patients proceed, is substantive theory. When this is linked to the concept of 'status passage' that can be applied to many different situations, it becomes formal theory. This type of theory has general applicability, that is, it holds true not just for the setting of the specific study but also for other settings and situations.

Glaser and Strauss (1967) maintain that grounded theory is superior to the *grand theory* of the sociologist Talcott Parsons and the *middle range theory* of Robert Merton. As these latter theories are not rooted in research, they are merely speculative. Good examples of substantive theory in nursing research are given in the book edited by Morse and Johnson (1991) in which five researchers develop grounded theories about the illness experience.

Example

A clear example is that given by Johnson (1991). She shows that individuals go through a process of regaining control after a heart attack, a control that is often affected by health professionals. Patients test their abilities constantly until they know that they have again achieved a sense of control.

In a small student project, it would be difficult to produce a formal theory with wide applications, but substantive theories can still be important and have general implications for the work of the nurse. Melia (1995), for instance, declares that she meets many nursing students today who recognise their own learning process from her research tracing student socialisation in the late 1970s and 1980s although this took place in a different system of nurse education.

Another example can be given from midwifery:

Example

Dodd (2001) carried out research to explore the skills that midwives consider they use to facilitate normal vaginal birth, especially in the second stage of labour. She used semi-structured interviews to examine the perspectives of eleven midwives and their experience of providing interpartum care. The emerging theoretical ideas demonstrate that the way in which midwives apply skills to the care of women, influences the outcome of labour and enables these professionals to facilitate normal vaginal birth.

Theoretical memos and fieldnotes

While going through the process of research, the researcher writes fieldnotes and memos. When observing and interviewing, the investigator writes fieldnotes from the beginning of the data collection. Certain occurrences or sentences seem of vital interest and they are recorded either during or immediately after data collection. They remind the researcher of events, actions and interactions and trigger thinking processes. There can be descriptions of the setting.

Example

One of our research students who explored patients' hospital experience wrote the following when a patient told her that time drags:

Date xx

Imagine missing something so fundamental. I am too aware of my own busyness to notice the time dragging for patients. Note Roth's classic work is called 'Timetables' (Excerpt from fieldnotes, Warren, 1995)

Strauss and Corbin (1998: 110) define memos as 'records of analysis, thoughts, interpretations, questions and directions for further data collection', and they should be dated and detailed. Every grounded theory researcher should write memos. They are meant to help in the development and formulation of theory. In theoretical memos the researcher discusses tentative ideas and provisional categories, compares findings, and jots down thoughts on the research. Initially, memos might contain notes to remind the researcher 'don't forget...' or 'I intend to...'. Later they encompass micro-codes, and later still, major emergent categories, hunches, implications and concepts from the literature; memos become more varied and theoretical. Ideas for follow-up, related issues and thoughts about deviant cases become part of these memos. Strauss (1987) gives a number of different types of memos. A complete list with examples is given in Strauss, 1987.

Strauss (1987) suggests that memos are the written version of an internal dialogue that goes on during the research. Diagrams in the memos can help to remind the analyst and structure the study. Writing memos continues throughout the whole of the research. It goes through stages and becomes more complex in the process. Memos and diagrams provide 'density' for the research and guide the researcher to base abstract ideas in the reality of the data. Eventually, memos become integrated in the writing.

Problems and pitfalls

Wilson and Hutchinson (1996) discuss some of the common mistakes made in GT. They list six of these:

(1)   Muddling method (or method slurring)
(2)   Generational erosion
(3)   Premature closure
(4)   Overly generic analysis
(5)   The importing of concepts
(6)   Methodological transgression

Some of these are discussed further in other chapters, as they are common to several approaches.

Norton (1999) describes some problems inherent in the use of GT, in particular the danger that description rather than theory might be the outcome of a grounded theory study. In fact, many of our students give good conceptual descriptions but do not develop a theory or even theoretical ideas. Becker (1993) also suggests that researchers produce good stories including categories or types but often neglect the underlying social processes and abstract concepts. She stresses the need for explanations in GT. This is confirmed by Strauss and Corbin (1994) who emphasise the difference between description and conceptualisation. It is not enough to describe the perspectives of the participant to develop a truly 'grounded' theory.

The term 'emerging categories' (or 'emerging theory') is problematised by Stern (1994) who states that these do not simply 'emerge' as if arising by magic. They have to be worked for and 'pulled' from the data. This problem is linked to theoretical sampling. Often researchers use selective (or purposive) sampling procedures. Coyne (1997) differentiates clearly between purposeful and theoretical sampling. While the researcher decides on purposeful sampling beforehand according to certain criteria, dimensions and settings, for grounded theory research this type of sampling is necessary but does not suffice. The decisions about theoretical sampling are not made on the basis of initial criteria but throughout on the basis of emerging concepts, because of the inductive–deductive nature of the research. Induction is linked to emerging theories which, according to Strauss and Corbin (1998), researchers must try to test through theoretical sampling.

Becker (1993) warns the grounded theorist about the use of computers. A number of good computer programmes for qualitative research do, however, exist (see Chapter 15). Becker feels that computers might prevent sensitivity to the data and the discovery of meanings. Computers distance researchers from the data. Although this need not be so, we realise that in nursing and midwifery research, where emotional engagement and sensitivity is necessary, the use of computers could be problematic. Charmaz (2000) also maintains that in a study in which the researcher is deeply involved with the participants, computer analysis has an undesirable distancing effect.

Generalisability and replicability of grounded theory research are often discussed. Of course, it is difficult to match the original situation and context. Each researcher has a personal approach and a relationship with the participants which cannot be exactly reproduced. However, if nurses and midwives make procedures explicit and clearly describe the original conditions and setting, others can follow the same rules and procedures and discover the same general scheme. Strauss and Corbin (1998) maintain that the findings of a grounded theory study become more generalisable if the study is systematic, relies on theoretical sampling and examination of special conditions and discrepancies. A range of similar theoretical concepts from a variety of sources can become cumulative.

Glaser's critique

Stern (1994) distinguishes between the main two schools of GT which share some common elements but have also major differences. The ideas of Strauss and Glaser have diverged in the last decade. In 1992 Glaser wrote a book in response to the book by Strauss and Corbin (1990), criticising the authors for distorting the procedures and meaning of grounded theory. Glaser claims that the book does not truly describe GT. He accuses the authors of 'forced conceptual description' (p. 5). He exhorts the researchers not to impose their research problem but start with an interest and a questioning mind so that they see their informants' perspectives with no preconceptions. Thus, the researcher does not start with a research question but with a research interest.

Although agreeing that Strauss and Corbin have described a research method, Glaser denies that its roots have much in common with the original 1967 volume. The new method, he claims, results in conceptual descriptions rather than in the emergence of concepts and formation of the links between them that explain variations in behaviour. The difference between the ideas in Strauss and Corbin's text and the original development lies in the way in which concepts are generated and relationships explained. Glaser states clearly that grounded theory should not be verificational but inductive, it does not move between inductive and deductive thinking (although the 1967 book clearly mentions verification). Deduction is rarely used except for reasons of conceptual guidance; this differs from the ideas of Strauss and Corbin who include the element of verification by suggesting that researchers test working propositions or 'provisional hypotheses' during their research.

Glaser also argues that participant observation does not suffice for a truly grounded theory; interviews which explain the meanings of the participants are always necessary (this would merit a debate as many researchers see interviews as an integral part of participant observation in any case). Another difference exists between the two camps. Annels (1997a) claims that Strauss and Corbin see theory as a construct 'cocreated' by the researcher and participants, while Glaser believes that theory is 'emerging' from the actual data. It is interesting that Glaser, who started out as a survey researcher, seems to have become more flexible and less structured over time, while Strauss develops a more prescriptive way of researching.

Glaser (1992) believes that any initial literature review would contaminate the data and denies the need for it because it might direct researchers to irrelevant ideas. This he had also stated in his earlier book (1978). However, he suggests that the literature can be integrated in the developing concepts. Discrepancies between concepts developed from the researchers' original data and the data from the literature may be discovered and the reasons for them investigated. Theoretical sensitivity helps to generate ideas and relate them to theory.

Charmaz (2000) criticises some of the early ideas in the GT approach and argues that it has developed from a more prescriptive and more positivist style of research to a more flexible way of thinking. She claims that the methods have developed in a number of different ways depending on researchers' perspectives. She sees this as developmental and she welcomes the move towards a more constructivist GT.

Researchers can make up their own minds which approach to adopt when doing grounded theory as long as they are knowledgeable about it. In any case, many researchers adapt methods during the process of research. For a study to be called GT research, the major features of GT should be used, most importantly a theory and theoretical ideas should be generated (Annels, 1997b).

Summary

Grounded Theory is a style of analysis where data collection and analysis interact.

- The aim of the GT approach is the generation or modification of theory.
- Data usually are collected through non-standardised interviews and participant observation.
- Researchers code and categorise transcripts from interviews or fieldnotes, sometimes by using the words of the participants, at other times by using their own interpretive or summarising labels.
- Relationships found between categories generate working hypotheses, eventually establishing a new theory, and through this, the storyline emerges.
- Relevant ideas from the literature and other documents can become part of the data.
- Throughout the analytic process, constant comparison and theoretical sampling takes place.
- Memos – theoretical notes – provide the researcher with developing theoretical ideas.
- The ideas and theory that emerge are grounded in the data.

References

Alvesson, M. & Sköldberg, K. (2000) *Reflexive Methodology: New Vistas for Qualitative Research*. London, Sage.

Annels, M. (1997a) Grounded theory method, part 1: within the five moments of qualitative research. *Nursing Inquiry*, **4**, 120–29.

Annels, M. (1997b) Grounded theory method, part 2: options for users of the method. *Nursing Inquiry*, **4**, 176–80.

Backman, K. & Kyngäs, H.A. (1999) Challenges of the grounded theory approach to a novice researcher. *Nursing and Health Sciences*, **1**, 147–53.

Becker, P.H. (1993) Common pitfalls in grounded theory research. *Qualitative Health Research*, **3** (2) 254–60.

Benoliel, J.Q. (1973) *The Nurse and the Dying Patient*. New York, Macmillan.

Benoniel, J.Q. (1996) Grounded theory and nursing knowledge. *Qualitative Health Research*, **6** (3) 406–28.

Blumer, H. (1971) Sociological implications of the thoughts of G.H. Mead. In *School and Society* (eds B.R. Cosin *et al.*), pp. 11–17. Milton Keynes, Open University Press.

Charmaz, K. (1991) *Good Days, Bad Days: The Self in Chronic Illness and Time*. Berkeley, University of California Press.

Charmaz, K. (2000) Grounded theory: objectivist and constructivist methods. In *Handbook of Qualitative Research* (eds N.K. Denzin & Y.S. Lincoln), 2nd edn, pp. 509–535. Thousand Oaks, Sage.

Chenitz, W.C. & Swanson, J.M. (eds) (1986) *From Practice to Grounded Theory: Qualitative Research in Nursing*. Menlo Park, Addison-Wesley.

Corbin, J. (1986) Qualitative data analysis for grounded theory. In *From Practice to Grounded Theory: Qualitative Research in Nursing* (eds W.C. Chenitz & J.M. Swanson), pp. 91–101. Menlo Park, Addison-Wesley.

Coyne, I.T. (1997) Sampling in qualitative research: purposeful and theoretical sampling: merging or clear boundaries? *Journal of Advanced Nursing*, **26**, 623–30.

Cutcliffe, J.R. (2000) Methodological issues in grounded theory. *Journal of Advanced Nursing*, **31**, 1486–4.

Denzin, N.K. (1989) *The Research Act: A Theoretical Introduction to Sociological Methods*, 3rd edn. Englewood Cliffs NJ, Prentice Hall.

Dey, I. (1999) *Grounding Grounded Theory: Guidelines for Qualitative Inquiry*. San Diego, Academic Press.

Dodd, P. (2001) *Facilitating normal birth for women with epidurals*. Unfinished MPhil study, Bournemouth University, Bournemouth.

Glaser, B.G. (1978) *Theoretical Sensitivity*. Mill Valley, CA, Sociology Press.

Glaser, B.G. (1992) *Basics of Grounded Theory Analysis*. Mill Valley CA, Sociology Press.

Glaser, B.G. & Strauss, A.L. (1965) *Awareness of Dying*. Chicago, Aldine.

Glaser, B.G. & Strauss, A.L. (1967) *The Discovery of Grounded Theory*. Chicago, Aldine.

Glaser, B.G. & Strauss, A.L. (1968) *Time for Dying*. Chicago, Aldine.

Hutchinson, S.A. (1993) Grounded theory: the method. In *Nursing Research: A Qualitative Perspective* (eds P.L. Munhall & C. Oiler Boyd), pp. 180–212. New York, National League for Nursing Press.

Johnson, J.L. (1991) Learning to live again: the process of adjustment following a heart attack. In *The Illness Experience* (eds J.M. Morse & J.L. Johnson), pp. 13–88. Newbury Park, Sage.

Layder, D. (1993) *New Strategies in Social Research: An Introduction and Guide*. Cambridge, Polity Press.

Mead, M. (1934) *Mind, Self and Society*. Chicago, University of Chicago Press.

Melia, K. (1987) *Learning and Working*. London, Tavistock.

Melia, K. (1995) Presentation at a Conference on Qualitative Health and Social Care, Bournemouth University, September 28–29.

Morse, J.M. (ed.) (1991) *Qualitative Nursing Research: A Contemporary Dialogue* (Rev. edn). Newbury Park, Sage.

Morse, J.M. (1995) Editorial: The significance of saturation. *Qualitative Health Research*, 5 (2) 147–9.

Morse, J.M. & Johnson, J.L. (eds) (1991) *The Illness Experience*. Newbury Park, Sage.

Norton, E. (1999) The philosophical bases of grounded theory and their implications for research practice. *Nurse Researcher*, 7 (1) 31–43.

Orona, C.J. (1990) Temporality and identity loss due to Alzheimer's disease. *Social Science & Medicine*, 30 (11) 1247–56.

Schatzman, L. & Strauss, A.L. (1973) *Field Research: Strategies for a Natural Sociology*. Englewood Cliffs NJ, Prentice Hall.

Smith, P. (1992) *The Emotional Labour of Nursing*. London, Macmillan.

Stern, P.N. (1980) Grounded theory methodology: its uses and processes. *Image*, 12 (1) 20–23.

Stern, P.N. (1985) Using grounded theory in nursing research. In *Qualitative Research Methods in Nursing* (ed. M. Leininger), pp. 149–60. Philadelphia, WB Saunders.

Stern, P.N. (1994) Eroding grounded theory. In *Critical Issues in Qualitative Research Methods* (ed. J.M. Morse), pp. 212–23. Thousand Oaks, Sage.

Strauss, A.L. (1987) *Qualitative Analysis for Social Scientists*. New York, Cambridge University Press.

Strauss, A. and Corbin, J. (1990) *Basics of Qualitative Research: Grounded Theory Procedures and Techniques*. Newbury Park, Sage.

Strauss, A. & Corbin, J. (1994) Grounded theory methodology: an overview. In *The Handbook of Qualitative Research* (eds N.K. Denzin & Y.S. Lincoln), pp. 173–285. Thousand Oaks, Sage.

Strauss, A.L. & Corbin, J. (eds) (1997) *Grounded Theory in Practice*. Thousand Oaks, Sage.

Strauss, A. & Corbin, J. (1998) *Basics of Qualitative Research: Techniques and Procedures for Developing Grounded Theory*, 2nd edn. Thousand Oaks, Sage.

Strauss, A., Fagerhaugh, S., Suczek, B. and Wiener, C. (1985) *The Social Organization of Medical Work*. Chicago, University of Chicago Press.

Thomas, W.I. (1928) *The Child in America*. New York, Alfred Knopf.

Warren, J. (1995) Fieldnotes. Personal communication.

Wiener, C.L. & Wysmans, W.M. (eds) (1990) *Grounded Theory in Medical Research*. Amsterdam, Swets and Zeitlinger.

Wilson, H.S. & Hutchinson, S.A. (1996) Methodologic mistakes in grounded theory. *Nursing Research*, 45 (2) 122–4.

Wuest, J. (1995) Feminist grounded theory: an exploration of the congruency and tensions between two traditions in knowledge discovery. *Qualitative Health Research*, 5 (1) 125–37.

CHAPTER 11

Phenomenology

What is phenomenology?

Phenomenology is an approach to philosophy, and as a method of inquiry it has often been misunderstood. Indeed, Caelli (2001: 275–6) argues: 'Because phenomenology is first and foremost philosophy, the approach employed to pursue a particular study should emerge from the philosophical implications inherent in the question'. To address this problem, we have traced the rather complex history of the philosophy of phenomenology and its adaptation as a qualitative research approach in nursing and midwifery. As a method of inquiry it is not often carried out at undergraduate level but is popular in postgraduate nursing studies. Researchers must be aware, however, that various ways of 'doing' phenomenology exist. They all have similar aims however, and their analytic procedures overlap. McLeod (2001) reminds researchers that the major aim of a descriptive phenomenological research approach is to generate an exhaustive description of a phenomenon of everyday experience to achieve an understanding of its essential structure while hermeneutic inquiry emphasises understanding more than description and is based on interpretation.

Essentially phenomenology has three major streams: the *transcendental* phenomenology of Edmund Husserl (1859–1938); the *hermeneutic* phenomenology of Martin Heidegger (1889–1976); and the *existentialist* phenomenology of Merleau-Ponty (1908–1961) and Jean-Paul Sartre (1905–1980). There are ongoing philosophical debates about the distinctions and overlaps between these streams, but the differing emphases indicated in this chapter generally remain.

Some researchers follow Husserl and his followers who advocate a descriptive phenomenology, others utilise the ideas of Heidegger and his colleagues who believe that phenomenology is interpretive. Neither approach is wrong; these phenomenologies merely approach the study of lived experience in different ways (Streubert and Carpenter, 1999).

The term 'phenomenology' derives from the Greek word *phainomenon* meaning 'appearance' (the term was first used by the philosopher Kant according to Spiegelberg). Phenomenological philosophy is partly about the epistemological question – about the theory of knowledge – of 'how we know', the relationship of the person who knows and what can be known (McLeod, 2001). It is also connected to the ontological question: 'what is *being*'. The ontological question is concerned with the nature of reality and our knowledge about it, 'how things really are'.

As philosophy in general, the study of phenomenology is not immediately understandable. It is however, necessary to focus on language, as it is a main tool for expressing meaning. Nurses have a long experience of tackling jargon from a number of disciplines. Medicine, for instance, is known for its complex language as are the social and behavioural sciences. Often nurses have to demystify medical language for patients and clients and find other words to describe diseases, investigations and treatments to facilitate patient and client understanding.

In general, to understand any new theory, conceptual framework or school of thought more fully, it is useful to trace its origins. The following section will outline the background of phenomenology from so-called 'continental philosophy', the subsequent ideas of Franz Brentano and Edmund Husserl, as well as the later development of the phenomenological movement and schools of phenomenology.

Intentionality and the early stages of phenomenology

Teichman and Evans (1991) describe two different approaches to the study of philosophy, namely *analytic* and *continental*. Analytic philosophy, as the word suggests, is about analysing and defining concepts that are usually abstract. The analytic tradition is the approach used mostly in the United Kingdom and English speaking countries. It is derived originally from the ancient philosophers Socrates, Aristotle and Thomas Aquinas in the Middle Ages. Continental philosophy, as the name suggests, is mostly found in continental universities but also in South America and parts of the United States. It is more cohesive and linked to such names as Heidegger and Habermas, the German philosophers.

Phenomenology begins with Husserl who was the core figure in the development of phenomenology as a modern movement. It is important however, to trace the earlier history of phenomenology in the influence of Franz Brentano (1838–1917) on the work of Husserl. Brentano was part of the preparatory phase of this movement (Cohen *et al.*, 2000).

The central theme of Brentano's philosophy is the notion of *intentionality*. Intentionality is a way of describing how in consciousness the mind directs its thoughts to an object. Priest describes the notion of intentionality as:

'…the property or characteristic of the mental of being "of" or "about" something. For example, it does not make sense to say there is perception but not perception of something or other (even if the perception is an illusion or hallucination). It does not make much sense to talk about there being thinking without there being thinking about something or other (even if what is thought about is imaginary).'

(Priest, 1991: 194)

The way Priest describes this feature in Brentano's concept of intentionality is both clear and logical. Yet importantly, he also documents the criticism of this view. For the purpose of this chapter, it is not possible to get involved in this debate. It is important to acknowledge that Husserl was a student of Brentano and was influenced by his doctrine of intentionality. He differed from Brentano, however, and claimed that to state that mental phenomena have an intentional object, establishes a relationship between the two. Questions need to be asked about this relationship. Then three things would arise: the mental act, the intentional object and the relationship. Husserl could not accept that a person is aware of two things at once:

'For example, suppose you are looking at a colour, what you are aware of is colour. You are not aware both of the colour and your awareness of the colour. There are not two items present to your consciousness but only one.'

(Priest, 1991: 206)

This critical statement concerning Brentano's notion of intentionality shows the complexity of any attempt to define the act of conscious thought. There is much puzzlement concerning the so-called mind–body problem. Philosophers, psychologists and natural scientists, including doctors and psychiatrists, neither agree nor have firmly established what exactly consciousness is, or what is the true relationship between mind and body. The ideas presented in this chapter cannot resolve the mind–body problem. However, it is useful to note that phenomenology is, in fact, one approach that attempts to do this. Priest places phenomenology within mind–body theories arising from the following.

- Descartes' dualism which separates mind and body.
- So called logical behaviourism: this is a belief that everything concerns behaviour. The mind is really observable behaviour.
- Notions of idealism: all that exists can be explained in terms of the mind.
- Materialism: everything in the universe can be explained in terms of matter.
- Functionalism: everything is a kind of cause and effect. The mind is given a stimulus and responds physically or behaviourally.
- So-called 'double aspect theory': the physical and mental are, in fact, merely aspects of something else, another reality, outside notions of the mental and the physical.
- The phenomenological view: this is an attempt to describe lived experiences, without making previous assumptions about the objective reality of those experiences.

Whilst these ideas are presented as theories, Priest points out that phenomenology is, in fact, also a practice. It is this practice that is so exciting for nursing, health and social care alike, because it offers the possibility of '...characterizing the contents of experience just as they appear to consciousness with a view to capturing their essential features' (Priest, 1991: 183).

Phases and history of the movement

As has already been stated, phenomenology has philosophical origins. In 1960, the first edition of Spiegelberg's review of the history of the phenomenological movement was published. He described what he termed three phases in the movement, the preparatory, the German and the French phases. Cohen (1987) summarises these in a paper giving her account of the history and importance of phenomenological research for nursing. The influence of Brentano in the so-called preparatory phase has been described (pp. 171–72).

The German phase

The German phase involved primarily Husserl and later Heidegger. Concerning Husserl's contribution to the movement, Cohen *et al.* (2000) highlight his centrality for phenomenology, his search for rigour, his criticism of positivism (all knowledge is derived from the senses – linked to scientific inquiry of observation and experiment) and his concepts of *Anschauung* (phenomenological intuition) and phenomenological reduction. In the former, a different kind of experience is apparent, closely involved with the imagination. Experience suggests a relationship with something real, such as an event, while *Anschauung* can also occur in imagination or memory. The latter is a process to suspend attitudes, beliefs and suppositions in order properly to examine what is present. Husserl termed this part of phenomenological reduction *epoché* (from the Greek, meaning 'suspension of belief'). Bracketing (a mathematical term) is the name given by Husserl to this process of suspending beliefs and prior assumptions about a phenomenon. For researchers this means examining their attitudes, beliefs and prejudices literally to bracket these out, and in a sense, remove them from influencing the research. Bracketing and phenomenological reduction are important features of the method, the actual 'doing' of Husserlian phenomenology (these features are discussed later in this chapter). The complex approach of various forms of phenomenology and the idea of bracketing in Husserl's and Heidegger's work has been debated in many books and articles explaining phenomenology to and for nurses, such as, for instance, Jasper (1994), Crotty (1996) and Paley (1997).

More recently, Koch (1995) has reviewed the influence of Husserl and Heidegger in so-called interpretive research. She argues that Husserl, in fact, maintained Cartesian dualism in his philosophy. For Koch, Husserl's major contribution centred on three features: intentionality, essences and phenomenological reduction (bracketing).

According to Cohen *et al.* (2000) two important elements of phenomenology were developed by colleagues and students of Husserl. These are notions of intersubjectivity and the idea of 'lifeworld' *(Lebenswelt)*. Intersubjectivity is about the existence of a number of subjectivities which are shared by a community, that is, by individual persons who share a common world. The intersubjective world is accessible because humans have empathy for others. The way of making sense of experience is essentially intersubjective (Schwandt, 2001).

The concept of lifeworld *(Lebenswelt)* is about the lived experience that is central to modern phenomenology. Human beings do not often take into account the commonplace and ordinary; indeed they do not even notice it. Phenomenological inquiry is the approach needed to help examine and recognise the lived experience that is commonly taken for granted.

The next stage in the German phase of phenomenology involved Heidegger who was at some point an assistant to Husserl. Due to the recent upsurge of interest (particularly in North America) in using the phenomenological framework for nursing and midwifery research, Heidegger is examined in the work of Cohen and Omery (1994), Leonard (1994), Ray (1994), Taylor (1994) and Koch (1995). Benner's (1984) phenomenological research uncovered excellence and power in clinical nursing practice, and she references, amongst others, Heidegger. Later she (1994) examines and reviews Heidegger's philosophy. Taylor (1994) points out that Heidegger's main break from Husserlian phenomenology occurred in the way he developed the notion of *Dasein* which is explained fully in his work *Being and Time* in 1927 and translated into English in 1962. Heidegger's concern was to ask questions about the nature of being and about temporality (being is temporal). In this sense he was interested in ontological ideas. Heidegger's notion of *Dasein* is an explanation of the nature of being and existence and, as such, a concept of personhood. Leonard (1994) makes five main points concerning a Heideggerian phenomenological view of the person. These are as follows.

(1) The person has a world, which comes from culture, history and language. Often this world is so inclusive that it is overlooked and taken for granted until we reflect and analyse.
(2) The person has a being in which things have value and significance. In this sense, persons can only be understood by a study of the context of their lives.
(3) The person is self-interpreting. A person has the ability to make interpretations about knowledge. The understanding gained becomes part of the self.
(4) The person is embodied. This is a different view from the Cartesian, which is about possessing a body. The notion of embodiment is the view that the body is the way we can potentially experience the action of ourselves in the world.

(5) The person 'is' in time. This requires a little more elaboration as outlined below.

Heidegger had a different notion from the one of traditional time, which is perceived to flow in a linear fashion, with an awareness of 'now'. According to Leonard (1994) he used the word 'temporality' which denotes a new way of perceiving time in terms of including the *now*, the *no longer* and the *not yet*.

As well as these ideas, Heidegger developed phenomenology into interpretive philosophy that became the basis for hermeneutical methods of inquiry (in classical Greek mythology Hermes was the transmitter of the messages from the Gods to the mortals). This often involved interpreting the messages for the recipients to aid understanding. Hermeneutics developed as a result of translating literature from different languages, or where direct access to authoritative texts, such as the Bible, was difficult. Hermeneutics became the theory of interpretation and developed into its present form as the theory of the interpretation of meaning. Text means language. Gadamer (1975) suggests that human beings' experience of the world is connected with language.

Linking the ideas of hermeneutics with phenomenology, Koch (1995: 831) states:

'Heidegger (1962) declares nothing can be encountered without reference to the person's background understanding, and every encounter entails an interpretation based on the person's background, in its "historicality". The framework of interpretation that we use is the foreconception in which we grasp something in advance.'

Heidegger's purpose is going beyond mere description into interpretation (Cohen and Omery, 1994).

Draucker (1999), in particular, mentions Heideggerian interpretive pheno-menology as a popular research approach in nursing. She stresses that this form of inquiry explores the meaning of being a person in the world. Rather than suspending presuppositions, researchers examine them and make them explicit.

The French phase

Cohen (1987) argues that Heidegger's major contribution to the phenomen-ological movement was his influence on French philosophy. She points out that the main figures in this phase were Gabriel Marcel (1889–1973), Jean-Paul Sartre (1905–1980) and Maurice Merleau-Ponty (1908–1961). Marcel did not call himself a phenomenologist but viewed phenomenology as an introduction to analysing the notion of *being*.

Jean-Paul Sartre was the most influential figure in the movement but again did not want the label phenomenologist; rather he was termed as an *existenti-alist*. Phenomenological concepts and terms are difficult to grasp and it is often difficult to find a starting point. A dictionary is useful in this process, and we offer a definition of 'existentialism' from Chambers Dictionary (1993) that follows:

'A term covering a number of related philosophical doctrines denying objective universal values and holding that people, as moral free agents, must create values for themselves, through actions and must accept the ultimate responsibility for those actions in the seemingly meaningless universe.'

Understanding of terminology can be obviously further enhanced in progression from general to specific. The *Collins Dictionary of Philosophy* is an example of more specific outlines and links 'existentialism' with phenomenology in this passage:

'In so far as existentialist thinking relies heavily on raw experience, it has made use of the work of PHENOMENOLOGY, which attempts to capture experience without imposing on it any prior theoretical views held by the observer. In a purely formal sense, existentialism seeks to emphasise that something is, rather than how it is: the fact of its being, rather than describing the features it has. This has been simply put in the tag that existence comes before ESSENCE. Existence (from Latin *ex(s)istere* to stand out there) is what we have as standing in the world, essence (from Latin *essentia*, the being of this or that kind) belongs to a description of us in terms of CONCEPTS.'

(Vessey and Foulkes, 1990: 109)

The idea of existence and essence are from Sartre; his famous and often quoted phrase is 'existence precedes essence'. This is Sartre's idea that a person's actual consciousness and behaviour (existence) comes before character (essence) (Cohen, 1987). In this sense research would focus on real and concrete thoughts and behaviour before imaginary or idealised qualities or essences. The notion of intentionality features also in Sartre's work.

Merleau-Ponty's interest in phenomenology focused on perception and the creation of a science of human being (for the purpose of this chapter it is not necessary to develop this further).

Another major figure in French phenomenology is Paul Ricoeur. Spiegelberg (1984) argues that Ricoeur's phenomenology is primarily descriptive and based on a Husserlian eidetic concern with essential structures. Ricoeur, like Gadamer, focuses on the intersubjective and on issues of language and communication.

There are then different approaches within phenomenology. Schwandt (2001: 191) stresses strongly that phenomenology is not 'a single, unified philosophical standpoint'. In the next stage of this chapter, we will examine the schools of phenomenology outlined by Cohen and Omery (1994).

Schools of phenomenology

It has been shown thus far that phenomenology is an approach within continental philosophy. For purposes of qualitative research however, phenomenology has also been adapted and used as a framework within the so-called interpretive tradition that broadly includes grounded theory and ethnography as Lowenberg (1993) points out. She states: 'Basic to all these approaches is the recognition of the interpretive and constitutive cognitive processes inherent in all social life' (p. 58) and shows that there are many 'quandaries in terminology' which lead to misinterpretations in the nursing and education research literature, and sometimes in social research. She argues that there is a problem with phenomenology, the distinctions between the assumptions that lie behind the theories (e.g. Husserl and Heidegger) and the actual method, the 'doing' of phenomenology. Part of the purpose of this chapter is to try to unravel these perplexities.

A useful outline of phenomenological philosophy, guiding research and describing the development of schools with different approaches, is presented by Cohen and Omery (1994). However, they do highlight that the broad goal in each school remains the same, that is, to gain knowledge about phenomena.

Three major schools can be found, but there is overlap and linkage between them. The first is the *Dusquesne* school, guided by Husserl's ideas about eidetic structure (so-called because its followers worked at one stage in time at Duquesne University). The second school is about the *interpretation* of phenomena (Heideggerian hermeneutics). The combination of both is found in the *Dutch* School of phenomenology.

The Duquesne School focuses mostly on the notion of description. Giorgi (1992) states that social scientists describe that which presents itself without adding or subtracting from it. His advice is to acknowledge the evidence and not go beyond the data. He does acknowledge however that 'description is never complete' (p. 122). The 'interpretation of phenomena' approach concentrates on taken for granted practices and common meanings, whilst the Dutch School aims to combine both description and interpretation.

Streubert and Carpenter (1999) argue that phenomenology is, in fact, an integral research approach that involves philosophical, sociological and psychological perspectives. It has been most often used by phenomenological psychologists in psychotherapy and clinical psychology. The authors also contend that, whilst it is a useful method for examining phenomena important to nursing – and, one would add, midwifery – it still remains relatively new. Lawler (1998) recognises the problem in applying a philosophical approach to a practice discipline. This means that new researchers are often uncertain of how to proceed when wishing to use phenomenological research. While developing ideas about the complementarity of different phenomenological approaches as a philosophical basis for nursing research, Todres and Wheeler (2001: 2) discuss some philosophical distinctions in the approach to human experience that need to be included when carrying out practical research. They approach three areas in which they show that phenomenology, hermeneutics and existentialism have a contribution to make to nursing inquiry: *grounding*, *reflexivity* and *humanisation*.

Grounding

Grounding means taking the life-world as a starting point. It includes the everyday world of common experiences. The life-world is more complex than that which can be said about it and contains inherent tensions. Lived experience for Husserl is the *ground* of inquiry. There is also a *need* for inquiry. The commonplace, taken for granted, becomes a phenomenon when it becomes questionable. The understanding of the life-world demands an open-minded attitude in which prior assumptions are bracketed so that descriptions can clarify meanings and relationships.

Reflexivity and positional knowledge

Hermeneutics has added certain dimensions to phenomenological research. Gadamer (1975) developed Heidegger's ideas about interpretation as integral to human existence. Human beings are self-reflective persons who are based in everyday life and personal relationships and experience in a temporal and historical context and their position in the world. Preconceptions and provisional knowledge are always revised in the light of experience and reflection. The text is always open to multiple interpretations because researchers or reflective persons are involved in their own relationships with the world and others.

Humanisation and the language of experience

Human beings cannot be separated from their relationships in the world. Heidegger's notion of *Dasein*, being-in-the-world, entails a relationship between being human and being-in-the-world. Researchers search for fundamental and general categories of human existence that illuminate experiences that reveal a world. Heidegger (Todres and Wheeler, 2001: 5) reflects on fundamental structures that characterise the essential qualities of being-in-the-world such as:

- The way in which the body occurs
- The way the co-constituting of temporal structures occurs
- The way the meaningful word of place and things occurs
- The way that the quality of interpersonal relationships occurs

This is how Heidegger shows that body, time and space reflect the qualities of human presence rather than being notions of quantitative measurement.

From these ideas Todres and Wheeler (2001) conclude that phenomenology *grounds* research and stays away from theoretical abstraction. They also claim that hermeneutics adds the notion of *reflexivity*, which makes researchers ask questions meaningful and relevant in cultural, temporal and historical contexts. Lastly these writers state that the ontological existential dimension *humanises* the research so it is not merely technical and utilitarian.

The phenomenological research process

Van Manen (1990: 5) outlines some important points that identify phenomenological research. Oiler Boyd (1993: 126–8) summarises these.

- Phenomenological research is the study of lived experience.
- Phenomenological research is the explication of phenomena as they present themselves to consciousness.
- Phenomenological research is the study of essences or meaning (depending on the specific approach).
- Phenomenological research is the description of the experiential meanings we live as we live them.
- Phenomenological research is the human scientific study of phenomena.
- Phenomenological research is the attentive practice of thoughtfulness.
  Oiler Boyd (1993: 127) describes this: 'The impetus for doing research is the researcher's everyday practical concerns in her or his orientation as nurse for example'.
- Phenomenological research is a search for what it means to be human.
- Phenomenological research is a poetizing activity.
  Oiler Boyd (1993: 128) summarises this: 'phenomenological description is then characterized by inspirational insight won through reflective writing. Research and writing are thus closely related.'

To begin the process of phenomenological inquiry, researchers obviously need an area of interest, puzzlement, concern or a gap in general or specific knowledge about a phenomenon.

'Practising science', as Giorgi (2000b) calls it, is distinctly different from 'doing philosophy'. Indeed he criticises researchers who write on nursing research, such as Crotty (1996) or Paley (1997) for not distinguishing between the two. Giorgi sees value in the use of phenomenological research in nursing but suggests that this means scientific work rather than doing philosophy. Giorgi's engagement with the ideas of Crotty and Paley is important but cannot be followed up here.

In all research approaches the researcher has a responsibility to justify the type of theoretical framework (e.g. symbolic interactionism, phenomenology or any other) and specify and outline the approach to data analysis (e.g. grounded theory for the former, or Colaizzi's (1978) and other writers' approaches as regards the latter). Baker, Wuest and Stern (1992) argue that there is a need to define the methodology clearly to avoid 'method-slurring'. This is particularly important in phenomenology because of its distinctive underlying philosophy.

In data analysis for phenomenological inquiry, the researcher aims to uncover and produce a description of the lived experience. The procedural steps to achieve this aim vary with the approach taken by the researcher in terms of the three main types of phenomenology previously outlined. Ray (1994) points out that data analysis in eidetic or descriptive phenomenology requires the researcher to make full use of bracketing (that is to suspend their past experience, knowledge or prediction of phenomena). Intuition and reflection are important in the data analysis process to help open up '...the meaning of experience both as discourse and as text' (Ray, 1994: 129). Various researchers have developed approaches to data analysis that follow the requirements of bracketing, intuition and reflection. One of these, Colaizzi (1978), outlined a seven-stage process of analysis. Although there has been criticism of pioneering work such as this (Hycner, 1985), this particular process of analysis for the eidetic approach of phenomenology is both logical and credible. Hycner (1985: 279) states, however, that 'there is an appropriate reluctance on the part of phenomenologists to focus too much on specific steps in research methods for fear that they will become verified as they have in the natural sciences'. There are, however, several interpretations of the data analysis process depending on the school of phenomenology chosen. For example Streubert and Carpenter (1999: 50) outline the different procedural steps from other authors, such as van Kaam (1959), Paterson and Zderad (1976), Colaizzi (1978), Van Manen (1984) and Giorgi (1985).

Procedures for data analysis

The phenomenological research studies reviewed by Beck (1994) appeared to be guided by the Duquesne School and used the approaches from one of the following authors: Colaizzi (1978), Giorgi (1985) or Van Kaam (1966). In consequence Beck outlines the different procedural steps for data analysis developed by them. Colaizzi advocates seven steps, Giorgi four and Van Kaam six but many of these steps are similar or overlap.

In selecting a school of phenomenology, the researcher will be guided by the approach to the most appropriate procedural steps in data analysis. For the purposes of this chapter, we outline and discuss those developed by Giorgi (1985; 2000b) and Colaizzi (1978). It is however, a decision for student and supervisor (novice or expert researcher) to select the approach best suited for the phenomenon under investigation and to utilise the appropriate literature to guide the research methodology and analysis.

Both Giorgi (1985; 2000b) and Colaizzi (1978) argue for a descriptive approach and provide a method for data analysis, for instance from transcribed tapes of interviews with participants. These are just examples of qualitative data analyses.

Giorgi's steps for analysis are as follows.

(1) The entire description is read to get a sense of the whole statement.
(2) Once the *Gestalt* has been grasped, the researcher attempts to differentiate between meaning units and centres on the phenomenon under study.
(3) Once the meaning units have been illuminated, the researcher expresses the insight that is contained in them.
(4) The researcher integrates the transformed meaning units into a consistent statement about the participant's experience. This is called the *structure* of experience.

Colaizzi's seven-stage process is another approach to data analysis for the researcher. The seven-stage process of analysis occurs as follows.

(1) Read all of the subject's [*sic*] descriptions (conventionally termed *protocols*) in order to acquire a feeling for them, and to make sense out of them.
(2) Return to each description and extract from them phrases or sentences which directly pertain to the investigated phenomenon; this is known as *extracting significant statements.*
(3) Try to spell out the meaning of each significant statement; these are known as *formulated meanings.*
(4) Repeat the above for each description and organise the aggregate formulated meanings into *clusters of themes.*
    (a) Refer these clusters of themes back to the original protocols in order to *validate* them.
    (b) At this point, discrepancies may be noted among and/or between the various clusters; some themes may flatly contradict others, or may appear to be totally unrelated to others. (The researcher is advised by Colaizzi to refuse the temptation to ignore data or themes which do not fit).
(5) The results of everything so far are integrated into an *exhaustive description* of the investigated topic.
(6) An effort is made to formulate the exhaustive description of the investigated phenomenon in as unequivocal a statement of *identification of its fundamental structure* as possible. This has often been termed as an essential structure of the phenomenon.
(7) A final validating step can be achieved by returning to each subject, and, in either a single interview session or a series of interviews, asking the subject about the findings thus far.

These are descriptions of procedural steps adapted from Colaizzi (1978: 59–61).

Colaizzi encourages researchers to be flexible with these stages, and we have found this to be useful. For example, we have encouraged students to take the exhaustive description back to informants, rather than the final, essential structure, because it appears to be more recognisable for them for comment. This ensures rigour.

Diekelman *et al.* (1989) who are nurse researchers described the following process including seven steps that they adopted:

(1) Reading interviews to gain a holistic impression
(2) Writing interpretive summaries and searching for potential themes
(3) Analysing transcripts as a group task for an interpretive team
(4) Returning to the text or participants to clarify certain issues
(5) Comparing texts to identify common meanings and shared practices
(6) Identifying patterns linking the themes
(7) Asking the interpretative group and other peers for suggestions on the final draft

It can be seen that many of the steps overlap in the analysis process of different writers on phenomenological research. All inquiry should go beyond these formal steps. When Todres (2000: 43) discusses a specific example of phenomenological research, he lists some signposts that go beyond mechanical stages, and they could become signposts for other researchers.

The presentation of his discoveries involve the following:

- It will go beyond a definition or a series of statements; it will reflect a narrative in a coherence
- It will tell us something that connects with universal human qualities so that the reader can relate personally to the themes
- It will tell a story with which readers can empathise in imaginative ways
- It contributes to new understanding
- It will clarify and illuminate the topic to help the reader make sense of it without wholly possessing it

These signposts are significant for phenomenological studies. They show that the search for the essence of a phenomenon and its meaning within a defined context is not merely a technique or a series of mechanical steps but an exploration of meaning.

Phenomenological research in nursing and midwifery

Streubert and Carpenter (1999) suggest that professional nursing orientation towards holistic care provides the background for deciding whether to undertake phenomenological research. We would argue 'holistic care involves a multi-dimensional understanding of health (and illness) that is concerned with physical, emotional and spiritual aspects of health' (Wheeler, 1995: 50). This holistic perspective, coupled with the study of lived experience, provides the foundation for phenomenological research. Streubert and Carpenter advise the researcher to ask several questions about the intended topic. For example: is there some need for clarity concerning a phenomenon? Has there been anything published in relation to this, or is there a need for further inquiry? If there is, the nurse researcher should question whether inquiry concerning the lived experience is the most appropriate approach to collecting data. As the accounts of those experiencing the phenomenon are the primary data, the researcher needs to consider that this will yield both rich and descriptive data. Streubert and Carpenter argue that researchers examine their own style, preference and ability to engage with this approach to research. Further considerations for the research process concern completion and presentation of the study to relevant audiences.

Topics for phenomenological approaches

Appropriate areas for phenomenological research include topics that are important to life experience such as happiness, fear and anxiety or what it means to be a nurse specialist or a community midwife. There are other health and illness-related topics such as the experience of having a myocardial infarction, an acute illness or chronic pain.

Beck (1994) points out that few published phenomenological studies existed in the 1970s, with a large increase in the latter part of the 1980s. This continued in the 1990s and recently there has been a proliferation of phenomenological studies in the health profession. The studies Beck found covered a range of topic areas including caring in nursing practice, and caring between nursing students and physically/mentally disabled children, meaningful life experiences to the elderly, women with advanced breast cancer, infertility in couples, postpartum depression, loss of a partner due to AIDS, chronic illness and relationships in health care, addiction, violence and therapeutic touch. The phenomenological approach can also be used in nursing and midwifery education. Diekelman (1993), for instance, carried out a phenomenological study in nurse education in which she investigated the lived experiences of students and teachers in nursing.

The following are other examples of phenomenological research.

Example of descriptive phenomenological research in nursing

Karen Halliwell is using a phenomenological approach to explore and present the lived experience of third year student nurses of learning through reflective processes. The sources of data are one-to-one interviews of third year nurses. She is using the procedural steps suggested by Giorgi (2001) to analyse the descriptive data generated from interviews with participants.

(Halliwell, 2001)

Example of hermeneutic research in nursing

In Sweden, Sundin *et al.* (2001) carried out a hermeneutic study exploring the experiences of nurses who cared for patients who had suffered a stroke and aphasia. The researchers based their empirical study on the philosophical ideas of Gabriel Marcel, Paul Ricoeur and others. Revealing the lived experience through an interpretation of narrative text, they attempted to grasp the meaning of the experience. They proceeded through three phases in their analysis. The naïve (and holistic) reading of the text (the interview), the structural analysis and comprehensive understanding of the meaning of the narratives.

Example of an existentialist study in nursing

Sadala and Mendes (2000) explored the lived experience of caring for brain-dead patients who were kept alive for organ donation by interviewing nurses working in intensive care units. They demonstrate in their study the contradictions, conflicts and ambiguities of this type of caring. The ideas of Merleau-Ponty formed the basis for their key concepts. The interpretation of data allowed the researchers to perceive the general structure of the phenomenon they studied. (The authors describe the research process in some detail.)

These examples illustrate the breadth of phenomenological research and the potential of this method of inquiry. Clarke and Wheeler (1992) discussed the phenomenon of caring in nursing practice. In 1994, Lodi interviewed six individuals with a chronic condition and used a phenomenological inquiry to examine the lived experience of multiple sclerosis. Caelli (2001) attempted to examine nurses' understanding of health and its transfer to nursing practice by describing their experience of health-centred care to their patients. In these studies, research participants were volunteers and the usual ethical issues were considered carefully. In this and other aspects of the research process, phenomenological research follows the same sequence as other qualitative inquiry.

For nurses and midwives, phenomenological research is a rewarding enterprise. It is not easy because researchers have to understand the underlying philosophies before carrying out a study and decide which type of phenomenological approach to use.

Summary

Phenomenology is primarily a philosophy but is sometimes applied as a research approach.

- There are three main phases in the phenomenological philosophical movement: preparatory, German and French. There is overlap and interaction of ideas between the phases.
- Writers developed different conceptual formulations, (very broadly) descriptive (Husserl), interpretive (Heidegger) and ontological-existential (Sartre) which have been adapted as methods of inquiry by researchers.
- Researchers in the different schools of phenomenology have formulated various methods of data analysis.
- The approach should never be mechanical but insightful and illuminate the phenomenon under study and capture its essence.

References

Baker, C., Wuest, J. & Stern, P.N. (1992) Method slurring: the grounded theory/phenomenology example. *Journal of Advanced Nursing*, **17**, 1355–60.

Beck, C.T. (1994) Phenomenology: Its use in nursing research. *International Journal of Nursing Studies*, **31** (6) 449–510.

Benner, P. (1984) *From Novice to Expert: Excellence and Power in Clinical Nursing Practice*. Menlo Park, Addison Wesley.

Benner, P. (ed.) (1994) *Interpretive Phenomenology: Embodiment, Caring and Ethics in Health and Illness*. Thousand Oaks, Sage.

Caelli, K. (2001) Engaging with phenomenology: Is it more of a challenge than it needs to be? *Qualitative Health Research*, **11** (2) 273–81.

Chambers Dictionary (1993) Edinburgh, Chambers Harrap.

Clarke, J.B. & Wheeler, S.J. (1992) A view of the phenomenon of caring in nursing practice. *Journal of Advanced Nursing*, **17**, 1283–90.

Cohen, M.Z. (1987) A historical overview of the phenomenologic movement. *Image: Journal of Nursing Scholarship*, **19** (1) 31–4.

Cohen, M.Z. & Omery, A. (1994) Schools of phenomenology: implications for research. In *Critical Issues in Qualitative Research Methods* (ed. J.M. Morse), pp. 136–56. Thousand Oaks, Sage.

Cohen, M.Z., Kahn, D.L. & Steeves, R.H. (2000) *Hermeneutic Phenomenological Research: A Practical Guide for Nurse Researchers*. Thousand Oaks, Sage.

Colaizzi, P. (1978) Psychological research as a phenomenologist views it. In *Existential Phenomenological Alternatives for Psychology* (eds R. Vallé & M. King), pp. 48–71. New York, Oxford University Press.

Crotty, M. (1996) *Phenomenology and Nursing Research*. Melbourne, Churchill Livingstone.

Diekelman, N.L. (1993) Behavioural pedagogy: a Heideggerian hermeneutical analysis of the lived experiences of students and teachers in baccalaureate nursing education. *Journal of Nursing Education*, **32** (6) 245–50.

Diekelman, N.L., Allen, D. & Tanner, C. (1989) *The NLN Criteria of Appraisal of Baccalaureate Programs: A Critical Hermeneutic Analysis*. New York, National League for Nursing Press.

Draucker, C.B. (1999) The critique of Heideggerian hermeneutical nursing research. *Journal of Advanced Nursing*, **30** (2) 360–73.

Gadamer, H. (1975) *Truth and Method*. (Originally published in 1960. Translated by G. Barden & J. Cumming; 2nd edn. 1989.) New York, Seabury Press.

Giorgi, A. (ed.) (1985) *Phenomenology and Psychological Research*. Pittsburgh, Duquesne University Press.

Giorgi, A. (1992) Description versus interpretation: Competing strategies for qualitative research. *Journal of Phenomenological Psychology*, **23** (2) 119–35.

Giorgi, A. (2000a) The status of Husserlian phenomenology in caring research. *Scandinavian Journal of Caring Science*, **14**, 3–10.

Giorgi, A. (2000b) Concerning the application of phenomenology to caring research. *Scandinavian Journal of Caring Science*, **14**, 11–15.

Halliwell, K. (2001) *Learning through the utilisation of reflective processes: a phenomenological study to explore the lived experience of final year nursing students*. Unfinished PhD research; Bournemouth University, Bournemouth.

Heidegger, M. (1962) *Being and Time*. (Translated from the original 1927 publication by J. Maquarrie and E. Robinson). New York, Harper and Row.

Hycner, R.H. (1985) Some guidelines for the phenomenological analysis of interview data. *Human Studies*, **8**, 279–303.

Jasper, M.A. (1994) Issues in phenomenology for researchers of nursing. *Journal of Advanced Nursing*, **19**, 309–14.

Koch, T. (1995) Interpretive approaches in nursing research: the influence of Husserl and Heidegger. *Journal of Advanced Nursing*, **21**, 827–36.

Lawler, J. (1998) Phenomenologies as research methods for nursing: From philosophy to researching practice. *Nursing Inquiry*, **5**, 111–19.

Leonard, V.W. (1994) A Heideggerian phenomenological perspective on the concept of person. In *Interpretive Phenomenology: Embodiment, Caring and Ethics in Health and Illness* (ed. P. Benner), pp. 43–63. Thousand Oaks, Sage.

Lodi, Y. (1994) *The lived experience of multiple sclerosis: A phenomenological inquiry*. Unpublished BSc study: Bournemouth University, Bournemouth.

Lowenberg, J.S. (1993) Interpretive research methodology: Broadening the dialogue. *Advances in Nursing Science*, **16** (2) 57–69.

McLeod, J. (2001) *Qualitative Methods in Counselling and Psychotherapy*. London, Sage.

Oiler Boyd, C. (1993) Phenomenology: the method. In *Nursing Research: A Qualitative Perspective* (eds P.L. Munhall & C. Oiler Boyd), pp. 99–132. New York, National League for Nursing Press.

Paley, J. (1997) Husserl, phenomenology and nursing. *Journal of Advanced Nursing*, **26**, 187–93.

Paterson, J.G. & Zderad, L.T. (1976) *Humanistic Nursing*. New York, Wiley.

Priest, S. (1991) *Theories of Mind*. London, Penguin Books.

Ray, M. (1994) The richness of phenomenology: philosophic, theoretic and methodologic concerns. In *Critical Issues in Qualitative Research Methods* (ed. J.M. Morse), pp. 117–35. Thousand Oaks, Sage.

Sadala, M.L.A. & Mendes, H.W.B. (2000) Caring for organ donors: The extensive care unit nurses' view. *Qualitative Health Research*, **10** (6) 788–805.

Schwandt, T.A. (2001) *Dictionary of Qualitative Inquiry*, 2nd edn. Thousand Oaks, Sage.

Spiegelberg, H. (1984) *The Phenomenological Movement: A Historical Introduction*, 3rd edn (1st edn 1960). The Hague, Martinus Nijhoff.

Streubert, H.J. & Carpenter, D.R. (1999) *Qualitative Research in Nursing: Advancing the Human Imperative*, 2nd edn. Philadelphia, J.B. Lippincott.

Sundin, K., Norberg, A. & Jansson, L. (2001) The meaning of skilled care with stroke and aphasia patients. *Qualitative Health Research*, **11** (3) 308–21.

Taylor, B.J. (1994) *Being Human: Ordinariness in Nursing*. Melbourne, Churchill Livingstone.

Teichman, J. & Evans, K.C. (1991) *Philosophy, A Beginner's Guide*. Oxford, Blackwell.

Todres, L. (2000) Writing phenomenological psychological descriptions: An illustration to balance texture and structure. *Auto/Biography*, **8** (1/2) 41–8.

Todres, L. & Wheeler, S. (2001) The complementarity of phenomenology, hermeneutics and existentialism as a philosophical perspective for nursing research. *International Journal of Nursing Studies*, **38**, 1–8.

Van Kaam, A. (1959) A phenomenological analysis exemplified by the feeling of being understood. *Individual Psychology*, **15**, 66–72.

Van Kaam, A. (1966) *Existential Foundations of Psychology*. Pittsburgh, Dusquesne University Press.

Van Manen, M. (1990) *Researching Lived Experience: Human Science for an Action Sensitive Pedagogy*. New York, State University of New York Press.

Van Manen, M. (1998) *Researching Lived Experience: Human Science for an Action Sensitive Pedagogy*, 2nd edn. New York, State University of New York Press.

Vessey, G. & Foulkes, P. (1990) *Collins Dictionary of Philosophy*. Glasgow, Collins.

Wheeler, S.J. (1995) Child abuse: the health perspective. In *Family Violence and the Caring Professions* (eds P. Kingstone & B. Penhale), pp. 50–76. Basingstoke, Macmillan.

CHAPTER 12

Action Research

What is action research?

Action research (AR) is a useful approach to organisational and professional change and has been increasingly applied to professional and organisational settings since the early 1990s. Community development is another area in which AR is often applied. It can involve both qualitative and quantitative methods but many researchers see it as 'the antithesis of experimental research' (see Hart and Bond, 1995: 39) and as essentially qualitative. Indeed AR is not a 'pure' research approach but a particular style of research, and researchers can use many of the well known methodologies and procedures. As the name implies, AR includes both research and action. It should fulfil a number of criteria, which will be discussed in this chapter.

Reason and Bradbury (2001) speak of 'a family' of approaches, which derive from various philosophical and psychological assumptions and have their basis in different traditions. AR is not distinguished from other types of research by the use of different research procedures; any of the conventional approaches may be carried out in its research phase. In general action researchers use qualitative methods, as this type of inquiry is a reaction against positivist approaches.

Although some agreement exists about the nature and features of AR, there are a number of definitions, some of which are quoted here. All involve the concepts of change, participation and action. In one of the definitions (Carr and Kemmis, 1986: 162) it is claimed that AR is 'a form of self-reflective inquiry undertaken by participants in social situations in order to improve the rationality and justice of their own practices, their understanding of these practices, and the situations in which practices are carried out'. Carr and Kemmis are educationists, and in the past AR has most often been used in education. Banister *et al.* (1994: 110) give Elliot's useful explanation (1980: 110): 'The study of a social situation with a view of improving the quality of action within it. The total process ... review, diagnosis, planning, implementation, monitoring effects, provides the necessary link between self-evaluation and professional development'. In nursing, AR addresses the theory–practice gap in particular, as this gap has long been seen as detrimental to clinical professional work.

Action research is more than mere production of knowledge about a problem, a topic or an area of study but involves situations where change is necessary or desirable to improve practice. Badger (2000) claims that AR stands within a continuum of definitions and philosophies and is not a single unitary approach.

Action researchers claim that AR differs from other research mainly because:

- It has different aims and conceptions
- Researchers collaborate with or are themselves participants in the setting
- The process integrates action as an essential element
- As well as research, it includes intervention and change in the situation under study
- It is research in the setting where the changes take place
- The findings can be of immediate benefit as solutions to problems can be implemented and assessed straight away

Because of its complexity, AR is more appropriate for small rather than large studies. The language used also differs from that of other approaches; it must be understood by all the participants and not be full of academic terminology or researcher jargon. Newman (2000) suggests that there is no 'right' way of carrying out AR, but that action researchers should modify their approach as they go through the process of planning, acting and evaluating.

The origins of action research

Action research does not have a very long history but started in the 1940s. It is still in its infancy in many disciplines, but in education it has been used often. Kurt Lewin (1946), the social psychologist, was one of the early researchers to develop AR although he used it differently from more recent action researchers. The concept of change, however, was already present in this type of research, and he wanted to employ AR to bring about change in behaviour. Lewin adopted a number of stages, which consisted of:

- Planning an initial step to change a setting or individuals' behaviours
- Implementing the change
- Evaluating the results of the change
- Modifying the actions in the light of the evaluation
- Starting the process all over again.

Although modern action researchers still use the stage approach, much has changed; in particular it has become much more democratic and participatory. Action researchers now take account of the power relationships inherent in a setting.

The Tavistock Institute of Human Relations set up organisational action research from the late 1940s onwards – although at this stage the type of research was not called AR. The members of the Institute, in general psychologists, developed a problem-solving approach. At a later stage this problem-solving approach was also used to help deprived communities to solve social and educational problems and ameliorate the 'cycle of deprivation'. Since the work of the Tavistock Institute, AR has been carried out in many disciplines including management, sociology, health care and other disciplines. Often it is inter-disciplinary and interprofessional.

Critical social theory

Many ideas of modern AR have their base in critical social theory and critical social science. Carr and Kemmis (1986) give an overview of critical theory and critical social science. We have summarised some of their ideas here.

Critical theory attempts to add to positivist and interpretive research. Critical theorists of the 1950s, such as Horkheimer, Adorno, Marcuse and others, criticised the dominance of positivist social science in the twentieth century which conformed to rigid rules and stifled critical and creative thinking although they did agree with the scientific aim of generating rigorous knowledge about social life. While retrieving for social science those elements that are connected with values and human interests, they also tried to integrate these into a new framework that included ethical and critical thought. Rigorous knowledge about social life, however, was still a requirement of social science.

Habermas (1974) discusses human behaviour in terms of interests and needs. He argues that knowledge consists of three constitutive interests, which he calls the *technical*, the *practical* and the *emancipatory*. The technical interest helps people to gain knowledge in order to achieve technical control over nature. This instrumental knowledge requires scientific explanations. Habermas suggests that, although this form of knowledge is necessary, not everything can be reduced to scientific explanations, and people need to grasp the social meanings of life to understand others. Another way of generating knowledge serves 'practical' interests in the form of interpretive methods, but this still does not suffice. Human beings need 'emancipatory' knowledge in order to achieve freedom and autonomy, overcome social problems and change power relationships. This will diminish alienation. Habermas's thinking (developed in his books in 1972 and 1974) is based in Marxist philosophy to some extent. Habermas' theories cannot be developed here; this section merely gives a hint of the thinking behind modern AR. He also discusses the relationship between theory and practice.

Educationists in the 1970s and 1980s developed ideas for AR, because they pressed for change in educational settings and society within a critical theory framework. The concept of 'conscientization' discussed by Freire (1970), the educationist, is also connected to critical social science. Freire believed that people become increasingly aware of the social and historical reality that influences their lives and are able to take action in order to change it. McTaggart and Kemmis (1982) developed guidelines in an action research planner. Although educational and community development studies are not directly connected to AR in nursing, the underlying ideas are important as nurses too desire the empowerment of patients who will be able to take control of their own lives and change their situation.

Action research in nursing

As AR focused on improving education and society, it was also seen as useful in nursing (although it has not been often used in midwifery as far as we know). In the words of Hart and Bond (1995:3): 'it represents a counter to positivism and can develop reflexive practice and general theory from this practice'. It is, in their view, a tool for practitioners as knowledge is vital for improving nursing practice; only those involved in the setting are fully able to apply this knowledge. Action research generates practical knowledge intended to assist in raising standards of care and delivery of service in general. It is not 'blue skies research'. Nurses do now use it frequently but do not always go back to its base and develop it merely on a practical level rather than taking into account its added importance in developing theory.

One of the aims of AR is bridging the theory–practice gap. Rolfe (1996) argues that engaging practitioners from the clinical setting to carry out research in their own practice area would help to overcome this gap and generate direct improvement in practice and generate nursing knowledge. This, after all, is one of the justifications for doing nursing research. In the health professions AR is also a useful way of attempting and evaluating change in order to improve settings and care in the clinical arena. Professionals are able – through AR – to undertake research into their own practices. Earlier deeply held assumptions might be questioned.

This is linked to the reasons McNiff (1988) gives for engaging in AR, and these can be applied to nursing. She suggests that the aims are political, professional and personal. Through AR nurses and midwives are able to make sense of the clinical situation and become aware of the impact of policies and practices imposed on them through the system. They will also recognise more clearly that the health services and guidelines for care and treatment should exist initially for the good of the patients and ultimately for the health of society.

As professionals, nurses and midwives make independent decisions while adopting procedures based on theory and research rather than being controlled by outside forces. Action research helps professionals to make decisions in the interest of their clients (Carr and Kemmis, 1996). Rather than accepting unsatisfactory decisions imposed on them, they observe and diagnose problems as well as plan and implement changes that are based on the knowledge gained through the research. Professionals need to adopt a thinking and self-critical stance towards their practice which enables them to justify what they do.

On a personal level, AR not only improves the situation for clients and patients, it also enlightens the practitioners themselves and enhances their lives through reflection and engagement in the situation. The clinical setting provides the opportunity for active involvement and personal satisfaction and hence for personal growth.

Example

One of the best known examples of AR in nursing is that by Titchen & Binnie (1993). They carried out research at the John Radcliffe Hospital in Oxford. The aim of the study was to help staff nurses on two wards to change from traditional to patient-centred nursing. The main participants were a researcher with a physiotherapy background and a senior sister. The latter involved ward sisters with whom she shared the identification of problems and decision-making processes. The changes were carried out by people in the setting who reflected on and evaluated them in collaboration with the researcher.

The main features of action research

Action research is more than just the generation or production of knowledge about an area of interest but involves situations in which change is seen as necessary or desirable to improve practice. Researchers carry out interventions in the setting to be investigated. The main features of good AR now include the following:

- AR draws data and information from a range of sources
- AR is cyclical and dynamic
- AR is collaborative and participatory
- The aim of AR is to devise solutions to practical problems and to develop theory
- Researchers and practitioners are critical, self-critical and reflective

Action research draws data from a range of sources and perspectives: for instance, data sources might be interviews and observation, documents or diaries. Action research is cyclical in the sense that it represents an action cycle consisting of planning, implementing action, observing and reflecting. Then the process starts again. Lewin (1946) already demanded these four stages which he called a 'spiral'. The difference between his and modern action research is that the research is no more imposed from outside the organisation or setting but planned and carried out by insiders, participants in the setting. Meyer (1993) points out that Lewin's (1946) stages still form the basis for action research, and Parahoo (1997) charts this process in nursing where the stages are similar, though the aims and character of action research are different now:

- Researchers identify a problem in practice
- They carry out research to assess the problem
- They plan and implement the change
- They evaluate the outcome
- After this, the cycle starts again

These stages will be developed further in the section on practical considerations (pp. 195–6). Waterman *et al.* (2001) see the cyclical process and the research partnership as 'fundamental' for AR.

Example

Webb (1993) was involved in a project to develop both nursing and management skills. She used a 'development ward' as a training base for these skills, so that nurses were able to transfer their learning to other wards in order to change and evaluate their own practice. She herself, as an experienced nurse and academic expert in research, worked alongside these nurses to help provide advice and support. Changes were introduced slowly and evaluated and modified. In her report Webb stresses the importance of voluntary participation rather than management selection in this AR project to motivate participants.

Action research is collaborative. It involves the individuals in the setting in the design, data collection and analysis and evaluation of the research as well as in its dissemination. This fulfils the criteria of empowerment and emancipation. As the research influences and intervenes in the participants' working lives, they should be included in decision making.

Once a problem or important issue has been highlighted and the need for change and improvement is clearly observed, participants develop the focus for the research as co-researchers. The research centres on the problem or issue in the situation in which they work or learn and on a specific location. Modern day AR is always collaborative and participatory. The researchers are often themselves involved in the system they study, but even when they are not, they work with practitioners and professionals to carry out the research.

The methodological continuum

There are different types of action research as suggested before and many of these are used depending on the intentions of the co-researchers. The most common in nursing are identified by Hart and Bond (1995) and Holter and Schwartz-Barcott

(1993), but the differences between them are not vast, and they overlap. Because the typology of the latter is inclusive, it will be discussed here.

Holter and Schwartz-Barcott distinguish between three approaches:

(1) Technical collaborative
(2) Mutual collaboration
(3) Enhancement

In the *technical collaborative* approach, the researcher acts as a professional expert who pre-plans the research, carries out the research with practitioners, advises on action and acts as facilitator. Whyte (1991) calls this an 'élitist model', and it does not reflect the spirit of AR. As it has a pre-specified framework and theory, it is rarely qualitative.

The *mutual collaborative* approach entails a more democratic process. The researcher(s) as facilitator and the practitioners collaborate to identify a problem. They plan intervention and change together, and they work as equal partners. Theory is developed rather than predetermined. This mode of AR is more flexible than the technical approach. It is designed to solve immediate and practical problems and needs quick decision making. There is the danger, however, that the practitioners will not continue when the facilitator leaves the clinical area.

The goals of the *enhancement approach* are first, to bridge the theory and practice to solve problems and explain them and second, to raise awareness so that practitioners can identify problems and make them explicit. While the mutual collaboration approach fosters mutual understanding, the enhancement approach leads to emancipation of all participants. Berg (2001) maintains that one of the aims of this approach is the creation of action-oriented policy which means that this type of AR continues after the facilitator leaves. The link between theory and practice generates empowerment because practitioners gain deeper understanding and are therefore able to apply it in different settings, not just in one location at a particular time.

Hart and Bond (1995) maintain that AR is not linked to just one approach but can involve a progression through the typology.

Example

Sturt (1999) showed that it is possible to use all three approaches described by Holter and Schwartz-Barcott (1993). She and her collaborators carried out research within a healthcare team, focusing on its members' health promotion practice and applied all three approaches.

Lax and Galvin (2002) describe the differences between action research and participatory action research (PAR), two terms that are often used inter-changeably. The focus in their research was the development of a working group for 'families and young children'. The action research approach was adopted to support the development of improved childcare. Although often used in community development, PAR has not often been used in nursing. Kemmis and McTaggart (2000) stress the significance of participation in PAR which has a stronger element of participation than other types of AR. They state that it usually has three main features of importance:

- *Shared ownership:* the projects are owned by all who take part in them
- *Community based analysis:* the collaborators investigate social problems that occur in a community
- *Orientation towards community action:* the findings will be acted upon among the participating group

Early developers of PAR include Reason (1988), Heron (1996) and Fals Borda (2001) who claim that it is a way by which participants can take power and control in the research. Its aim is empowerment, emancipation and the generation of knowledge that benefits them directly. The researchers in this type of action research are much more aware of the elements of power and control.

Practical considerations

We will now describe the practical steps which researcher-practitioners take while going through an action research cycle in clinical or educational practice.

(1) Researchers and practitioners carefully observe what is happening in the setting. Before starting the action research, all participants should agree on their participation in the project; and they jointly formulate the research question (Berg, 2001). This entails a number of meetings in which procedures will be discussed. These meetings also include managers and policy makers who need to give permission for the project to proceed and for access to all the participants. Initially there is a critical assessment of all the aspects of current practice and a review of its effectiveness, quality and cost-effectiveness.

(2) Researcher-practitioners identify problem areas that they want to improve and thoroughly examine the practices that seem to need change and intervention. They discuss these identified problems with their colleagues and others interested in the project, including clients, and ask for their ideas and confirmation of the areas in need of improvement. Observations, interviews and brainstorming and focus group sessions take place to ascertain the problem.
    At this stage, researchers plan changes and interventions and implement them in the practice setting.

Planning includes drawing up a budget, suggesting a timescale, giving details of procedures happening.

(3) During the implementation of change or intervention an evaluation process takes place, which carefully monitors all the steps and procedures. This is done through a number of meetings with others in the setting as well as observation and interviewing.

(4) In the light of this careful evaluation practitioners modify their practices to improve on the intervention or change.

The action and monitoring process continues until practitioners are satisfied with the level of improvement. Throughout the whole process there will be meetings and discussions. The number of meetings depends on the size and duration of the project. Record keeping too, is of major importance, and participants write progress reports and give account of their actions to each other and to their managers. Stringer (1999) advocates the use of focus groups, meetings and discussions not only to develop the research but also to share the results of the project.

Example

Dowswell *et al.* (1999) report on their participatory process in developing a collaborative stroke training programme. Nursing staff, physiotherapists and managers were asked to identify training needs. They observed and interviewed practitioners and gave an account of what needed to be done. At the end of the research phase their reports were used to inform the content of the training course and its structure. The professionals interviewed were also involved in the development, implementation and evaluation of the training course.

Much useful action research can be carried out with patients, users of the services and lay carers.

Dowswell *et al.* (1999: 751) advise researchers on the stages of action research while describing their own project. The following are some excerpts from their account and demonstrate what needs to be done by other researchers.

- *Preliminary stage:* All participants are involved in the proposal and understand the reasons for the project. It is important that they all agree and willingly take part in it.
- *Assessment phase:* Ethical issues are clarified and anonymity ensured. Aims and limitations are truthfully described.
- *Planning phase:* Participants find innovative ways of solving problems and carry out agreed tasks and reflect on decision making.
- *Implementation phase:* All participants, regardless of ability, must be comfortable with the materials and incorporate both theory and practice.

- *Evaluation phase:* Interviews, observations and written reviews are used to evaluate the project.

Trustworthiness in AR

The criteria for validity or its equivalent have been discussed and developed by several nursing researchers, among them Titchen (1995) and Waterman (1998) (see also Chapter 16). Titchen's discussion overlaps with other arguments about trustworthiness in qualitative research while Waterman claims that an unquestioning acceptance of general criteria for qualitative research does not suffice and describes three types of validity:

(1) *Dialectical validity:* tensions and processes
(2) *Critical validity:* moral responsibilities
(3) *Reflexive validity:* valuing ourselves

First, Waterman (1998) points to the importance of examining the inherent tensions of an action research project. It implies attention to and description of details in the ongoing process as well as the conflicts and tensions between practice, theory and research. Second, she describes the moral responsibility of researchers who have to be aware and take account of the problems of people in the setting. Decision making not only includes action but also knowing when not to take action. Waterman goes on to say that researchers have the responsibility to give reasons for their decisions and argue their cause, as the ultimate aim is 'to improve people's lives'. Third, the reflexive nature of AR is acknowledged. The final report of an AR project should reflect the variety of perspectives that were examined. There is the important dilemma of the multiple roles of researchers who are, in the same study, research participants, change agents and evaluators of change. This position needs a reflexive stance by researchers on their own practices and assumptions. Whilst 'valuing themselves' researchers must also be aware of their own biases and limitations. Another important aspect for judging AR is the existence of more than one cycle. Some researchers who maintain they have used AR do not go further than a single cycle.

Whatever the criteria for trustworthiness, all those involved in the study must agree on the issues. For a project to be truly based on action research, they should reflect collaboratively on data collection, analysis and other methodological and procedural issues because reflection on action is inherent in this approach. Schön (1987), too, demands the element of reflection; he sees 'practice as inquiry' with a reflective stance as a way to gain knowledge about and to change the process of practice.

Guidance on assessment of the quality of AR projects and proposals can be found in Waterman *et al.* (2001: 43).

Problems and critique

Of course, action research can be problematic for a number of reasons. First, it is obvious that not everybody may wish to be involved. It takes diplomacy and persuasion to recruit reluctant participants. While undertaking the research, practitioners may be in conflict with each other. Managers too, may make objections especially if the process takes too much time or is expensive.

Action research is not always appropriate. Morton-Cooper (2000: 25) suggests certain situations in which it should not be used:

- If the policy or service to be implemented is forced on the people in the setting, especially when managers have already made their own decisions about this
- If the procedures and methodology used have not met the same quality criteria as other clinically based studies
- If the members of the team giving care, treatment or service do not work well together
- If the researchers want to enhance their own status and reputation

We would have to add that AR takes time because of its cyclical nature.

Meyer (1993) also notes some problems and limitations of action research. She identifies the problem of defining stages in AR when it is difficult to describe them before the start of the research as they develop during its process. This also means that informed consent is problematic because the stages are unknown beforehand. She warns researchers that the members of the participating team – which may consist of practitioners and facilitators as experts in research – have to be able to collaborate willingly and with a common aim rather than by edict and selection of management. Power relationships may also have inherent problems: research experts from outside have to negotiate rather than using their expertise as control. Waterman *et al.* (2001) suggest, among other problems, that the familiarity of co-researchers with the setting might 'cloud understanding'. Again, this means that they have to become 'professional strangers' or naïve observers.

Some health professions still do not see AR as a respectable, scientific type of research because it is not generalisable. It is, however, increasingly used in nursing because it can offer practical solutions to problems and enhancement of theory. Morrison and Lilford (2001) describe the dilemma inherent in AR. Action researchers have developed innovative and imaginative ways of developing practice and theory that could be applied in all research approaches. In their enthusiasm, however, they maintain that a major difference from traditional research (or mainstream research) exists. In fact, so Morrison and Lilford argue, many of the tenets of AR could be applied to mainstream research. There is only one major difference: that AR takes account of its unique social context. However, one might argue that this is true for much qualitative research which is context bound, meaning that the specific context in which it takes place has to be taken into account. This does not necessarily indicate that the findings of one specific context cannot be applied in other contexts, or that the theoretical advances are not useful in other settings. The researcher should also be able to apply what is learnt from one situation to another setting. Action research is, nevertheless, of most use in a specific context in which a local problem needs a solution or where actions and thinking need improvement. This supports the claim by Waterman *et al.* (2001) about AR as 'real world research'.

This chapter does not tell researchers how to carry out the research, as the research strategies may include many types of qualitative (and indeed, occasionally quantitative) approach. Data collection and analytic procedures can be found in the other chapters of this book.

Summary

The aim of action research is to improve practice and to extend theory.

- AR draws data from a range of sources
- Researchers can apply a number of different approaches
- AR bridges the theory–practice gap and is 'real world' research
- AR is most often used where a problem needs a solution
- AR includes planning, action and evaluation
- It is cyclical, reflective and dynamic

References

Badger, T.G. (2000) Action research: change and methodological rigour. *Journal of Nursing Management*, 8, 201–207.

Banister, P., Burman, E., Parker, I., Taylor, M. & Tindall, C. (1994) *Qualitative Methods in Psychology*. Buckingham, Open University.

Berg, B.L. (2001) *Qualitative Research for the Social Sciences*. Boston, Allyn and Bacon.

Carr, W. and Kemmis, S. (1986) *Becoming Critical: Education, Knowledge and Action Research*. London, The Falmer Press.

Clarke, J.E. (2000) Action Research. In *The Research Process in Nursing* (ed. D. Cormack), pp. 183–97. Oxford, Blackwell Science.

Dowswell, G., Forster, A., Young, J., Sheard, J., Wright, P. & Bagley, P. (1999) The development of a collaborative stroke training programme for nurses. *Journal of Clinical Nursing*, 8, 743–52.

Elliot, J. (1980) Action research in schools: some guidelines. *Classroom Action Research Bulletin 4*. Norwich, University of East Anglia.

Fals Borda, O. (2001) Participatory (action) research in social theory. In *Handbook of Action Research: Participatory Inquiry and Practice* (eds P. Reason & H. Bradbury), pp. 27–37. London, Sage.

Freire, P. (1970) *Cultural Action for Freedom*. Cambridge, Mass, Centre for the Study of Change.

Habermas, J. (1972) *Knowledge and Human Interest* (translated by J. Shapiro). London, Heinemann.

Habermas, J. (1974) *Theory and Practice* (translated by J. Viertel). London, Heinemann.

Hart, E. & Bond, M. (1995) *Action Research for Health and Social Care: a guide to practice*. Buckingham, Open University Press.

Heron, J. (1996) *Co-operative Inquiry*. London, Sage.

Holter, I.M. & Schwartz-Barcott, D. (1993) Action research: what is it? How has it been used and how can it be used in nursing? *Journal of Advanced Nursing*, **18**, 298–304.

Kemmis, S. (1993) Action research. In *Educational Research: Current Issues* (ed. M. Hammersley), pp. 177–90. London, Open University/Paul Chapman.

Kemmis, S. & McTaggart, R. (2000) Participatory action research. In *Handbook of Qualitative Research* (eds N.K. Denzin & Y.S. Lincoln), pp. 567–605. Thousand Oaks, Sage.

Lax, W. & Galvin, K. (2002) Reflections on a community action research project: Inter-professional issues and methodological problems. *Journal of Clinical Nursing*, **11**, 1–11.

Lewin, K. (1946) Action research and minority problems. *Journal of Social Issues*, **2**, 34–46.

McNiff, J. (1988) *Action Research: Principles and Practice*. London, Routledge.

McNiff, J., Lomax, P. & Whitehead, J. (1996) *You and your Action Research Project*. London, Routledge.

McTaggart, R. & Kemmis, S. (1982) *The Action Research Planner*. Geelong, Deakin University Press.

Meyer, J.E. (1993) New paradigm research in practice: the trials and tribulations of action research. *Journal of Advanced Nursing*, **18**, 1066–72.

Morrison, B. & Lilford, R. (2001) How can action research apply to health services? *Qualitative Health Research*, **11** (4) 436–49.

Morton-Cooper, A. (2000) *Action Research in Health Care*. Oxford, Blackwell Science.

Newman, J.M. (2000) Action research: A brief overview. *Forum Qualitative Sozialforschung/Forum Qualitative Research* (On-line journal), **1** (1). Available at http://www.qualitative-research.net/fqs

Parahoo, K. (1997) *Nursing Research: Principles, Process and Issues*. Basingstoke, Macmillan Press.

Reason, P. (ed.) (1988) *Human Inquiry in Action: Developments in New Paradigm Research*. London, Sage.

Reason, P. & Bradbury, H. (eds) (2001) *Handbook of Action Research: Participatory Inquiry and Practice*. London, Sage.

Rolfe, G. (1996) Going to extremes: action research, grounded practice and the theory–practice gap in nursing. *Journal of Advanced Nursing*, **24**, 1315–20.

Schön, D. (1987) *Educating the Reflective Practitioner*. San Francisco, Jossey-Bass.

Stringer, E.T. (1999) *Action Research: A Handbook for Practitioners*, 2nd edn. Thousand Oaks, Sage.

Sturt, J. (1999) Placing empowerment research within an action research typology. *Journal of Advanced Nursing*, **30**, 1057–72.

Titchen, A. (1995) Issues of validity in action research. *Nurse Researcher*, **2** (3) 38–59.

Titchen, A. & Binnie, A. (1993) Research partnerships: collaborative action research in nursing. *Journal of Advanced Nursing*, **18**, 858–65.

Waterman, H. (1998) Embracing ambiguities and valuing ourselves: issues of validity in action research. *Journal of Advanced Nursing*, **28** (1) 101–105.

Waterman, H., Tillen, D., Dickson, R. & de Koning, K. (2001) Action research: a systematic review and guidance for assessment. *Health Technology Assessment*, **5** (23).

Webb, C. (1993) Action research: philosophy, methods and personal experiences. In *Nursing: Art and Science* (ed. A. Kitson), pp. 120–33. London, Chapman and Hall.

Whyte, W.P. (ed.) (1991) *Participatory Action Research*. Newbury Park, Sage.

CHAPTER 13

Narrative Inquiry

The nature of narratives

Narratives are reflections and tales of people's experience. Narrative research is neither more nor less appropriate than other types of inquiry but is a useful way of gaining access to feelings, thoughts and experience. Many researchers apply the terms 'narrative' and 'story-telling' interchangeably, although others make a distinction: a narrative is seen as the account of an individual's experience while story-telling is its retelling by others. For instance, illness narratives are accounts of the progress of people's illness and suffering; the retelling of the experiences by the researcher in an article or in a report is considered story-telling; in fact the story is 'a legitimate research product' in Koch's view (Koch, 1998). Riessman (1993) claims that the term narrative is ambiguous. Researchers refer to life stories or narratives, but Labov (1972), one of the first sociologists to carry out research through narratives, sees the term as more specific – as events in the past that are being retold. First person narratives provide much material for research. It must be remembered, however, that their content emerges from memory, and that people's memories are selective (Skultans, 1998). Nevertheless, the remembered events, as well as the experiences people choose from their vast store of memory, focus on the significant aspects of their social reality.

Narrating helps people to make sense of their experience. It unveils the intentions of human beings and allows them to see the effects of their actions and to change direction if they wish (Richardson, 1990). Individuals remember an experience, they often tell the story sequentially as it happened and seek explanations for events and actions while interpreting and reflecting on them. However, narrators prioritise; some events and experiences carry more importance than others.

> ## Examples of narrative
>
> Sparkes (1996, 1998, 1999) explores body narratives of athletes and physical education teachers (including his own story) which are not only tales of identity but also studies of disruption and fragmentation when events occur that disturb the physical image of self. These narratives become the means through which individuals make sense of their suffering and disrupted lives, but they also help the listener or reader to gain insights into bodily experience. Storytellers reveal aspects of their identities to others through narratives while the researcher re-tells the story in the research report. Together they give an account of the narrator's experience.

Frank (1995) uses the concepts of story and narrative differently: He cites the term 'story' when discussing the tales people tell, and narrative when referring to 'general structures' that encompass a number of particular stories. However, the line between storytelling and narrative is blurred, and we shall occasionally use these terms interchangeably. Even Frank admits that a distinction between the two is difficult.

Narrative research is a broader term than many of the other qualitative approaches, indeed it can incorporate them – a narrative study may be an ethnography, take a phenomenological approach or use discourse analysis. It refers to 'any study that uses or analyses narrative material' (Lieblich *et al.*, 1998: 2). Narratives are not only used in research but also in psychotherapy and in clinical and developmental psychology, mostly in the form of life stories. In sociology and anthropology too, narrative is seen as useful for examining culture, society or social and cultural groups. Lieblich *et al.* maintain that it is natural for people to tell stories. Researchers can use this talent to elicit stories from their participants. Participants affirm their identities through narratives. Ricoeur (1984, 1991) also affirms the ability of human beings to integrate actions and thoughts into a coherent narrative and create a link between past, present and future. Narrators create and affirm their identities through telling their tale. Frank (1995: 61) notes that Ricoeur shows 'how the self only comes to be in the process of the life story being told'.

While sociologists such as Arthur Frank and Julius Roth and others have written portrayals of their own illness and told their own story, lay people such as journalists (for instance John Diamond (1998) and Ruth Picardie (1998)) also told of the process and progress of their condition.

Narratives in nursing research

Although the use of narratives for research purposes has gone on in an informal way for very long and has had its place in nursing and medical practice, it is relatively recent in nursing research (Frid *et al.*, 2000).

Narrative accounts in health care can be obtained from a number of different groups:

- Patients or clients
- Caregivers and relatives
- Colleagues and other professionals

Patients, for instance, might tell their experience of an illness or a chronic medical condition or of care and treatment by professionals. Narratives from the point of view of the patient can be seen in several ways. Ill people tell stories to show what it means to be sick. New mothers tell stories about the meaning of childbirth. Old people tell stories about the meaning of old age in the context of this society. Narratives can also be a reaction to nursing/midwifery care and medical treatment, or as a counterperspective to that of health professionals. Through narratives and narrative interpretations, patients and clients may also attempt to justify their own actions and behaviour. As long as patients tell their stories, they might feel that they have some control. In addition, they use these narratives to achieve an attempt at normality: they compare their ill selves to their normal social, physical and psychological condition.

Example

Wenneberg and Ahlström (2000) examined the lifetime illness narrative of the post-polio syndrome in 15 individuals who narrated the stages of their experience. The researchers showed that these people managed to restore normal work and family life. Wenneberg and Ahlström claim that through knowing the history of the participants' condition, nurses are better able to understand the needs of this group and improve their care.

McCance *et al.* (2001) use narrative methodology to explore caring in nursing practice. They use it as a means to 'tap into the patient experience'. It is not easy to gain access to people's feelings and thoughts but eliciting a narrative may help in this process. Telling stories about specific experiences rather than giving general accounts or thinking in general terms is 'real' for patients; they often tell the story sequentially along temporal dimensions. Greenhalgh and Hurwitz (1998: 45) claim that narratives used in healthcare research can:

- Set a patient-centred agenda
- Challenge received wisdom
- Generate new hypotheses

Through their stories, patients help health professionals to focus on their perceptions and experiences rather than applying a professional framework immediately. If professionals truly listen to patients, they might also hear the unexpected and will be able to change their own assumptions if necessary.

Relatives are narrators of their care-giving experience as it happened and seek explanations for their own behaviour, for the patient's reactions and for professional care and treatment. Through this they are able to justify their own thoughts and actions to professionals and researchers. Caregivers of patients with Alzheimer's disease, for instance, tell the sequence of events and discuss the behaviour of their relatives and their own reaction towards them. Essentially, caregivers attempt to share what caring means to them.

Researchers and health professionals use patient narrative to locate the sufferer at the centre of his or her illness. They see the narrative as a useful device in the understanding of sick people and the illness experience, as interpreted by patients in a specific cultural framework. Professionals – be they individual professionals in interaction with particular patients or professional groups who define specific conditions or illnesses within a biomedical framework – give different versions from patients. Both versions are valid and together might give the full picture. Sakalys (2000), in particular, addresses the question of culture in a discussion of narratives and claims that the social and cultural interpretation defines the illness experience and the sick role for the individual. Narratives also demonstrate the conflicts and dilemmas between individual meanings and healthcare ideologies.

In professional education and practice, narrators might tell the story of interaction in specific situations and of learning or teaching experiences. The researcher's aim is the understanding of the essence of that experience in the context of the participants' lives. Josselson (1995) claims that empathy and narrative show the way to people's reality, and understanding of this can only be achieved through qualitative research. Kleinman (1988) also urges 'empathic listening'. Nurses and midwives need both empathy for and stories from their clients. Nurse and midwife teachers often use narratives to teach students reflection and clinical decision making.

The role of narrative in nursing and midwifery research

Narratives develop and increase nursing and midwifery knowledge, and through the acquisition of knowledge they can improve care. Stories enable professionals to understand their clients and gain access to their experience and the interpretations of this experience. For clinical and professional practice it means 'the focus of narrative will enable nursing [and midwifery] knowledge to be grounded in concrete situations' (Frid *et al.*, 2000: 3). It is not easy for health professionals to abandon their own assumptions and focus on the stories of ill people. Frank (2000) gives examples of this. He refers to the difficulty for professionals in listening to the voice of patients to hear what is relevant to those who suffer, because professionals have more skills to respond to patients as 'medical subjects' rather than 'ill persons'.

Types of narrative and story

Jovchelovitch and Bauer (2000) list the two dimensions of narrative and story-telling: the chronological dimension where narratives are told in sequential form with a beginning, a middle and an end, and the non-chronological, which is a plot constructed as a coherent whole from a number of events – small tales which combine into a big story. It depends on the storyteller what he or she wishes to communicate to others or what to leave out of the story. People organise their experience through narratives and make sense of them, not least by relating them to time. Narratives allow access to a person's perceived reality in many different ways. Richardson (1990) describes many of these types of stories:

(1) Everyday stories
(2) Autobiographical stories
(3) Biographical stories
(4) Cultural stories
(5) Collective stories

Many narratives contain a number of overlapping stories. We shall illustrate these by examples (real, but not literal, comments):

The everyday story

In the everyday story, people tell how they did everyday things and carry out their normal tasks: '... And then I went out into the garden and did some work, and then I came inside and sat down.' Most patients import these everyday stories into the history of their condition, care and treatment. When researching people's experience in hospital, one of our students found that their narratives always tended to start well before they arrived. 'We were watching television, I had just made a cup of tea when it happened ... and then my wife called the ambulance, I could hardly walk, and then they went through the night with all lights blazing and a lot of noise.'

Autobiographical stories

In an autobiographical story people link the past to the present and future: 'I used to go dancing, but now I can't dance any more, I shall probably never dance again because of my pain.' Through autobiographical stories people also legitimate and explain their actions: 'Because I had such an awful pain in my back I could not have regular work.' In autobiographies in which individuals tell their illness history, they demonstrate that they see their own stories as unique and quite separate from those of others. The storyteller can link together various disparate events through narrative (Polkinghorne, 1995): '... And then I went into the garden, and I did some work, and then my back went ... and that's why I am unemployed now.'

Biographical stories

Biographical stories, however, link individuals with each other. Reading and listening to biographical stories enables them to share and compare their experiences. The stories guide beyond the subjective to intersubjective under-standing and empathy by living in a shared world. By writing accounts of others' stories, researchers help readers understand the feelings and vulnerability of others. An element of the autobiographical or biographical tale is the victory story in which individuals demonstrate how they overcame adversity by describing their feelings and actions (Sandelowski, 1996).

Cultural stories

Through the cultural story participants tell, they make visible and demonstrate meanings in a particular cultural context, for instance the meaning of death or the understanding of disease: 'I had epilepsy. In our society people don't understand that, and I was labelled as not quite normal.' Or 'My back pain is invisible, nobody believes that it exists, if I had a broken leg I would not be labelled lazy or work shy.' Or 'Everybody wants you to have the baby in hospital, in an earlier time, you could have it at home. Luckily times are changing again.' Wengraf (2001) also claims that narratologists focus on unconscious assumptions of individuals and cultural groups.

Collective stories

In research the collective story is significant. By retelling a number of stories, for instance of patients, professionals or students, researchers reflect the thoughts and paths of a group or collective of people with similar experiences and give a portrayal of a condition or patterns of experience. This creates a *Gestalt* or whole picture of the condition or experience. For nurses and mid-wives this means that they might recognise the needs of the group members and improve their care.

Illness narratives

Kleinman's *The Illness Narratives* (1988) is probably the best known example of narrative in the health and illness arena. Frank (1991) tells his own story of the illness from which he suffered. The most famous researcher into illness tales, of course, was Sigmund Freud who used his psychoanalysis on individual narratives and narrators.

Patients use narratives to seek meaning and make sense of their suffering, and they want to share this with 'significant' others. The researcher on the other hand, tells stories to give voice about participants' feelings and thoughts. It is questionable, however, that the account is always the authentic voice of the participants because researchers translate and interpret the narrators' tales. Sandelowski (1996: 122) criticises the naïve notions of stories as either true or false. Nevertheless, researchers make an attempt to represent the ideas of the participants. Although the narration may be true in its meaning, it is not always based on fact or objective reality but is a social construction and perception of what has happened to the narrator. At a time when people have little power to act – for instance when they have experienced an illness, breaking up of a relationship or another trauma in their lives – they attempt to explain this in a different language from that of those in power. To paraphrase Bruner (1991: 11): the patient tells the tale in 'life talk' (that is, in ordinary language) while the professional listens to it and translates it into professional language.

People often tell stories about their illness, particularly when the condition threatens their lives such as in an acute illness or when it restricts their daily activities and intrudes on normal life. Through illness and suffering, individuals often have an impaired sense of self. They are also used to telling the tale to doctors and nurses or other professionals, to their relatives and friends and their employers and work colleagues (Frank, 1995), and they adopt different ways of telling. Illness narratives differ from other stories in that they have an altered temporality; while in ordinary tales the present connects effortless to the past and future. The future of those telling about their illness is sometimes uncertain and occasionally nonexistent. Ruth Picardie (1998), for instance, knew that she had no future.

Frank (1995) proposes three different forms that narratives can take:

(1) The *restitution* narrative
(2) The *chaos* narrative
(3) The *quest* narrative

Frank's justification for differentiating between narratives is to create 'listening devices' – the wish to sort out narrative threads in order to help listeners attend these stories, not to question the uniqueness of an individual's tale nor to give a unifying view of experience. In any case, most stories combine elements of all three forms of narrative. Each of these forms is a reflection of both culture and the person of the storyteller.

The restitution narrative

The restitution narrative permeates the tale of those who have been ill. This includes the wish to get well soon. It can be connected with the concept of

Parsons' (1951) sick role. The person is sick – she receives treatment and care – it is seen as her duty to get better – she will be better in the future. People emphasise not only their desire to get better, but they often claim that they are well and have achieved the state of normality: 'I am OK now'. Most restitution tales reflect Parsons' ideas about the sick role: the person inhabiting the role is not at fault; the patient is exempt from normal role responsibilities; he or she is expected to ask for expert help, comply with the advice and make every attempt to get better.

Excerpt from restitution tale

My husband did all the housework
Because I couldn't
I had to leave my paid employment
I was in such pain
But I went to the doctor's
He told me not to stay in bed all the time
He prescribed some painkillers
And then it got better
Very slowly (paraphrased and condensed)

The restitution narrative reflects the predominant Western culture. Indeed, Frank claims that 'it is the culturally preferred narrative'. It takes the machine as a model: the machine breaks down, one takes it to a repair shop, and it is repaired. It is reconstructed, almost 'as good as new'. It also implies that people have control over their bodies and minds, and that the future is, to some extent, predictable.

The chaos narrative

The chaos narrative suggests that the person will not ever get well again and encompasses his or her suffering in words and silences. This tale is not always tolerated in the predominant culture that focuses on cure (the 'machine' can be fixed or repaired). Perhaps a chaos narrative is easier to listen to for nurses because they focus on care. It has no order and little structure, and it is told by people who have a serious chronic condition, or a life-threatening or terminal illness. This tale is more difficult to understand because it is never linear; it does not have a proper beginning, middle and end nor does it follow the same direction.

For the story to be effective, the storyteller must have some distance from it as the person in the middle of an experience finds it difficult to talk about it. There is iteration with narrators going backwards and forwards much of the time. The chaos narrative implies the narrators' lack of control over their lives. The illness generates complete 'biographical disruption'. Frank claims that health professionals should not hurry patients on when they are telling the tale as this denies the patients the right to their experience. He advises professionals to have tolerance for chaos within a story.

Excerpts from chaos narratives

I have no expectations for the future
I think I'll just carry on going
You don't feel your life is yours
It's controlled by other people

I can't see what my life
what my future is
       Both from Holloway *et al.*, 2000

The quest narrative

The quest narrative is told by people who are on a mission, who accept the challenge to learn something from their experience and feel that they are on a journey during which they change their identity. People think they must transmit to others what they have learned. They tell the story chronologically. Disability stories often contain the element of challenge and mission. We have all read of people with a serious illness who tell their story to the newspapers or on television 'to help others'. They often maintain that the illness has transformed them; the narrative has a moral dimension. Even though the condition may not improve, the ill person has control over his or her life.

Excerpt from a quest narrative

This has happened
I just get on with it
I was in control – then I wasn't
Now I am again!
It's all a learning experience
       Excerpt from Holloway *et al.*, 2000

Narrative interviewing

To obtain a narrative from participants, researchers use narrative interviews in which individuals can tell of their experience. The tale is not the experience itself but a representation of the experience as it is stored in the memory of the individual. Ochs and Capps (2002: 127) suggest 'remembering is a subjective event', but participants see it as true although it cannot necessarily be corroborated or verified. Nevertheless, the perception of the 'truth' of the event, treatment or care determines, or at least influences, both perception and action.

Narrative interviewing does not break a story into pieces and take it out of context, which other types of interview do; they 'often fracture the text' (Riessman, 1993: 3). Narrative interviewing has a main focus of deep interest to participant and researcher. This stimulus provides the trigger for the story. Riessman does stress that narratives differ distinctly from other types of discourse such as question and answer interviews.

Jovchelovitch and Bauer (2000) state that the topic area must not only be familiar but also experiential to the participant. The initial question must be broad enough to trigger a long story. For instance, 'Tell us about your time in hospital' might encourage patients into narrating a lengthy tale about what happened to them in the hospital setting. If the interviewer interrupts this story continually, it cannot flow. When the narrative is completed, however, the interviewer might ask some questions to develop the story by including the words of the participant. For instance: 'You said to me that time hung heavily while you were in hospital, can you tell me more about that?' Narrative interviews, like all other forms of interview, are affected by the relationship between the researcher and the participant, perhaps even more so as the researcher does not just ask questions to receive some answers but gives the participants control of the interview and as much time as they need to tell their story. Narrative interviews sometimes contain elements of question and answer exchange as well as sections of narrative. It is not always possible to draw boundaries and discover where the narrative starts and finishes.

Narrative interviews often focus on life histories or life stories as they show development of experience and perspective over time. For instance, Paris and Bradley (2001), in their narrative approach to women who were alcoholic, show that alcohol misuse and rehabilitation processes are linked to experiences and developmental stages. These processes are also closely connected to the identities of the participants.

Problematic issues

The narratives of people and the storytelling by the researcher can be problematic. On the one hand, Lieblich *et al.* (1998) state that narratives are often seen more as art than as science because they are rooted in intuition and experience. On the other, they argue for a structured and coherent approach to storytelling. Koch (1998), also asks the question whether the researcher's storytelling is science or not.

Atkinson (1997), highlights three major issues:

(1) Narratives of health and illness play an important part in medical sociology and anthropology (and, we would add, in nursing and midwifery)
(2) Sometimes these narratives are based on inappropriate assumptions and on mistaken methodological and theoretical claims
(3) Narrative analyses must be systematic and should not be seen as single solutions to problems

Atkinson criticises the unexamined assumptions that underlie these narratives in which researchers take a simplistic view of this form of research; the link between narratives and experiences is complex and they should not be seen as individualistic and romantic constructions of self but located within the context of interaction and social action. They are no more 'authentic' (a favourite word of narrative researchers), he claims, than other forms of research. Readers of narratives need 'thick description' of socio-cultural settings in which the narratives are embedded.

Frank (2000) answers Atkinson by explaining some of the issues important in narrative. He makes five major points.

(1) He suggests that, although narrative and story are used interchangeably, people tell stories, they are not telling narratives. Narratives contain structures on which stories are based. Storytellers use these but are not fully aware of them.
(2) People share their stories with the listener, and through this sharing of the story the listener becomes part of a relationship in which the story is told.
(3) Stories create distance between storytellers and the threats they experience. They do perform the 'recuperative role' that Atkinson attributes to them.
(4) Stories are not just the data for analysis to be transformed into text. They affirm the purpose of the story, namely forming relationships.
(5) The stories of illness need to be heard. Frank (2000: 355) refutes 'Atkinson's dichotomy' between storytelling and story analysis; he maintains that 'any good story analysis accepts its place in relations of storytelling' and researchers can only listen inside a relationship with ethical and intellectual responsibilities.

Ultimately Frank sees storytelling in a different way from Atkinson. Frank (2000: 355) states emphatically: 'Storytellers do not call for their narratives to be analysed; they call for other stories in which experiences are shared, commonalities discovered and relationships built'.

The debate about the purpose of narrative and story-telling goes on. Regardless of the stance of nurse and midwifery researchers, they should be aware of the ongoing debate.

Narrative analysis

This whole chapter is about narrative analysis and what it implies. Riessman (1993) does not acknowledge a 'standard set of procedures' for analysing the data. The actual data analysis of narratives is similar to that in other types of qualitative research and depends on the methodological framework, be it phenomenology, ethnography or other types of approach. Polkinghorne (1995: 15) defines narrative analysis as 'the procedure through which the researcher organizes the data elements as into a coherent and developmental account'. The main steps include data transcription and reduction. The first step is the verbatim transcription of the narrative data (see the section on Transcribing and sorting, in Chapter 15).

There are different approaches to analysing narrative data which we will call holistic and sequential analysis.

Holistic analysis

The researcher analyses a narrative as a whole. In this type of analysis it is important to identify the main statements – the core of the experience that reflects and truly represents the narrators' accounts, even though they might not have given the story in a sequential and ordered way. The units of text in the transcription are reduced to a series of core sentences or ideas. The core statements of the experience integrate its various elements. This essence of experience is highly auditable in the examples below.

Statement of some participants in a pain experience study

Your life is pain
It stops you doing?
Going out
Just trying to be a normal person

I don't feel like doing anything
All you want to do is to dwell on your own suffering

Pain becomes an obstacle
To any type of performance

The essence of these statements and the core of the experience is that 'the pain takes over'. Other themes can be linked to this statement. Exhaustive description is used in phenomenological narrative (see Chapter 11).

Sequential analysis

The researcher can instead code and categorise the text starting with breaking it down and coding it. Codes are collapsed into key concepts or categories. Similar categories are linked and clustered into themes. Coding can also be done in phrases. Themes developed from the narrative of one individual are compared to those emerging from other narratives and an overall pattern emerges from which the researcher constructs a coherent story of the participants' experiences (see Chapter 15).

Conclusion

Sparkes (1994) demonstrates that the research 'product' is not just the participants' story but a presentation and articulation of their ideas. It includes an interpretation by the researcher. Although researchers interpret and edit the thoughts and ideas of the participants, 'even edited stories remain true' (Frank, 1995: 22). The 'good' research report entails collaboration between researcher and participant. The narrators, the researcher and the readers of the final account together construct the whole story of all participants. The social and cultural world of the narrators is not simple, however, but complex and always influences the story. This means that narratives are not the only way to gain access to this socially constructed reality.

Summary

Narratives are tales of experience.

- Narratives are rarely simple or linear, and they consist of many different stories
- Illness narratives are expressions of illness, suffering and pain
- Health professionals gain knowledge of the illness experience from their patients which assists in understanding the condition and the person
- The analysis of narrative data depends on the research methodology used
- In narrative inquiry the final story is constructed by participant, researcher and reader
- Illness and professional narratives must be located in the socio-cultural context

References

Atkinson, P.A. (1997) Narrative turn or blind alley? *Qualitative Health Research*, **7** (3) 325–44.

Bailey, P.H. (1996) Assuring quality in narrative analysis. *Western Journal of Nursing Research*, **18** (2) 186–94.

Bruner, J. (1991) The narrative construction of reality. *Critical Inquiry*, **18**, 1–21.

Cortazzi, M. (1993) *Narrative Analysis*. London, The Falmer Press.

Diamond, J. (1998) C: *Because Cowards Get Cancer Too*. London, Vermilion Press.

Fagermoen, M.S. (1997) Professional identity: values embedded in meaningful practice. *Journal of Advanced Nursing*, **25**, 434–41.

Frank, A.W. (1991) *At the Will of the Body: Reflections on Illness*. Boston, Houghton Mifflin.

Frank, A.W. (1995) *The Wounded Storyteller: Body, Illness, and Ethics*. Chicago, University of Chicago Press.

Frank, A.W. (2000) The standpoint of storyteller. *Qualitative Health Research*, **10** (3) 354–65.

Frid, I., Öhlen, J. & Bergbom, I. (2000) On the use of narratives in nursing research. *Journal of Advanced Nursing*, **32** (3) 695–703.

Greenhalgh, T. & Hurwitz, B. (1998) Why study narrative? In *Narrative Based Medicine* (eds T. Greenhalgh & B. Hurwitz), pp. 3–16. London, BMJ Books.

Hatch, J.A. & Wisniewski, R. (eds) (1995) *Life History and Narrative*. London, The Falmer Press.

Holloway, I., Sofaer, B. & Walker, J. (2000) The transition from well person to 'pain afflicted' patient: the career of people with chronic back pain. *Illness, Crisis and Loss*, **8** (4) 373–87.

Josselson, R. (1995) Imagining the real: empathy, narrative and the dialogic self. In *Interpreting Experience: The Narrative Study of Lives* (eds R. Josselson & A. Lieblich), pp. 27–44. Thousand Oaks, Sage.

Josselson, R. & Lieblich, A. (eds) (1999) *Making Meaning of Narratives*. Thousand Oaks, Sage.

Jovchelovitch, S. & Bauer, M.W. (2000) Narrative interviewing. In *Qualitative Interviewing with Text, Image and Sound* (eds M.W. Bauer & G. Gaskell), pp. 57–74. London, Sage.

Kleinman, A. (1988) *The Illness Narratives: Suffering, Healing and the Human Condition*. New York, Basic Books.

Koch, T. (1998) Storytelling: is it really research? *Journal of Advanced Nursing*, **28** (6) 1182–90.

Labov, W. (1972) The transformation of experience in narrative syntax. In *Language in the Inner City* (ed. W. Labov), pp. 354–96. Philadelphia, University of Pennsylvania Press.

Lieblich, A., Tuval-Mashiach, R. & Zilber, T. (eds) (1998) *Narrative Research: Reading, Analysis and Interpretation*. Thousand Oaks, Sage.

McCance, T.V., McKenna, H.P. & Boore, J.R.P. (2001) Exploring caring using narrative methodology: an analysis of the approach. *Journal of Advanced Nursing*, **33** (3) 350–56.

Mitchell, R.G. & Charmaz, K. (1996) Telling tales, writing stories. *Journal of Contemporary Ethnography*, **25** (1) 144–66.

Ochs, E. & Capps, L. (2002) Narrative authenticity. In *Qualitative Research Methods* (ed. D. Weinberg), pp. 127–32. Malden, Mass, Blackwell.

Paris, R. & Bradley, C.L. (2001) The challenge of adversity: Three narratives of alcohol dependence, recovery and adult development. *Qualitative Health Research*, **11** (5) 647–67.

Parsons, T. (1951) *The Social System*. New York, Free Press.

Picardie, R. (1998) *Before I Say Goodbye*. Harmondsworth, Penguin.

Polkinghorne, D.E. (1995) Narrative configuration in qualitative analysis. In *Life History and Narrative* (eds J.A. Hatch & R. Wisniewski), pp. 5–23. London, The Falmer Press.

Richardson, L. (1990) Narrative and sociology. *Journal of Contemporary Ethnography*, **19** (1) 116–35.

Ricoeur, P. (1984) *Time and Narrative*, Vol. 1. Chicago, Chicago University Press.

Ricoeur, P. (1991) *Time and Narrative*, Vol. 2. Chicago, Chicago University Press.

Riessman, C.K. (1993) *Narrative Analysis*. Newbury Park, Sage.

Sakalys, J.A. (2000) The political role of illness narratives. *Journal of Advanced Nursing*, **31** (6) 1469–75.

Sandelowski, M. (1991) Telling stories: narrative approaches in qualitative research. *Image*, **23** (3) 161–6.

Sandelowski, M. (1996) Truth/storytelling in nursing inquiry. In *Truth in Nursing Inquiry* (eds J.F. Kikuchi, H. Simmons & D. Romyn), pp. 111–24. Thousand Oaks, Sage.

Skultans, V. (1998) Anthropology and narrative. In *Narrative Based Medicine* (eds T. Greenhalgh & B. Hurwitz), pp. 225–33. London, BMJ Books.

Sparkes, A. (1994) Life histories and the issue of voice: reflections on an emerging relationship. *Qualitative Studies in Education*, **7** (2) 165–83.

Sparkes, A. (1996) The fatal flaw: a narrative of the fragile body-self. *Qualitative Inquiry*, **2** (4) 463–94.

Sparkes, A. (1998) Athletic identity: an Achilles heel to the survival of self. *Qualitative Health Research*, **8** (5) 644–64.

Sparkes, A. (1999) Exploring body narratives. *Sport, Education and Society*, **4** (1) 17–30.

Wengraf, T. (2001) *Qualitative Interviewing: Biographic Narrative and Semi-Structured Methods*. London, Sage.

Wenneberg, S. & Ahlström, G. (2000) Illness narratives of persons with post-polio syndrome. *Journal of Advanced Nursing*, **31** (2) 354–61.

CHAPTER 14

Additional Approaches

Feminist research

Feminist inquiry is research that focuses on the experience, ideas and feelings of women in their social and historical context. Researchers adopt a gender perspective to the phenomenon under investigation. Feminist approaches do not prescribe methods of analysing research but suggest ways of thinking about it. The intention is to make women visible, raise their consciousness and empower them. As Oleson (2000) states: 'It is research *for* rather than *about* women'. Because qualitative research has affinity with the ideas of feminists, it is used more often than quantitative approaches (although feminist researchers also see the latter as valid).

Feminist research is important for nurses and midwives, as they are still mainly female professions. We refrain from giving a great deal of space to this standpoint because it is not a specific approach to qualitative research although it more often adopts qualitative than quantitative methods (this does not detract from its importance). Some feminists believe in a separate and distinctive feminist research methodology, and that this type of inquiry is not merely a variation or branch of qualitative research (Stanley and Wise, 1993). Many researchers maintain (for instance Harding, 1987) that a distinctive feminist method does not exist, but that feminist researchers address certain epistemological and methodological issues related to gender. One major element of feminist research is critical theory. Feminist researchers often see women as an oppressed group controlled by the media, the political and economic systems and ultimately by men. Feminists believe that women are economically exploited and suffer social discrimination. Hearing the voices of women and raising their consciousness through research may therefore assist in overcoming inequalities.

The most common form of feminist research is the narrative or life history, because it gives women the chance to tell their own stories in their own way, 'letting the women speak'. Feminist research and cooperative inquiry share many of their most important features such as complete equality between researcher and participant and a democratic non-judgemental stance (though one might say this about all qualitative research).

The feminist approach to research gives women the opportunity to voice their concerns and interests, and is not merely concerned with the technical details of data analysis. The latter depends on the field in which researchers work and on the specific research question, although methods, too, reflect the feminist principles of equality between researcher and participant and focus on women's experiences and their empowerment. Taking into account the requirements of feminist research, researchers use grounded theory, ethnography and other types of data analysis. The focus on the 'lived experience' and the affective elements in the participants' lives mean that phenomenological approaches are often taken in feminist qualitative research.

The term 'feminist standpoint research' is used. It is a less specific term than feminist methodology and carries with it the implication that feminist research uses a specific type of analysis. Feminist standpoint researchers recognise that their view of the world is distinctive and different. There should be a fit, they suggest, between the worldview of feminism and the methods adopted for research.

The origins of feminist methodology

Feminist methodology has its roots in feminist theory. Writers such as Millett (1969), Mitchell (1971) and Oakley (1972) as well as others, particularly in the US and Britain, were the pioneers who helped to direct the focus on women's interests and ideas. Early feminist writers in the professions in Britain include Stanley and Wise (1993) in social work and Webb (1984) in nursing.

A number of major issues emerge in thinking and doing research within a feminist methodological framework. Initially feminist research was a reaction against positivist research and traditional strategies which were seen as male-dominated and androcentric. Problems in the lives of women had been discussed in the light of male experience and the interest of men promoted and those of women subordinated (Lennon and Whitford, 1994). Feminist writers used consciousness-raising as a methodological tool to empower women. It also becomes a tool for narrowing the distance between researchers and participants by generating reciprocity and collaboration. This affects all participants and gives individuals – including researchers – a sense of their identity. Women, so feminists believe, become aware of their position through the research process and relationships, they aim to change their situation and become more powerful.

Feminist researchers emphasise an alternative social reality and value women's lives and experience. Researchers intend to contribute to the improvement of the lives of women who will learn to control their own lives through this. Feminists are concerned with the importance of women's lives and their position in the social structure. They claim that unequal relations are not only embedded in the structure of society but have taken part in the construction of social relationships.

Travers (2001) claims that feminism has been one of the most important movements in the late twentieth century. The aversion to 'male-stream' research which was often seen as embodied in positivism has helped feminist researchers to value qualitative research though they do not use it exclusively; indeed Oakley (2000) stresses the importance of 'scientific' quantitative research.

Feminist thought and methodology

Even before feminism, disenchantment with natural scientific methods had emerged which led to a critique of positivism. Researchers who took the approach of natural science believed that objectivity was possible, that to use the scientific method was the best way to examine social reality and would be neutral and objective. Feminists question the notion of value-neutral research and agree with other qualitative researchers who react against the positivist and neo-positivist approach.

Traditional research is also described as male-dominated (Westkott, 1990). Feminist critics of this approach maintain that it is often stripped of its context while questions and answers are predefined and controlled by researchers who, whilst claiming objectivity, impose their own subjective framework. Feminists believe that researchers cannot achieve complete objectivity. They can only state their bias or assumptions and demonstrate the value bases from which they come; that is, they are reflexive. They criticise the differentiation between the objective and subjective and put an emphasis on the relationships and realities of everyday life through which social structures can be understood.

Women explain their social reality in personal accounts of their lives, and these accounts emerge from their shared experiences. The researcher listens to these accounts and, while interpreting them, gives a faithful picture of the personal histories and biographies of women. Feminist research aims to raise the consciousness of people in general and of the women participants specifically. Consciousness of their reality can guide women to an understanding and helps them to change their lives and empower them. Research makes emotions, personal values and the thoughts of participants legitimate topics of research.

The relationship between researchers and women participants

The research relationship follows that of other types of qualitative research but collaboration and equality between the researcher and women participants is stressed even more. Empathy with women may be easier to achieve by female researchers because of their gender (though feminists do not claim that men cannot have empathy, nor that research supports a woman's perspective just because it is done by a woman). The personal experience and values of the researcher become important in feminist research. Feminists often describe and integrate their own feelings while recounting and analysing women's experiences, pains and passions. Sometimes they study women's conditions or problems that they have experienced in their own lives. Feminist qualitative research allows for interactive interviewing where participants can ask professional as well as personal questions.

There are considerable variations in feminist research that we do not intend to discuss here. New books on feminist research appear every year. We believe, however, that this can be a useful perspective in nursing and midwifery, where women are still presently in the majority.

Case studies

The term 'case study' is used for a variety of research approaches, both qualitative and quantitative. Stake (2000) states that much qualitative research is case study research but argues that case study research is very specific, 'a bounded system' and both a process as well as a product of the inquiry. A case study is an entity studied as a single unit, and it has clear boundaries and a specific focus. Merriam (1988: 9) defines it as 'An examination of a specific phenomenon, such as a program, an event, a person, a process, an institution, or a social group'. The boundaries of the case should be clarified in terms of the questions asked, the data sources used and the setting and person(s) involved. Although different authors have their own definitions and ideas about the nature of the case study, they also agree on many issues (Platt, 1988).

Case studies can be quantitative, qualitative or both, but we shall summarise here the main features of the qualitative case study which tends to be more common in nursing research. It is often combined with action research (Webb, 1989).

Background

The case study is used in a number of disciplines such as anthropology, sociology or geography, though not all studies of limited cases are case studies. It has been most popular in business studies, but is also used in social work and nursing.

The best known writer on this type of research, Robert Yin, has discussed case studies in a number of books and articles (for example, Yin, 1993, 1994). Although his writing, on the whole, focuses on the quantitative framework, he sees the qualitative approach as valid.

Example of case study

One of the most famous early case studies is that of Whyte (1943) in which he studied a neighbourhood gang in Chicago. Other researchers who used ideas from this study found that it was a 'typical case', meaning that theories emerging from this work could be applied to their research.

Features and purpose of case study research

Generally nurse researchers who develop case studies are familiar with the case they study and its context before the start of the research. Nurses study cases because they may be interested in it for professional reasons or because they need the knowledge about the particular case.

As in other types of qualitative research, the case study is a way of exploring the phenomenon or phenomena in their context. The researchers therefore use a number of sources in their data collection, for instance observation, documentary sources and interviews so that the case can be illuminated from all sides. Observation and documentary research are the most common strategies used in case study research. It does not have specific methods for data collection or analysis; for instance, the researcher can apply ethnographic or phenomenological approaches. The analysis of qualitative case studies involves the same techniques as that of other qualitative methods: the researcher categorises, develops typologies and generates theoretical ideas.

Studies focus on individuals such as a patient or a group which might consist of individuals with common experiences or characteristics, a ward or a hospital. Life histories of individuals would also be interesting examples of cases.

Examples

In the community, a researcher might shadow District Nurses throughout the day and explore their interaction with a specific group such as patients with leg ulcers.

In a children's ward, the nurse researcher could explore all specialist nurses' work and their interaction with children at the time of the doctor's round.

In nursing studies with a psychological emphasis, cases often focus on individuals and an aspect of their behaviour, while the nurse sociologist is more interested in groups. Kent (1992) sees an institution as a case. She examined multiple cases, organisations which provided midwifery education. Her 'case' focused on both the physical and social elements in the setting.

As in other qualitative research, case studies explore the phenomenon or phenomena under study in their context, indeed Platt (1988) states that case studies are holistic and contextual. The lines of division between the phenomena and the context, however, are not always clear (Yin, 1994).

Case studies can be exploratory devices, for instance as a pilot for a larger study or for more quantitative research, and they could also illustrate the specific elements of a research project. One of our students demonstrated all the ideas she obtained from informants by writing up the case of one single participant. Usually the case study stands on its own and involves intensive observation. The description of specific cases can make a study more lively and interesting.

Case study research is used mainly to investigate cases that are tied to a specific situation and locality, and hence this type of inquiry is even less readily generalisable than other qualitative research. Therefore researchers are often advised to study 'typical' and multiple cases (Stake, 1995). Atypical cases may, however, sometimes be interesting because their very difference might illustrate the typical case. It is important though that the researcher does not make unwarranted assertions on the basis of a single case.

Meier and Pugh (1986) argue that clinical knowledge improves through focusing on individual cases that nurses collect, be they about responses of the individual to illness or to treatment and interventions. Meier and Pugh stress the importance of a detailed decision trail so that other cases can be studied in the light of the findings of a single case.

Critical incident technique

The critical incident technique is a type of data collection designed to solve problems in practice or educational settings. In the past, it was not often used in the health arena, but recently it has been seen as appropriate for nurses. Midwives would also find it useful. It is not a methodology but a means of developing questions, focusing on people's behaviour in critical situations in order to solve problems in task performance. A critical incident is an observed event that is perceived as particularly significant. Researchers examine those events that are significant for a particular process. They collect examples of critical incidents in the situation under study, and participants give an account of the way in which they act in critical situations or times of crisis.

Flanagan (1954) suggests that, to be critical, an incident has to occur in a situation with definite consequences and effects. Generally researchers ask about the critical event and gain a perspective on effective and ineffective behaviour in specific decisive and important situations.

The critical incident technique was initially developed as a result of the Aviation Psychology Program in the United States to collect information from pilots about their behaviour when flying a mission. In particular, the psychologists asked for reports about critical incidents that helped or hindered the successful outcome of the mission. Through analysis of these reports, a list of components for successful performance was generated from the data.

Flanagan (1954) developed and refined the procedure for industrial psychology to assess the outcomes of task performance, in personnel selection and in identifying motivation and factors in effective counselling (Woolsey, 1986). Although the method was neglected after the 1950s, it can be a useful, effective and qualitative approach to studying critical events in order to improve task performance and is thus very useful for the health professions. Flanagan (1954: 335) states that the technique is 'a procedure for gathering certain important facts concerning behaviour in defined situations'.

Woolsey (1986) lists four stages in the process of critical incident technique. Cormack (2000) mentions six. The stages of both authors overlap:

(1) The researchers decide on the aim of the research
(2) They design and plan the research
(3) The data are collected
(4) The data are analysed

It can be seen that this type of inquiry follows the traditional path of data collection and analysis in qualitative research.

The critical incident approach is very useful and relevant in particular for research in the professional arena of nurses and midwives. Cormack (2000) quotes several examples for nursing. It is a type of data collection that focuses on people's behaviour in critical situations in order to solve problems in task performance. Researchers examine those events that are significant for a particular process. They collect examples of critical incidents in the situation under study, and participants give an account of the way in which they act in critical situations or times of crisis. Generally the researchers ask about the critical event and gain a perspective about effective and ineffective behaviour in specific decisive and important situations.

The process of critical incident technique

The first step consists of stating a clear aim. The aim of the technique is to obtain information about each specific incident. This will include choosing the type of events on which researchers wish to focus, generally critical events or incidents in care or educational settings. The second stage involves selecting a purposive sample of incidents and people from which to collect data. The sample size depends on the number of critical incidents, not on the number of people interviewed or observed (Kemppainen, 2000). Generally researchers find out about critical incidents through incidental and casual observation, or they collect data through focused or semi-structured interviews and reports. The data are analysed in a similar way as other qualitative data. There is however, a slight difference: researchers choose a more defined frame of reference in this type of research as they wish to focus on particular events.

Example

An accident has happened on a ward for elderly people in spite of the many precautions taken. The researcher observes for similar occurrences and interviews the patients involved and the nurses who saw or dealt with these accidents. From this and other nurses' and patients' observations the researcher describes the events that led to the accident, the way nurses dealt with these accidents and the effects of the behaviour on all those involved.

The aim of the researcher is to investigate a recurring problem and to find a solution to it. To examine the critical incidents, the nurse or midwife has to be familiar with the setting and the nursing or midwifery tasks that are performed. Kemppainen (2000) claims that the responses of the participants to the researcher's questions must be specific and accurate and not vague or unclear. Direct observation is also part of the technique.

Conversation analysis

Within the great variety of qualitative methods, some emphasise language and language use. Any professional–client interaction relies on the use of language as a major communication device. Conversation(al) analysis (CA) is a form of discourse analysis that examines the use of language and asks the question of how everyday conversation works (Nunan, 1993). This type of inquiry focuses on ordinary conversations and on the way in which talk is organised and ordered in speech exchanges. While researchers primarily examine speech patterns, they also analyse non-verbal behaviour in interaction such as mime, gesture and other body language. As Nofsinger (1991:2) explains: 'If we are to understand interpersonal communication, we need to learn how this is accomplished so successfully'.

The origins of conversation analysis

Harold Garfinkel, Harvey Sacks, Emmanuel Schegloff and others initially developed CA in the 1960s and 1970s in the United States. While other types of discourse analysis have their roots in the field of linguistics, CA originates in ethnomethodology, a specialist direction of sociology and phenomenology. Ethnomethodology focuses in particular on the world of social practices, interactions and rules (see Turner, 1974). Garfinkel attempted to uncover the ways in which members of society construct social reality. Ethnomethodologists focus on the 'practical accomplishments' of members of society, seeking to demonstrate that these make sense of their actions on the basis of 'tacit knowledge', their shared understanding of the rules of interaction. Goodwin and Heritage (1990: 283) summarise this: 'Through processes of social interaction, shared meaning, mutual understanding and the coordination of human conduct are achieved'.

The use of conversation analysis

Conversation analysis focuses on what individuals say in their everyday talk, but also on what they do (Nofsinger, 1991). Through conversation, movement and gesture, we learn of people's intentions and ideas. The sequencing and turn taking in conversations demonstrate the meaning individuals give to situations and show

how they inhabit a shared world. Body movements too, are the focus of analysis. Conversation analysts do not use interviewing to collect data but analyse ordinary talk, 'naturally occurring' conversations. Most sections of talk analysed are relatively small, and the analysis is detailed. According to Heritage (1988: 130), CA makes the assumptions that talk is structurally organised, and each turn of talk is influenced by the context of what has gone on before and establishes a context towards which the next turn will be oriented. There are two other fundamental tenets of CA according to Heritage: sequential organisation and empirical grounding of analysis. Talk happens in organised patterns, the action of the member who takes part in the conversation is dependent on and makes reference to the context, and researchers should avoid generalities and premature theory building (Silverman, 2001).

Conversation analysis is more often used in sociological or education studies rather than in nursing. We think, however, that it could contribute a valuable research approach in nursing and lead to changes in the interaction between nurses and patients or other health professionals. Researchers generally audio or videotape these interactions and transcribe the conversations in a particular way (see transcription techniques in Nofsinger, 1991 or, in more detail, in Button and Lee, 1987) largely developed by Gail Jefferson.

Example of CA

A good example for the use of CA is given by Couchman (1995) who used a piece of action research to train staff working with people who have learning difficulties. Videotaping staff and clients in day centres, she found that staff had underestimated the responsiveness of clients and did not always notice their readiness for interaction. When shown the tapes staff became more aware of clients' needs and responded quickly.

There are examples in nursing of doctor–patient or nurse–patient interaction which show how talk is generated and organised by the participants and follows an orderly process in which a turn-taking system exists (Sharrock and Anderson, 1987; Bergstrom et al., 1992). Tapes show what actually takes place in a setting.

Example

Mallett (1990) explored the interaction between nurses and post-anaesthetic patients. She videotaped dental patients post-operatively. Verbal and non-verbal communication was observed. Mallett found that nurses varied in the ways in which they engaged with patients, depending on their needs and level of consciousness. She highlighted some of the difficulties in the situation and indicated how the analysis of nurse–patient interactions could illustrate potential problems and could be used as a teaching aid for novices.

The analysis of CA includes the discovery of regularities in speech or body movement, the search for deviant cases and the integration with other findings without over-generalisation (Heritage, 1988). One of the disadvantages is the way in which conversation analysts emphasise the formal characteristics of interaction at the expense of content, but they do focus on the dynamic aspects in which interaction takes place (Leudar & Antaki, 1988).

Conversation analysis is difficult, highly complex and very detailed. Researchers may not find it easy, and we do not recommend it to novice researchers.

Discourse analysis

Gill (2000) suggests that the term 'discourse' is complex, as people use it in different ways. Some of these are discussed here but not elaborated in detail. Discourse in general is applied to talk and text, such as conversations, interviews or documents.

Discourse analysis (DA) in psychology is an analysis of text and language drawing on 'accounts' of experiences and thoughts that participants present. This type of discourse analysis has been carried out mainly by psychologists. Accounts consist of forms of ordinary talk and reasoning of people, as well as other sources of text, such as historical documents, diaries, letters or reports. Discourse analysis is not only a method but also a specific approach to the social world and research (Potter, 1996a). It focuses on the construction of talk in social action. In common with other types of qualitative inquiry, discourse analysts initially use an inductionist approach by collecting and reviewing data before arriving at theories and general principles. The way people use language and text is taken for granted within a culture (Gill, 1996). Discourse analysis as the structural analysis of discourse, is often used in media and communication research (Van Dijk, 1985) to analyse 'message data'. An example would be an analysis of the speeches of politicians. Language itself, and reality are socially constructed. Potter (1997) and Silverman (2001) suggest that early DA identified 'discourses' in which participants attempt to define themselves and their moral status. The vocabularies which individuals and groups use are located in interpretive 'repertoires' that are coherent and related sets of terms.

It is important to read the documents and transcripts carefully before interpreting them. The first step in the analysis is a verbatim transcription of the interview and a close look at other documents. The relevant documents are read and re-read until researchers have become familiar with the data. Immersion in the data, after all, is a trait of all qualitative research. Important issues and themes can then be highlighted. The analysis proceeds like other qualitative research: analysts code the data, look for relationships and search for patterns and regularities that generate tentative hypotheses. Through the process, they always take the context into account and generate analytical notes as in other forms of qualitative inquiry.

Like other qualitative research, the findings from discourse analysis are not instantly generalisable; indeed researchers are not overly concerned with generalisability, because the analysis is based on language and text in a specific social context. There are a number of similarities between conversation analysis and discourse analysis: both CA and DA focus on language and text. While discourse analysis generally considers the broader context, CA emphasises turn-taking and explains the deeper sense of interaction in which people are engaged, particularly 'naturally occurring' talk, while discourse analysts look mainly at interview material, although they can also use records, newspaper articles or reports of meetings, etc.

Discourse analysts are interested in the ways through which social reality is constructed in interaction and action. DA is based on the belief that language does not just mirror the world of social members and cultures but also helps to construct it. Indeed there is not just one but many 'languages' (Banister *et al.*, 1994). In Potter and Wetherell (1987) and Potter (1996b: 130, 131), there is developed the notion of 'interpretative repertoires' which they see as a set of related concepts 'organised around one or more central metaphors'. These provide researchers with commonsense concepts of a group or a culture. Language is 'action oriented': it is used so people can 'do'. It is shaped by the cultural and social context in which it occurs. Social groups possess a variety of repertoires and use them appropriately in different situations. The integrated discourses of people about various specific areas in their lives generate a text (Banister *et al.*, 1994). Discourse analysts must therefore be aware of the context in which action takes place so that the context can be analysed as well. The same text can be interpreted in different ways: different versions of reality exist in different contexts. The discourse analysis of psychologists and linguists focuses on text. Readers can make judgements about this type of research because they themselves possess knowledge of everyday discourse and its construction.

McHoul and Grace (1995) differentiate between Foucauldian and non-Foucauldian discourse. Michel Foucault, the French historian and philosopher, made the concept of discourse famous while describing the links of language with disciplines and institutions. For him, discourses are bodies of knowledge, by which he means both academic scholarship and institutions, which exist in disciplines. Indeed, he claims that discourse reproduces institutions. Social phenomena are constructed through language. Specific language is connected with specialist fields, for instance 'professional discourse', 'scientific discourse' or 'medical discourse'. In Foucault's works, discourses as specialist languages are linked to power. Discourse analysis discovers the language that operates within the particular discourse under study. For instance, professionals use particular types of discourse to impose their own or the official version of reality on their clients.

Other approaches

The approaches mentioned above are not exclusive; other styles of qualitative research do, of course, exist, but they are less common in nursing. *Historical research* is used frequently and *repertory grid methods* are occasionally adopted, the latter particularly in nurse education.

Historical research can be qualitative; it often starts without firm assumptions and preconceived ideas. Researchers might, for instance, study a particular era in history or attempt to find out how a particular condition was treated or perceived by society over time.

Historical research generally means analysing contemporary texts and documentary sources and books by experts who discuss the period of history or the condition under study. Newspapers and archives too, supply useful information. Primary sources provide the best data and first-hand accounts (Fitzpatrick, 1993); they have not undergone the same process of interpretation, although the originator, too, has influenced what is written. Often the researcher attempts to develop a comparison between past and present. It is useful in nursing to apply the insights gained through studying the past.

The psychology of personal constructs, or the repertory grid technique is sometimes seen as qualitative. George Kelly, a psychologist, was the originator and developer of this approach (Kelly, 1955, 1986). The emphasis is on the idea of 'man [*sic*] the scientist', that is, individuals themselves give meaning to their action and make sense of the world, and on this basis they predict that something will or will not happen. Kelly argues that people are unique in building a framework of constructs on the dimensions of similarity and differences. This approach has been used especially in nurse education, psychiatric nursing and clinical psychology (Rawlinson, 1995; Banister *et al.*, 1994).

Conclusion

This chapter gives an overview of some qualitative research methods such as case study research that can be both qualitative and quantitative but are often adopted by nurse and midwife researchers. Conversation and discourse analysis are used rarely in the disciplines. Historical approaches and personal construct methods are more often seen as positivist approaches but are sometimes used or seen as qualitative research.

References

Feminist research

Harding, S. (ed.) (1987) Introduction. In *Feminism and Methodology*, pp. 1–14. Bloomington, Indiana Press.

Lennon, K. & Whitford, M. (1994) Introduction. In *Knowing the Difference: Feminist Perspectives in Epistemology* (eds K. Lennon & M. Whitford), pp. 1–9. London, Routledge.

Millett, K. (1969) *Sexual Politics*. London, Abacus.

Mitchell, J. (1971) *Women's Estate*. Harmondsworth, Penguin.

Oakley, A. (1972) *Sex, Gender and Society*. London, Temple Smith.

Oakley, A. (2000) *Experiments in Knowing: Gender and Method in the Social Sciences*. Cambridge, Polity Press.

Oleson, V. (2000) Feminisms and qualitative research at and into the millennium. In *Handbook of Qualitative Research* (eds N.K. Denzin and Y.S. Lincoln), 2nd edn, pp. 215–55. Thousand Oaks, Sage.

Stanley, L. & Wise, S. (1993) *Breaking Out Again*. London, Routledge.

Travers, M. (2001) *Qualitative Research through Case Studies*. London, Sage.

Webb, C. (1984) Feminist methodology in nursing research. *Journal of Advanced Nursing*, **9**, 249–56.

Westkott, M. (1990) Feminist criticism of the social sciences. In *Feminist Research Methods: Exemplary Readings in the Social Sciences* (ed. J.M. Nielsen), pp. 58–68. London, Westview Press.

Case studies

Kent, J. (1992) An evaluation of pre-registration midwifery education in England. *Midwifery*, **8**, 69–75.

Meier, P. & Pugh, E.J. (1986) The case study: a viable approach to clinical research. *Research in Nursing and Health*, **9**, 195–202.

Merriam, S.J. (1988) *Case Study Research in Education*. San Francisco, Jossey-Bass.

Platt, J. (1988) What can case studies do? *Studies in Qualitative Methodology*, **1**, 2–23.

Stake, R.E. (1995) *The Art of Case Study Research*. Thousand Oaks, Sage.

Stake, R.E. (2000) Case studies. In *The Handbook of Qualitative Research* (eds N.K. Denzin & Y.S. Lincoln), pp. 435–54. Thousand Oaks, Sage.

Travers, M. (2001) *Qualitative Research through Case Studies*. London, Sage.

Webb, C. (1989) Action research: philosophy, methods and personal experiences. *Journal of Advanced Nursing*, **14**, 403–10.

Whyte, W.F. (1943) *Street Corner Society: The Social Structure of an Italian Slum*. Chicago, University of Chicago Press.

Yin, R.K. (1993) *Applications of Case Study Research*. Newbury Park, Sage.

Yin, R.K. (1994) *Case Study Research*, 2nd edn. Thousand Oaks, Sage.

Critical incident technique

Cormack, D.F.S. (2000) The critical incident technique. In *The Research Process in Nursing* (ed. D. Cormack), 4th edn, pp. 327–35. Oxford, Blackwell Science.

Flanagan, J. (1954) The critical incident technique. *Psychological Bulletin*, **51**, 327–58.

Kemppainen, J.K. (2000) The critical incident technique and nursing care quality research. *Journal of Advanced Nursing*, **32** (5) 1264–71.

Woolsey, L. (1986) The critical incident technique: an innovative qualitative method of research. *Canadian Journal of Counselling*, **20** (2) 242–54.

Conversation analysis

Antaki, C. (ed.) (1988) *Analysing Everyday Explanation: A Casebook of Methods*. London, Sage.

Beck, C.S. & Ragan, S.L. (1992) Negotiating interpersonal and medical talk. *Journal of Language and Social Psychology*, **11**, 47–61.

Bergstrom, L., Roberts, J., Skillman, L. & Seidel, J. (1992) You'll feel me touching you, sweetie: vaginal examination during the second stage of labour. *Birth*, **19**, 11–18.

Button, G. & Lee, J.R.E. (eds) (1987) *Talk and Social Organisation*. Clevedon, Multilingual Matters.

Couchman, W. (1995) Personal communication.

Goodwin, C. & Heritage, J. (1990) Conversation analysis. *Annual Review of Anthropology*, **19**, 283–307.

Heritage, J. (1988) Explanations as accounts: a conversation analytic perspective. In *Analysing Everyday Explanation: A Casebook of Methods*, pp. 127–44. London, Sage.

Leudar, I. & Antaki, C. (1988) Completion and dynamics in explanation seeking. In *Analysing Everyday Explanation: A Casebook of Methods*, pp. 145–55. London, Sage.

Mallett, J. (1990) Communication between nurses and post-anaesthetic patients. *Intensive Care Nursing*, **6**, 45–53.

Nofsinger, R.E. (1991) *Everyday Conversation*. Newbury Park, Sage.

Nunan, D. (1993) *Discourse Analysis*. London, Penguin English.

Sharrock, W. & Anderson, R. (1987) Work flow in a paediatric clinic. In *Talk and Social Organisation* (eds G. Button & J.R.E. Lee). Clevedon, Multilingual Matters.

Silverman, D. (2001) *Interpreting Qualitative Data: Methods for Analysing Talk, Text and Interaction*, 3rd edn. London, Sage.

Turner, R. (ed.) (1974) *Ethnomethodology*. Harmondsworth, Penguin Books.

Weijts, W., Houtkoop, H. & Mullen, P. (1993) Talking delicacy: Speaking about sexuality during gynaecological consultations. *Sociology of Health and Illness*, **15**, 295–314.

Discourse analysis

Banister, P., Bruman, E., Parker, I., Taylor, M. & Tindall, C. (1994) *Qualitative Methods in Psychology: A Research Guide*, pp. 92–107. Buckingham, Open University.

Gill, R. (1996) Discourse analysis: practical implementation. In *Handbook of Qualitative Research in Psychology and the Social Sciences* (ed. J.T.A. Richardson), pp. 141–56. Leicester, BPS Books.

Gill, R. (2000) Discourse analysis. In *Qualitative Researching: with Text, Image and Sound* (eds M.W. Bauer & G. Gaskell), pp. 172–90. London, Sage.

McHoul, A. & Grace, W. (1995) *A Foucault Primer: Discourse, Power and the Subject.* London, UCL Press.

Nunan, D. (1993) *Discourse Analysis.* London, Penguin English.

Potter, J. (1996a) *Representing Reality: Discourse, Rhetoric, and Social Construction.* London, Sage.

Potter, J. (1996b) Discourse analysis and constructionist approaches: theoretical background. In *Handbook of Qualitative Research in Psychology and the Social Sciences* (ed. J.T.A. Richardson), pp. 125–40. Leicester, BPS Books.

Potter, J. (1997) Discourse analysis as a way of analysing naturally occurring talk. In *Qualitative Research: Theory, Method and Practice* (ed. D. Silverman), pp. 144–60. London, Sage.

Potter, J. & Wetherell, M. (1987) *Discourse and Social Psychology: Beyond Attitudes and Behaviour.* London, Sage.

Silverman, D. (ed.) (2001) *Interpreting Qualitative Data: Methods for Analysing Talk, Text and Interaction*, 3rd edn. London, Sage.

Van Dijk, T.A. (ed.) (1985) *Discourse and Communication: New Approaches to the Analysis of Mass Media Discourse and Communication.* Berlin, Walter de Gruyter.

Wetherell, M., Taylor, S., Yates, S.J. (eds) (2001) *Discourse as Data: A Guide for Analysis.* Milton Keynes, The Open University.

Other approaches

Banister, P., Bruman, E., Parker, I., Taylor, M. & Tindall, C. (1994) *Qualitative Methods in Psychology: A Research Guide*, pp. 92–107. Buckingham, Open University.

Beail, N. (ed.) (1985) *Repertory Grid Technique and Personal Constructs: Applications in Clinical and Educational Settings.* Buckingham, Croom Helm.

Fitzpatrick, M.L. (1993) Historical research: the method. In *Nursing Research: A Qualitative Perspective* (eds P. Munhall & C. Boyd), pp. 359–71. New York, National League for Nursing Press.

Kelly, G. (1955) *A Theory of Personality: The Psychology of Personal Constructs* (2 Vols). New York, Norton.

Kelly, G. (1986) *A Brief Introduction into Personal Construct Theory.* London, Centre for Personal Construct Theory.

Rawlinson, J.W. (1995) Some reflections on the use of repertory grid technique in studies of nurses and social workers. *Journal of Advanced Nursing*, **21**, 334–9.

PART FOUR

Data Analysis and Completion

CHAPTER 15

Data Analysis: Procedures, Practices and Computers

Features and process of data analysis

Data analysis in qualitative research is not a linear process, nor do all qualitative forms of inquiry take the same approach to data analysis, as discussed in the chapters on individual approaches. Indeed, grounded theory and phenomenology have very distinct ways of analysing data. Data reduction, description and/or interpretation are common to many types of qualitative data analysis although the approach to these procedures is flexible and creative. There is no rigid prescription as long as the story has its roots directly in the data generated by the participants, but there are distinctive and different approaches to analysis.

Data analysis is a complex, time-consuming and iterative activity. Researchers must remember this in order to allocate and segment their time appropriately. Nurses and midwives often lack time at the end of their study to carry out the appropriate data analysis, because they do not foresee the complexity of the data and the length of time needed for analysing them. The iterative character of qualitative research also makes it more time consuming.

It is important to remember that qualitative researchers usually collect and analyse the data simultaneously, unlike those involved in quantitative inquiry who complete collection before starting analysis. Indeed in grounded theory, data collection and analysis interact (see Chapter 10). Even when recording and transcribing data, researchers reflect upon them and so start the process of analysis at an early stage.

The process of analysis goes through certain stages common to most approaches:

- Transcribing interviews and sorting fieldnotes
- Organising and ordering the data
- Listening to and reading the material collected over and over again

Other stages depend on the approach taken by the qualitative researcher:

- Coding and categorising (this is particularly appropriate in interpretive methods)

- Building themes
- Describing a cultural group (in ethnography)
- Describing a phenomenon (this is appropriate in phenomenology)

Silverman (2001) repeats a warning about the status of interview data in particular, which must be taken into account before the process of data analysis can start. These data are rarely raw but have been processed through the mind of the interviewer and can only be seen in context. In observations too, fieldnotes do not always show how the environment, for instance the presence or absence of certain people, the work climate and other factors, has shaped interaction.

Transcribing and sorting

The fullest and richest data can be gained from transcribing all interviews verbatim. We advise that, if possible, students transcribe their own tapes because this way they immerse themselves in the data and become sensitive to the issues of importance. Transcription takes a long time: one hour of interviewing takes between four and six hours to transcribe. For those who are not used to audio-typing, it can be much longer. Transcription is very frustrating and can take time that researchers often lack. A typist using a transcription machine could do it more quickly, but this would be expensive. On the other hand, it would give more time to the researcher to listen and analyse. The decision about this depends on the researcher. Any outsider who transcribes must, of course, be advised on the confidentiality relating to the data.

Initial interviews and fieldnotes should be fully transcribed so that the researcher becomes aware of the important issues in the data. Novice researchers should transcribe all interviews, while more experienced individuals can be more selective in their transcriptions and transcribe that which is linked to their developing theoretical ideas. It is always better that the interviews or fieldnotes are fully transcribed by the researchers themselves if they have the time. There is danger that researchers who fail to record the interviews will overlook significant issues, which they would uncover on reflection when listening to the tape or considering the transcript. Pages are numbered, and the front sheet should contain date, location and time of interview as well as the code number or pseudonym for the informant and important biographical data (but no identifier). Many researchers number each line of the interview transcript so that they can find the data quickly during analysis. It is useful to keep the right or left half of the page free for analysis or notes and comments.

A minimum of three copies (usually more) should be made of the transcripts and a clean copy without comments for locking away in a safe place in case other copies are lost or destroyed.

Taking notes

Some researchers use the tape-recorder and take notes during the interview so that participants' facial expression, gestures and interviewers' reactions and comments can be recorded. Making notes might disturb the participant. We would suggest this only when taping is not feasible or if interviewees do not wish to be tape-recorded. This can be done immediately after the interview.

When participants deny permission for recording or when it seems inappropriate – for instance in very sensitive situations – interviewers generally take notes throughout the interview, and these notes reflect the words of the participants as accurately as possible. As interviewers can only write down a fraction of the sentences, they select the most important words or phrases and summarise the rest, and this might distort meaning. Patton (1990) advises on conventions in the use of quotation marks while writing notes. Researchers use them only for full, direct quotations from informants. Patton suggests that researchers adopt a mechanism for differentiating between their own thoughts and informants' words. When reading transcripts and writing memos, researchers should also collect a series of pithy quotes, which are representative of the thoughts of the participants and the phenomenon or phenomena under study.

Another method of recording is to take notes after the interview is finished. This should be done as soon as possible after the interview to capture the flavour, behaviour and words of the informants and the concomitant thoughts of the researcher. It should not be done in the presence of the participants.

The process of listening to the tapes will sensitise researchers to the data and uncover ambiguities or problems within them. At this time, any theoretical or other ideas that emerge should be written down in the field diary.

Writing analytical memos

During the process of analysis researchers write analytical memos or notes containing ideas and thoughts about the data as well the reasons for grouping them in a particular way. Sometimes researchers draw diagrams to demonstrate this, and these diagrams can be taken directly into the report when they discuss the methods and the decision trail. Researchers might develop concepts in the memos or ask analytic questions of the data, or elaborate ideas from the literature that link directly with the data. There are different ways of keeping memos: in field journals or diaries, or on a computer. This all helps 'tacking', that is, going back and forth between the data and theoretical ideas, between codes and themes. This is called 'iteration'.

Phenomenologists do not code or categorise because they wish to perceive the essence of the phenomenon as a whole, a *Gestalt*. Breaking the data into codes may lose this holistic view of the phenomenon and fragment the ideas contained in the data (phenomenological analysis is discussed in Chapter 11).

Ordering and organising the data

Bryman (2001) reminds researchers that qualitative researchers generate large amounts of data consisting of narratives, fieldnotes and documents, as well as a variety of memos about the phenomenon under study. Some even use the literature linked to the research as data.

Through organisation and management, the researcher brings structure and order to the unwieldy mass of data. This will help eventual retrieval and final analysis. All transcripts, fieldnotes and other data should have details of time, location and specific comments attached. The use of pseudonyms or numbers for participants prevents identification during the long process of analysis when the data might fall into the hands of individuals other than the researcher. Everything has to be recorded, crosschecked and labelled. Then the material has to be stored in the appropriate files for later retrieval.

From the very beginning of the study nurses and midwives will recognise significant ideas and themes in the material they generated. On listening to tapes, reading transcriptions and other documents or looking at visual data common themes and patterns will begin to emerge and become crystallised.

Borkan (1999) discusses the initial process of analysis and describes two strategies from which researchers can choose depending on their approach, namely *horizontal* and *vertical* 'passes' of the data. The horizontal pass involves:

- Reading the data and looking at themes, emotions and surprises, taking in the overall picture
- Reflective and in-depth reading of the data to find supporting evidence for these themes
- Re-reading for elements that might have been overlooked
- Searching for possible alternative meanings
- Attempting to link discrepancies together

Vertical passes involve:

- Concentrating on one section of the data and analysing it before moving on
- Reflecting on and reviewing the data in the section
- Looking for insights and feeding them back into the data collection process

The horizontal is more holistic than the vertical pass. However, researchers not only analyse according to the methods they adopt, but they also have different personal styles, which demand different ways of looking at the data.

Analytical styles

Different approaches to research have different types of data analysis. Even within one approach, researchers adopt a variety of analyses. Phenomenologists, for instance, use a variety of analytic styles (see, for instance, Van Kaam, 1959; Colaizzi, 1978; Giorgi, 1985; Diekelman *et al.*, 1989, in nursing). They all involve the steps of listening to and gaining a holistic view of the data as well as dividing them into units of meaning. Dahlberg *et al.* (2001) ask that each part of the transcribed text, analysed for meaning, should be understood in relation to the whole of the text and the whole understood in terms of its parts.

Moustakas (1994) modifies the analysis styles and comes up with overlapping steps in which researchers carry out the following:

- They reflect on each transcript and search for significant statements
- They record all relevant statements
- They list those statements that are non-repetitive and non-overlapping – the invariant constituents or meaning units – and organise them
- They link and relate these into themes
- Including verbatim quotes from the data, they integrate the themes into a description of the texture of the experience as told by the participants
- They reflect on this and their own experiences
- They construct a description of the essences and meanings of the experience

There is a more detailed discussion of analytic procedures in phenomenology in Chapter 11.

Coding and categorising

Coding is an early stage in analysis. Codes, in the words of Punch (1998: 204) are 'tags, names or labels given to sections of data'. Coding proceeds towards the development of categories, themes or major constructs (the nomenclature depends on the language of the specific approach). It breaks the data into manageable sections.

Line-by-line coding identifies information which both participant and researcher consider important. In their initial coding, many researchers single out words or phrases that are used by participants – these are called *in vivo* codes. This type of coding prevents researchers from imposing their own framework and ideas on the data, because the coding starts with the words of the participants.

Example of *in vivo* coding

A transcript might contain the sentence 'I was really shocked when the doctor told me that I suffered from cancer'. The *in vivo* code might be: *shocked when told about cancer*. At a later stage, of course, this would have to be refined by the words of the researcher but still seen from the perspective of the participant. It might become: *shock on receiving the diagnosis*.

In the beginning, line-by-line and *in vivo* coding can be useful, but it would be difficult to carry out in all transcriptions of the interviews and sets of fieldnotes. It does, however, help researchers discern important ideas in the data initially until they become used to coding.

Initial or *open* coding gives a name to specific pieces of data. The codes may be words, expressions or other chunks of data. Researchers might start with a mass of codes and reduce them so that each of them represents a concept. These concepts are *units of meaning*. Once simple coding has been completed, researchers group together the codes with similar meanings which are linked to the same phenomenon. If different terms are applied to the same concept, the best label is used as a name for the concept. Rather than coding line by line or sentence by sentence, many researchers code paragraph by paragraph. Others search for meaningful statements in the text.

There are some problems with coding and categorising. One is the loss of the holistic view or *Gestalt* of the phenomenon (Todres, 2002), which is the aim of phenomenologists. The other, according to Silverman (2000), is the loss of important information, because it does not 'fit' the code or category, hence the importance of the search for discrepant and alternative ideas.

When analysing data from different data sources, for instance from observation, interviews and documents, researchers search for similarities and differences. All the material that has conceptual links is grouped together for later categorisation. Some researchers actually cut up the data and keep them in a file, after pasting them on pages of paper and putting them into a ring binder, others use coloured pencils or pens to identify closely linked material.

Computers can of course, carry out the process much more quickly – even when researchers don't use a computer package for the analysis of data. There are, however, arguments both for and against computer use in qualitative research (see the section on computer-aided analysis later in this chapter).

Inferential leaps and 'premature closure'

As part of the process of data analysis, researchers should check against *inferential leaps*. In our early days of research supervision it became apparent that students would infer conclusions from the data too quickly. In their haste to make sense of the data and develop a picture, students can too readily make inferential leaps. It seems that nurse and midwifery researchers remember concepts or frameworks previously learned or discovered as a background to the research, and they try to fit these to the data. The researcher has to return to the data continually, checking and verifying so that inferential leaps are not made. This is closely connected with the warning against *premature closure* (Glaser, 1978) that is one of the problems of qualitative research. Often novice researchers decide on a theme or category at an early stage of the research process. In grounded theory in particular, the danger exists that once researchers have generated some theoretical ideas, they then sit back and decide that they arrived at full explanations for the phenomenon under study. Sometimes there has been no full investigation of the data; sometimes they close their minds to new ideas. Morse (1994) claims that premature closure can lead to inadequate theory.

Collaboration in the process of analysis and interpretation

In all types of qualitative data analysis it is important that researchers stay as close to the data as possible and look at everything connected with the phenomenon under study.

A completed study is never a mere description of the participants' experience. It is important to remember that the final product of research depends on the collaborative effort of participants and researcher. While those observed and interviewed are active agents in their world rather than passive participants and construct their social reality, researcher and participant also construct meaning together. The reader of the study too, will eventually be involved in construction of meaning.

Computer-aided analysis of qualitative data

Computers have been used in the analysis of qualitative data mainly since the 1980s. The type of approach influences the programme for analysis of qualitative data. Computers can be useful and make the process of qualitative research less cumbersome. Managing a large volume of data by hand is boring and tiring because the search for specific ideas, words, incidents or events takes time. Glesne and Peshkin (1992: 145) call the computer 'a tool for executing the mechanical or clerical task of qualitative research'. In the past, researchers depended for their analysis to a large extent on cutting, sorting and pasting bits of paper. This meant that the researcher was left with a mass of paper cuttings, a great many boxes and envelopes and/or an elaborate card system. Computers have changed all this.

Several types of computer aided qualitative data analysis software (CAQDAS) exist, of which the best known are NUDIST (Non-numerical Unstructured Data Indexing, Searching and Theorising) Ethnograph, ATLAS.ti and HyperResearch (for a list and advice for best uses of the various programs see Fielding and Lee, 1998). Ethnograph is one of the earliest packages and NUDIST is one of the most widely used (perhaps because of its name). The packages have slightly different functions. Holland (2001) suggests that ATLAS.ti is easy to learn and best used in simple projects, while QSR NU*DIST is a good tool for more complex studies but difficult to learn.

Since the early 1980s, when the journal *Qualitative Sociology* (1984, 7 (1) 2) published a special edition on the use of computers in qualitative research, new ideas and packages have been developed. Some programs are more sophisticated than others. Each has its own technical traits depending on the choice of the designer. For researchers who wish to use this software, it is essential to become familiar with it.

For further information and details on particular programs, we advise researchers to look at the text books by Tesch (1990), Dey (1993) Weitzman and Miles (1994)), Kelle (1995, 1997), Fielding and Lee (1991, 1998), and the various writings of Richards and Richards who are strong advocates of CAQDAS and the developers of the NUDIST packages. In these books, programs and addresses can also be found. For complete beginners an examination of relevant chapters in Bryman (2001) or Fetterman (1998) might be useful.

The reasons for computer use

Tesch (1993) lists a variety of tasks, formerly done manually, which can now be performed by computers, some of which we list as the most important:

- Storing, annotating and retrieving texts
- Locating words, phrases, and segments of data
- Naming or labelling
- Sorting and organising
- Identifying data units
- Preparing diagrams
- Extracting quotes

Storing, annotating and retrieving texts

Storing and retrieving texts such as interview transcripts, fieldnotes or diaries is the most common use of computer programs in qualitative research. Data are easily accessible – for instance interview transcripts and fieldnotes can be stored in separated files and memos attached to the category to which they belong – and can be called upon when needed. Researchers must always label and date these files to keep order among them. NB: Copies of files should be made on floppy disks and stored safely in different locations.

Locating words, phrases or segments of data

Researchers may want to find particular words or phrases and the context in which they occur as well as their frequency. Sentences, paragraphs and specific key words can be recalled. These can indicate the importance, which informants and researcher attach to particular words or concepts (though it is dangerous to rely on the number of instances rather than an in-depth examination of each instance).

Naming or labelling

These labels are key words that define an idea, or they can be summaries of the content of data. Categorising starts here and is based on this labelling. Categories are concepts attached to a topic emerging from the data and a step in their interpretation. Researchers give the appropriate label to each segment of data or to instances that belong together. Revision of names in the light of further analysis then becomes less difficult. The creation of categories from the data is a step towards theory building.

Sorting and organising

Sorting and organising the data segments and topic units according to the named categories or key words attached to them is one of the procedures undertaken during the analysis process. Organising data into segments (bits, chunks or strips as they are sometimes called), means dividing them into discrete units (although these can sometimes overlap with each other). All segments with the same inherent themes or categories can be grouped together.

Identifying data units

Researchers identify data units relevant to several categories and discover relationships between them. They always try to see a structure and links between categories. While working with the data these links can be found more easily in and across particular files. This helps in the development of working hypotheses, models or typologies. Of course, the computer does none of these processes; they are based on the researcher's theoretical considerations and decision making but are helped by the machine. Each proposition can be checked out. For instance, a nurse researcher may infer from examining the data that women prefer male to female doctors. This can be checked quickly through viewing the categories and the links between them.

Preparing diagrams

Diagrams illustrate the relationship between themes or categories. The graphic display can enhance the story line and help to convey its meaning. Many of our students clarify their findings by showing links and connections through diagrams.

Extracting quotes

Quotes can be extracted from the informants' words or fieldnotes for insertion in the final story. Qualitative researchers use quotes from participants or excerpts from fieldnotes when they write up their study. These are excerpts from the data to give evidence that their discussion has its basis in the data themselves. The quotes enhance the story line, that is, they make the story more lively and interesting.

Approaches to qualitative computer analysis

Tesch (1991) describes three main approaches to qualitative data analysis (described below) but acknowledges that these groupings and their subgroups are not neat and discrete; they overlap and do not reflect reality. Both the content of the text and the process of communication are seen as important.

Language oriented

These types of analysis are used by researchers who are primarily interested in language and its meaning – examples are conversation and discourse analysis as well as ethnography. These approaches focus not only on words and verbal interaction but also on the way in which people make sense of their world.

Descriptive/interpretive approaches

These deal with narratives and give descriptions of feelings and actions. Examples are life histories and certain types of ethnography as descriptions and interpretations of a culture. Researchers tell stories and provide interpretations of meanings that participants in the research attach to their experiences.

Theory building

In theory building, the researcher finds patterns and links between ideas and attempts to build theory. From insights generated by the data general principles often emerge. This is more explanatory than other approaches. Grounded theory represents this type of research. Richards and Richards (1994) stress that the process of theory building is not mechanical but demands creativity from the researcher.

The practicalities of using computer aided analysis

Most students already use word processors for entering and storing data. It is essential for the small minority who do not do so to learn word processing skills because changing a text by correcting, cutting and pasting on the machine takes much less time than rewriting by hand or typewriter. Word processing programs create and revise text and can therefore be helpful to researchers in the transcription of interviews, fieldnotes and in writing the report.

Many researchers would like to learn the use of computers for qualitative analysis, but the practicalities of this must be sorted out before starting a project. The usefulness of computers depends on the researchers' initial knowledge of computers as well as the time span and size of the project. Some of our students started learning to use the computer for data analysis and found it impossible to do so within the allocated time.

Miles and Weitzman (1994) speak of levels of computer skills. Level 1 users have limited knowledge of computers. They use a word processing program efficiently, including creating, cutting and pasting text. We would suggest that the students who have a short time to finish a project might be better advised to start the process of analysis manually, using the computer knowledge they already possess rather than learning new and complex processes. Most undergraduate students generally only have between nine and twelve months for their project, and the time is too short for mastering a complex package; effort and energy are better expanded in listening to tapes, organising the data and thinking about them. PhD students with several years' research work ahead would do well to learn computer skills to help in the management of qualitative data. There is the likelihood that it will be possible for them to apply their knowledge in future research projects. Level 1 researchers interested in using computers are advised to consider user friendly programs and get help from others who have some expertise.

Level 2 users can cope with a variety of programs, and they should select one which is appropriate to their research. If they are planning a long-term project, they can choose a complex package. Miles and Weitzman (1994) advise researchers to consult experienced users of qualitative data analysis packages, but some guidelines and textbooks on the use of computers in qualitative research also detail the practical processes.

Researchers at level 3 are interested and knowledgeable computer users and quickly acquire expertise in the programme they need for their research. Level 4 computer users – individuals who are never far away from their machine – have expert knowledge and experience of computing and computer packages. They will have no difficulties dealing with programmes for qualitative research. We would advise the use of a computer programme for analysis if the nurse researcher has a large sample (for a qualitative research project, more than 40 interviewees for instance, would be a large sample) and a long time span, because the data can be managed more efficiently.

We found it difficult to learn the use of computer packages for qualitative analysis from manuals, although some people seem to be able to do so. It is always easier to let expert users teach rather than relying on a manual, but one must be aware that very experienced individuals might be too far advanced to use beginners' terms and explain the skills in a simple way. They take the language and skills needed for computers for granted. It is far better to have a teacher who is just a few steps ahead.

Russell and Gregory (1993) point out that researchers perform both mechanical and conceptual roles in the analysis of data. Not only do researchers store and retrieve data, actions that are mechanical activities, but they also group, code and categorise, tasks that involve conceptual activity. These two types of activities are always linked to each other and can both be helped by the use of computers.

Advantages of computer use

Researchers use computers as tools for facilitating processes that were done manually in the past; but it is a fallacy to believe that data can be analysed more quickly by computer programs, because it takes time to learn their use. Once learnt though, they can save time and help researchers to be more organised and systematic and facilitate planning. Data are more accessible and fewer hours are spent sorting and coding the data (however, this implies that all approaches use coding and categorising, and that, of course, is not so).

Cutting and pasting is easy when computers are used, and more time can be given to thinking through the analysis. Researchers should remember to back up their data by storing copies on floppy disks or other computers in several locations and update them regularly. Webb (1999) considers some of the advantages of using CAQDAS. She notes the hope of qualitative computer analysts that this analysis might be more systematic and objective. Large amounts of data can be more easily analysed. Webb does advise that not all qualitative analysis is appropriate for computers.

Tesch (1993) states that the introduction of computers in qualitative research does not mean a complete change in the process of analysis, but the new tool can make it easier and more flexible. While decisions and judgements are still made by the researcher, searching, cutting and pasting is done by machine. Computers cannot formulate categories or interpret the data, but they might make the analysis more accurate and comprehensive. Those nurse and midwife researchers who are not familiar with computer analysis when starting research, should not attempt computer analysis unless they are able to extend their project over a lengthy time period.

Problems and critique

Certain problems emerge, however, when using computers. Seidel (1991: 107), one of the major proponents of computer use in qualitative analysis, warns of 'analytic madness' and states that the use of technology may be a problem that can interfere with appropriate qualitative analysis. He discusses a number of issues. Researchers may be tempted to collect and manage more data than necessary, especially when they have mostly used quantitative methods in the past. The overload of data might prevent them from looking for the most interesting and significant ideas. Instead of searching for deeper meaning in the data, they try to make up for the lack of depth by focusing on the volume of data. There is also the issue of the relationship between researchers and data. This might become mechanistic if analysts do not see the need to examine and evaluate the data carefully. The number of instances of a code or category is often seen as more important than a single significant occurrence just because counting is easy. The lack of scrutiny might prevent the researcher from seeing the real meaning of the phenomenon under study. This also happens occasionally when the data are analysed manually, but the danger becomes greater through the use of computers.

Some researchers believe that computing skills are not only unnecessary but that their use could make qualitative research mechanistic and rigid, the very characteristics which might change its lively humanistic nature. Even now there are some who think this. For instance, Becker (1993) warns the grounded theorist about the use of computers; she feels that computers might prevent sensitivity to the data and the discovery of meanings. Computers might distance researchers from the data. In nursing and midwifery research where emotional engagement and sensitivity is necessary, the use of computers could be problematic.

The distancing of the researcher from the data is another problem in the use of computers. The involvement with a file on a computer or a printed sheet of paper, which is coded by machine, seems less personal than coding and categorising by hand. Coffey *et al.* (1996) suggest that rigid and mechanistic procedures might prevent researchers from getting close to the data or becoming engaged with them.

In spite of these potential problems many well known qualitative researchers use computer programs when conducting a major piece of research. Seidel himself is the developer of the much used computer package *Ethnograph* that helps researchers to identify and retrieve text from documents.

Computers have largely been accepted in qualitative research. In our experience some funding agencies are impressed by computer packages because their members are used to computers in survey research and often worry about the scientific value of qualitative research. (Computer packages do not, of course, confirm or deny the scientific value or quality of qualitative research as computer aided analysis is merely an instrument and as good or bad as the thinking and judgement of the researcher who uses it.) The greatest help from computers lies in the management of data, because 'good analysis requires efficient management of one's data' (Dey, 1993:74), but it is important for researchers not to distance themselves from the data.

Depending on their own stance towards the use of computer aided analysis, or their individual needs and skills, nurses and midwives can, of course, choose whether or not to use computer aided data analysis.

Summary

There are a number of different ways in which data are analysed depending on the research question and the approach.

- Many approaches use coding and categorising which proceeds from a basic to a more abstract level, others apply a more holistic approach and focus on the description of a phenomenon.
- Data analysis is not rigid or prescriptive although there are certain commonalities in most approaches
- Computers may be a useful tool in the analysis of data, especially in some areas of retrieval, organisation and management, but they should be used with caution.

References

Barry, C.A. (1998) Choosing qualitative data analysis software. *Sociological Research Online*, **3** (3). http://www.socresonline.org.uk/socresonline/3/3.html

Becker, P.H. (1993) Common pitfalls in grounded theory research. *Qualitative Health Research*, **3** (2) 254–60.

Borkan, J. (1999) Immersion/crystallisation. In *Doing Qualitative Research* (eds B.F. Crabtree & W.L. Miller), 2nd edn, pp. 179–94. Thousand Oaks, Sage.

Bryman, A. (2001) *Social Research Methods*. Oxford, Oxford University Press.

Coffey, A., Holbrook, B. & Atkinson, P. (1996) Qualitative data analysis: technologies and representations. *Sociological Research Online*, **1** (1). http://www.socresonline.org.uk/sorcresonline/1/1/4.hmtl

Colaizzi, P. (1978) Psychological research as a phenomenologist views it. In *Existential Phenomenological Alternatives for Psychology* (eds R. Vallé & M. King), pp. 48–71. New York, Oxford University Press.

Dahlberg, K., Drew, N. & Nyström, M. (2001) *Reflective Lifeworld Research*. Lund, Studentlitteratur.

Dey, I. (1993) *Qualitative Data Analysis*. London, Routledge.

Diekelman, N.L., Allen, D. & Tanner, C. (1989) *The NLN Criteria of Appraisal of Baccalaureate Programs: A critical hermeneutic analysis*. New York, National League for Nursing Press.

Fetterman, D.M. (1998) *Ethnography: Step by Step*, 2nd edn. Thousand Oaks, Sage.

Fielding, N.G. & Lee, R.M. (eds) (1991) *Using Computers in Qualitative Research*. London, Sage.

Fielding, N. & Lee, R. (1998) *Computer Analysis and Qualitative Research*. London, Sage.

Giorgi, A. (ed.) (1985) *Phenomenology and Psychological Research*. Pittsburgh, Duquesne University Press.

Glaser, B.G. (1978) *Theoretical Sensitivity*. Mill Valley, CA, Sociology Press.

Glesne, C. & Peshkin, A. (1992) *Becoming Qualitative Researchers: An Introduction*. New York, Longman.

Holland, M. (2001) Computer aided qualitative analysis software (CAQDAS) In *Qualitative Research in Public Relations and Marketing Communications* (eds C. Daymon & I. Holloway). London, Routledge.

Kelle, U. (ed.) (1995) *Computer-Aided Qualitative Data Analysis: Theory, Methods and Practice*. London, Sage.

Kelle, U. (1997) Theory building in qualitative research and computer management for the management of textual data. *Sociological Research Online*, **2** (2). http://www.socresonline.org.uk/socresonline/2/2.html

Lee, R.M. & Fielding, N.G. (1991) Computing for qualitative research: options, problems and potential. In *Using Computers in Qualitative Research* (eds N.G. Fielding & R.M. Lee), pp. 1–13. London, Sage.

Miles, M.B. & Weitzman, E.A. (eds) (1994) Choosing computer programs for qualitative data analysis. In *Qualitative Data Analysis* (eds M.B. Miles & A.M. Huberman), 2nd edn, pp. 311–30. Thousand Oaks, Sage.

Morse, J. (1994) 'Emerging from the data': The cognitive processes of analysis in qualitative inquiry. In *Critical Issues in Qualitative Research Methods* (ed. J.M. Morse), pp. 23–43. Thousand Oaks, Sage.

Moustakas, C. (1994) *Phenomenological Research Methods*. Thousand Oaks, Sage.

Patton, M. (1990) *Qualitative Evaluation and Research Methods*. Newbury Park, Sage.

Punch, K.F. (1998) *Introduction to Social Research: Qualitative and Quantitative Approaches*. London, Sage.

Richards, T.J. & Richards, L. (1994) Using computers in qualitative research. In *Handbook for Qualitative Research* (eds N.K. Denzin & Y.S. Lincoln), pp. 445–62. Thousand Oaks, Sage.

Russell, C.K. and Gregory, D.M. (1993) Issues for consideration when choosing a qualitative data management system. *Journal of Advanced Nursing*, **18**, 1806–16.

Seidel, J. (1991) Method and madness in the application of computer technology to qualitative data analysis. In *Using Computers in Qualitative Research* (eds N.G. Fielding & R.M. Lee), pp. 107–18. London, Sage.

Silverman, D. (2000) *Doing Qualitative Research: A Practical Handbook*. London, Sage.

Silverman, D. (2001) *Interpreting Qualitative Data: Methods for Analysing Talk, Text and Interaction*, 3rd edn. London, Sage.

Tesch, R. (1990) *Qualitative Research: Analysis Types and Software Tools*. London, Falmer Press.

Tesch, R. (1991) Software for qualitative researchers. In *Using Computers in Qualitative Research* (eds N.G. Fielding & R.M. Lee), pp. 16–37. London, Sage.

Tesch, R. (1993) Personal computers in qualitative research. In *Ethnography and Qualitative Design in Educational Research* (eds M.D. LeCompte & J. Preissle with R. Tesch), 2nd edn, pp. 279–314. Chicago, Academic Press.

Todres, L. (2002) Personal communication.

Van Kaam, A. (1959) A phenomenological analysis exemplified by the feeling of being understood. *Individual Psychology*, **15**, 66–72.

Webb, C. (1999) Analysing qualitative data: computerised and other approaches. *Journal of Advanced Nursing*, **29** (2) 323–30.

Weitzman, E.A. & Miles, M.B. (1994) *Computer Aided Qualitative Data Analysis: A Review of Selected Software*. New York, Center for Policy Research.

CHAPTER 16

Ensuring Trustworthiness and Quality

Truth value

All types of inquiry are rightly open to scrutiny from their readers. Nurse and midwife researchers too must consider the truth value of their research and demonstrate that it is credible and valid for professional practice. Qualitative research has its own criteria by which it can be evaluated. Bryman (2001: 276) suggests, however, that 'a simple application of the quantitative researcher's criteria of reliability and validity is not desirable . . .'.

There are three distinct perspectives on addressing the quality of qualitative research (Murphy *et al.*, 1998; Cutcliffe and McKenna 1999). Different groups of writers believe that:

- Qualitative and quantitative research should be evaluated by the same criteria
- Qualitative research should be evaluated by criteria that have been specially developed for it
- Criteriology should be rejected

One group, for instance Maxwell (1996), Hammersley (1998), Silverman (2001), argues for the retention of the criteria of reliability and validity while suggesting, at the same time, that these criteria cannot be directly 'translated' from quantitative to qualitative research. Wolcott (1994) and Stake (1995) reject many evaluative criteria as inappropriate for qualitative inquiry and believe that a specific research project should not be decontextualised.

Another school chooses alternative terms. Proponents of this are Lincoln and Guba (1985; Guba and Lincoln 1989) and Erlandson *et al.* (1993) who developed the concepts of trustworthiness and authenticity as parallel and alternative criteria. Researchers will come across both groups of terms during their reading and therefore will have to know about them regardless of the terms they themselves apply. However, a simplistic stance is sometimes taken. Different qualitative approaches often take a variety of viewpoints on criteria of quality (Whittemore *et al.*, 2001). Sparkes too (2001), claims that there is no shared understanding on what is 'good' qualitative research. Researchers find difficulty agreeing on how to judge the 'validity' of qualitative research or how to present convincing evidence of its trustworthiness.

Conventional criteria

We will here give the traditional criteria generally used in quantitative research, their meaning in qualitative inquiry and their alternatives. The latter are more often used than validity and reliability in qualitative health care research in nursing and midwifery, and are discussed in detail later in the chapter.

- Rigour–trustworthiness
- Reliability–dependability
- Validity–credibility
- Generalisability (external validity)–transferability
- Objectivity–confirmability

> Whatever labels health professionals apply, they have to demonstrate that their research has truth value, and they should be consistent in the terms and methods used to demonstrate this.

Rigour

Although quantitative researchers would say that rigour was a concept that has no real place in qualitative research, it has been defined by qualitative researchers as 'the means by which we show integrity and competence' (Aroni *et al.*, 1999).

Sandelowski (1986; 1993) has written two articles on rigour in qualitative research, and Koch (1994) too, has grappled with this concept that as mentioned might be better placed in quantitative research owing to its particular connotations with measurement and objectivity. Sandelowski's latter article recognises that the term rigour could imply inflexibility and rigidity, and that researchers should not be too preoccupied with it. Instead she advises they should create 'evocative, true-to-life and meaningful portraits, stories and landscapes of human experience...' (p. 1), and she criticises 'the reduction of validity to a set of procedures' (p. 2).

Reliability

Reliability in quantitative inquiry refers to the consistency of the research instrument. It is also linked to replicability, that is, the extent to which the study is repeatable and produces the same results when the methodology is replicated in similar circumstances and conditions. As the researcher is the main research instrument in qualitative inquiry, the research can never be wholly replicable. The researcher's characteristics and background will influence the research. Other investigators will have different emphases and foci, even when they adopt the same methods and select a similar sample and topic area.

Validity

Validity in quantitative research is seen as the extent to which an instrument measures what it is supposed to measure. In qualitative research the concept is more complex. Maxwell (1996: 87) maintains that it is 'the credibility of description, conclusion, explanation, interpretation, or other sort of account'.

To the term validity Hammersley (1998) adds that of *relevance* as a criterion for evaluating qualitative research. Relevance means that explanatory factors should have significance related to the purpose of the research and in solving the problems of practitioners in the discipline. The research must not only be meaningful but also useful for those who undertake it.

A number of threats to validity exist. These must be dealt with in the *description*, *interpretation* and *theory* (Maxwell, 1996). One of the threats to description is in collecting incorrect or incomplete data. The field diary must therefore be detailed and extensive. In interpretation, researchers are in danger of imposing their own ideas or distorting the meaning of the participants' accounts. Therefore it is important for the researcher to let the participants speak and listen to their voices. Researchers set aside their own thoughts and preconceptions about the phenomenon under study. Threats to theory emerge when alternative and rival explanations have not been taken into account. Although researchers can never be fully certain that all threats to validity have been eliminated, awareness of these threats helps produce a valid piece of research.

Internal validity is the extent to which the findings of a study are true, and whether they accurately reflect the aim of the research and the social reality of those participating in it. This can be established to an extent by taking the findings back to the participants (see the section entitled 'Member check' towards the end of this chapter). The researchers can compare their own findings with the perception of the people involved and explore whether they are compatible. *External validity*, also called generalisability, is described in the next section.

Generalisability or external validity

This is the most contentious concept linked to validity. For some authors such as Wolcott (1994) and Stake (1995) generalisability is not an issue to be discussed at length for they believe it is not relevant as they speak of specific situations and cases. For others however it is problematic. Most funding agencies and research committees in the UK National Health Service demand that the proposed research be generalisable, and this is understandable. If large amounts of money are given to researchers, funding bodies wish to know whether the outcomes are of general use in clinical practice and not just the results of 'blue skies' research undertaken for its own sake.

Generalisability exists when the findings and conclusions of a research study can be applied to other similar settings and populations. The term has its origin in quantitative research with its random statistical sampling procedures. Random sampling ensures that the results of the research are representative of the group from which the sample was drawn. It is clear that this type of generalisability cannot be achieved in qualitative research in which sampling is purposeful or, in grounded theory, theoretical.

Generalisability is difficult to achieve in qualitative research. Positivist and interpretive research differ in the sense that positivists seek law-like generalities while interpretivists focus on unique cases (see Chapter 1). As much quantitative research – though by no means all – is carried out in the positivist tradition and uses deductive methods, it can be more easily generalised. Many qualitative researchers, however, do not aim to achieve generalisability as they focus on specific instances or cases not representative of other cases or populations. The case(s) may even be atypical. Indeed the concept of generalisability might be irrelevant if only a single case or a unique phenomenon is examined. For instance, a nurse or midwife may want to examine a particular phenomenon important for local practice and patients in a particular area rather than of interest to the whole country. However, the study can still be successful, because it highlights specific non-typical features that can be related and compared to those of other, more typical cases.

Many qualitative researchers attempt to achieve some generalisability how-ever, because they feel that their research should be useful beyond their own study. Strauss and Corbin (1998) speak of the representativeness of concepts and applicability of theory to other situations. This means that qualitative research can have external validity through 'theory-based generalisation'. Morse (1994) claims that theory contributes to the 'greater body of knowledge' when it is 'recontextualised' into a variety of settings. It involves the application of theo-retical concepts found in one situation to other settings and conditions. If the theory developed from the original data analysis can be verified in other sites and situations, the theoretical ideas are generalisable.

Objectivity

This is a term often used in quantitative research. This means that the research is free of biases and relatively value neutral. Qualitative researchers do not find this concept very useful. Objectivity and neutrality are difficult to achieve; in fact, the values of researchers and participants become an integral part of the research, and they must openly acknowledge their own subjectivity. They do not conceal it but examine and then set it aside. Reason and Heron (1995) use the term 'critical subjectivity' (originally coined by Carr and Kemmis (1986)). They claim that although subjective experience is the basis for knowledge, it should not be accepted in a simplistic way but rooted in critical consciousness.

Validity and phenomenology

The concept of validity is used in phenomenological research, but its meaning and the way in which it is ensured is less precise and prescriptive than in other forms of qualitative research. Dahlberg *et al.* (2001) state that the research report should not contain any internal contradictions if the researcher wants it to be seen as valid.

Research can be valid through intersubjective knowledge. Moustakas (1994) speaks of 'intersubjective truth'. He states (p. 57) that according to Husserl 'each can experience and know the other, not exactly as one experiences and knows oneself but in the sense of empathy and copresence'. Initially truth is based in the unique perspective of unique individuals and their self-knowledge. As individuals inhabit the world of self and others, there is also communication with others. This enhances intersubjective understanding. If the research is to have validity, its readers will have learnt something of the human condition as well as recognised and grasped the essence of the phenomenon under study. This form of 'validity' is similar to, though not the same as, the concept of ontological authenticity described by Guba and Lincoln (1989) or that of 'thick description' by Geertz (1973).

An alternative perspective

It can be seen that the conventional terms used in quantitative research have different meanings in qualitative inquiry. Guba and Lincoln (1989), as stated before, go further than this and develop alternative terms and criteria. We will show how nurse and midwife researchers can attempt to demonstrate trustworthiness in the last section of this chapter.

Trustworthiness

Trustworthiness in qualitative research means methodological soundness and adequacy. Researchers make judgements of trustworthiness possible through developing dependability, credibility, transferability and confirmability. The most important of these is credibility.

Dependability

Lincoln and Guba (1985; Guba and Lincoln 1989) use the term dependability instead of reliability. If the findings of a study are to be dependable, they should be consistent and accurate. This means that readers will be able to evaluate the adequacy of the analysis through following the decision-making processes of the researcher. The context of the research must also be described in detail. To achieve some measure of dependability an audit trail is necessary. This helps readers follow the path of the researcher and demonstrates how he or she achieved their conclusions. It also guides other researchers wishing to carry out similar research. Although the study cannot be replicated, in similar circumstances with similar participants, it might be repeated.

Credibility

Credibility corresponds to the notion of internal validity (see p. 252). This means that the participants recognise the meaning that they themselves give to a situation or condition and the 'truth' of the findings in their own social context. The researcher's findings are, at least, compatible with the perceptions of the people under study.

Transferability

Lincoln and Guba use transferability instead of generalisability. This means that the findings in one context can be transferred to similar situations or participants. The knowledge acquired in one context will be relevant in another, and those that carry out the research in another context will be able to apply certain concepts originally developed. It seems to us that the concepts of transferability and generalisability are not too different.

Confirmability

Confirmability has taken the place of the term objectivity. As the research is judged by the way in which the findings and conclusions achieve their aim and are not the result of the researcher's prior assumptions and preconceptions, Lincoln and Guba demand 'confirmability'. This again needs an audit or decision trail where readers can trace the data to their sources. They follow the path of the researcher and the way he or she arrived at the constructs, themes and their interpretation. For this, both details of the research and the background and feelings of the researcher should be open to public scrutiny. When confirmability exists, readers can trace data to their original sources. Dahlberg *et al.* (2001) also demand intellectual honesty and openness from the researcher, as well as sensitivity to the phenomenon under study thus incorporating the idea of the audit trail although they do not explicitly call it this.

Authenticity

Trustworthiness, which relies on the methodological adequacy of the research, does not suffice according to Guba and Lincoln (1989), and they add the concept of authenticity. A study is authentic when the strategies used are appropriate for the true reporting of the participants' ideas. Authenticity consists of the following.

(1) *Fairness:* The researcher must be fair to participants and gain their acceptance throughout the whole of the study. Continued informed consent must be obtained. The social context in which the participants work and live also need to be taken into account.

(2) *Ontological authenticity:* This means that those involved, both readers and participants, will have been helped to understand their social world and their human condition through the research.

(3) *Educative authenticity:* Through understanding, participants improve the way in which they understand other people.

(4) *Catalytic authenticity:* Decision making by participants should be enhanced by the research.

(5) *Tactical authenticity:* The research should empower participants.

A study is authentic when the strategies used are appropriate for the true reporting of the participants' ideas, when the study is fair, and when it helps participants and similar groups to understand their world and improve it. It means that there is new insight into the phenomenon under study. A clear discussion of the terms can be found in Erlandson *et al.* (1993).

Trustworthiness and authenticity are achieved by the same strategies that all qualitative researchers are asked to follow. Indeed Lincoln and Guba developed and systematised these within their writing. Lincoln (1995, 2000) is still working on these concepts.

Strategies to ensure trustworthiness

There are a number of ways in which qualitative researchers can check and demonstrate to the reader whether the research is trustworthy. The most common strategies are the following (although not all of these are accepted by all qualitative researchers):

- Member checking
- Searching for negative cases and alternative explanations
- Peer review (also called peer debriefing)
- Triangulation
- The audit or decision trail

- Thick description
- Reflexivity

It is more likely that the study is trustworthy if researchers have been involved in the setting for a lengthy period of time as this may eliminate the reactivity of participants, because they learn to trust and are more likely to tell the truth, and also because their own assumptions can be examined in the process of prolonged engagement, persistent observation and immersion in the setting. This does not seem problematic for health professionals who are deeply involved with clinical practice. However, they occasionally bring preconceptions to the research and it is important to be aware of these.

Member checking

Throughout interviews and observations a check is needed on the understanding of the data with the people who are studied. Researchers do this by summarising, repeating or paraphrasing the participants' words. They then ask whether the participants feel that the interpretation is a true and fair representation of their perspective. This is called a *member check* (Lincoln & Guba, 1985) or *member validation*. The main reasons for member checking are the feedback of participants, their reaction to the data and findings, and their response to the researcher's interpretation of the data.

The specific purposes of member checking are:

- To find out whether the reality of the participants is presented
- To provide opportunities for them to change mistakes which they feel they might have made
- To assess the researcher's understanding and interpretation of the data
- To give the participants the opportunity to challenge the ideas of the researcher

Feedback from others ensures the trustworthiness of the research, and a member check is one of the strategies for achieving this. The procedure will help avoid misinterpretation or misunderstanding of the participants' words or actions. If a member check is carried out, it is more likely that the researcher presents the participant's point of view. After all, the aim of the study is to give a 'convincing account' (a term used by Seale, 1999) of the participants' different perspectives.

There are a number of ways to carry out member checks:

(1) The researcher presents participants with a transcript of their interview or fieldnotes of observations and asks them to comment on the contents. This is a very time-consuming process, and research participants cannot comment on the researcher's interpretations of their perspectives. Although this is an acceptable procedure, we would not advise undergraduates to do this, because of the time it takes.

(2) The interviewer can give the participants a summary of their interview, and his or her own interpretation of their words and the fieldnotes that were collected. This is a more useful way of confirming the ideas and the meaning of the account. The interviewers can discuss their own interpretations and discuss the meaning of the participants' words and actions. It is a check on the understanding of the account. Participants may change meaning and correct errors. The check may also add clarity or trigger and extend ideas that go beyond the original interview. The comments can be included in the final report.

(3) The researcher might present the final copy or substantial sections of the report and ask the participants to comment on the contents. Again, this is a lengthy process that demands time commitment and thought from participants, which they may not be able or willing to give. Although all or any of these procedures could be employed, we would suggest the second strategy as the most practical. Member checks do not only help in achieving validity in the study, but they also empower participants and give them control to confirm their words and actions and thus some control in the research itself. Member checking demands a large time commitment from both participant and researcher.

However rigorous and detailed the member check, some problems are inherent in it:

- The researcher's and participant's perspectives may be different
- The reactions of participants may be defensive
- The close relationship with the researcher may prevent the participant from adopting a critical stance
- Perceptions may change over time
- The researcher develops second-order concepts and theories

Sandelowski (1993) sees member checking as problematic and complex. She points to the fact that participants and researchers have a different agenda. Members are more interested in their own unique experiences. Researchers wish to portray 'multiple realities', while still representing the experience of each participant. Some of the issues related to member checks pose ethical dilemmas for the researcher. Participants might become aware and anxious that they have disclosed ideas that might be judged as unacceptable by the researcher or a reader of the report. In contrast to this they might hesitate to disagree because they have built up a close relationship with the researcher whom they see as a friend. Also, if the member check does not take place at an early stage after collection or analysis of the data, the participants might have changed their perceptions, and the researcher has to start again. Change over time is, of course, one of the reasons, why several interviews are better than one, and why prolonged engagement in the setting is useful.

Bryman (2001) sums up the problematics of member checking. He claims that researchers write for a readership of scholars and peers. This means that they always take the research to the level of developing concepts, an etic view which includes but goes beyond the participants' perspectives.

Searching for negative cases and alternative explanations

It enhances the validity of the research if the researchers identify data that do not easily fit into the developing theory or their own ideas. There may also be contrary occurrences that don't easily fit into developing patterns. These may provide alternative explanations. In the critical analysis researchers may find notions and events that do not fit their explanations and challenge the themes and patterns arising from the data. It means thinking about other possibilities, and whether they are grounded in the data. Maxwell (1996) suggests the basic principle of examining both supporting and alternative data. Researchers will have to explore whether conclusions from them are appropriate. Indeed, even if there is just one case that does not fit into the emergent theory, they should try to revise the working propositions so they can become confident that the explanations or interpretations derived from the data are the most valid and plausible and can account for the alternative case.

Erlandson *et al.* (1993) state that 'negative case analysis involves addressing and considering alternative interpretations of the data', especially those which may be contrary to their own view of reality. Working hypotheses or propositions and search for alternative explanations can then be revised. Single or few 'dissenting voices' included in the final report demonstrate the complexity of the research. Negative case analysis always presents challenges. It is not easy to become aware of discrepant data and negative or alternative cases, but at some stage researchers must stop searching when they feel they have exhausted the alternative possibilities and can account for the alternative cases.

Peer review

It is also useful to employ the strategy of peer review or 'peer debriefing' as Lincoln and Guba (1985) call it. This means that some colleagues who are competent in qualitative research procedures re-analyse the raw data, listen to the researcher's concerns and discuss them. Peers can be given the draft copy at the end of the research. They might detect bias or inappropriate subjectivity and try alternative explanations to the researcher's own working propositions and warn them against the attempt to 'fit' interpretations and explanations that cannot be substantiated by the data.

Example of peer debriefing

Walker, Sofaer and Holloway carried out research with people who had chronic back pain. After the collection of the data, they analysed them individually and then got together and decided to use those categories that in their collective view best described the experience of the participants.

Walker *et al.*, 1999

The example cited above shows that peer review is not problematic when colleagues who review have been involved in the research. Morse (1994) states that it can become more difficult if peers have not had any direct connection with the study, as they are less able to judge from the outside. Angen (2000) claims, however, that peers can make an assessment of the persuasiveness and coherence of the research.

Triangulation

Another important strategy to establish validity is to adopt triangulation procedures. Triangulation is the process by which the phenomenon or topic under study is examined from different perspectives. Triangulation in research means that the findings of one type of method (or data, researcher, theory) can be checked out by reference to another. This will provide a way of establishing whether there is generalisability in the research although researchers do not necessarily aim for this. Denzin (1989) differentiates between several types of triangulation as listed below.

- *Data triangulation*, where researchers use multiple data sources and obtain their data from different groups, settings or at different times (multiple sources of data).
- *Investigator triangulation*, when more than one expert researcher is involved in the study.
- *Theoretical triangulation*, when the researcher employs several possible theoretical interpretations in the study. Competing explanations or interpretations are developed and tested against each other to find the one which is most likely to describe or explain the phenomenon.
- *Methodological triangulation*, when researchers use two or more methods in one study to answer a similar question (observations, interviews, documents, questionnaires).

The last method in the list is most often used in a small-scale dissertation. Researchers might consider confirming findings using one method with the findings of another. It is not always necessary, though occasionally desirable, to use quantitative methods to confirm qualitative findings, that is, using 'between-method' triangulation. Morse (2001: 210) gives a number of possibilities for triangulation, each of which has different emphases. Studies using quantitative and qualitative methods can be used simultaneously or sequentially depending on the main direction of the research and its underlying assumptions. Morse claims (p. 209) that they may generate 'a more complete understanding'.

Example of between-method triangulation

A student nurse investigated attitudes of student nurses towards the subject of passive euthanasia. In this study the researcher decided to combine qualitative and quantitative approaches to investigate attitudes and thereby triangulate (use evidence from different sources). The qualitative part of this research concerned undertaking four in-depth interviews with student nurses to gain an initial insight into their perceptions, thoughts and feelings, towards passive euthanasia. The interview data provided a precursor for developing the research. The themes and categories that emerged in the analysis were linked with the subsequent literature. Certain hypotheses were constructed from these data and tested by constructing vignettes. The quantitative part of the research concerned presenting those vignettes to a further sample of student nurses using a questionnaire that incorporated a Likert scale for rating responses.

Ingram, 1994

NB: *This example is very sophisticated and undergraduates are not expected to develop a complex research project such as this.*

However, it is more common to check observations with answers from interviews or documents and thus stay within the same methodology; this is called 'within-method' triangulation.

Example of within-method triangulation

Joy Warren conducted a study on patients' hospital experience. As a research nurse in a nursing research unit, she carried out participant observation and the insights gained from observation guided her in-depth interviews of patients. Within-method triangulation was carried out because two qualitative strategies were employed: participant observation and in-depth interviews.

Warren *et al.*, 2000

Triangulation only takes place when the same phenomenon has been examined in different ways or from different perspectives. Triangulation does not, of course, automatically demonstrate validity. (See Chapter 1 for more detail.)

The audit or decision trail

All research should have an audit trail by which others are able to judge, to some extent at least, the validity of the research. Halpern (1983) discussed the inquiry audit in qualitative research, and Lincoln and Guba (1985) developed the concept of the audit trail. The audit trail is the detailed record of the decisions made before and during the research and a description of the research process. Rodgers and Cowles (1993) suggest four types of documentation:

(1) Contextual
(2) Methodological
(3) Analytic
(4) Personal response

The *contextual* documents should contain excerpts from fieldnotes of observation and interviewing, the description of the setting, people and location. The political and social context must also be described. Rodgers and Cowles suggest that *methodological* documents include methodological decision making and the rationale for these decisions. *Analytic* documents consist of reflections on the analysis of data and the theoretical insights gained. *Personal response* documents describe the thought processes and demonstrate the self-awareness of the researcher. This self-examination is part of 'reflexivity' discussed later in this chapter. Koch (1994) shows how to incorporate the decision trail into the research process by describing thought processes and decision making.

Thick description

Thick description too, helps to establish the truth value of the research and is linked to the audit trail. A term coined originally by Geertz (1973), it means a detailed description of the process, context and people in the research, inclusive of the meaning and intentions of the participants and the researcher's conceptual developments. Thick description provides a basis for the reader's evaluation of quality.

Thick description is an account of the complex processes in a specific context and a rich and 'holistic' and even 'artistic' portrayal of the phenomenon under study. Readers of the research report should feel that they were present when the researcher carried out the study, saw, heard and felt what he or she did, and draw similar conclusions (Geertz 1988). There is a chance, however that the research is not seen as useful if the reader cannot transfer the insight gained from the research to other settings, particularly in the healthcare arena. If the contextual description is rich and the analytical language comprehensive enough to enable readers to understand the processes and interactions involved in the context, it might be possible to generalise to the extent of stating that people in other settings have a similar way of understanding.

Reflexivity

Reflexivity means that researchers critically reflect on their own preconceptions and monitor their relationships with the participants and their own reactions to participants' accounts and actions. As the main tool of the research, researchers are part of the phenomenon to be studied and must reflect on their own actions, feelings and conflicts experienced during the research. If they adopt a self-critical stance to the research and their own role, relationships and assumptions, the study will become more credible and dependable. Koch and Harrington (1998) make a case for this. They claim that the research should be 'many-voiced' and not just include the narcissistic reflection and introspection of the person who carries it out. A self-critical position throughout the inquiry process and a location in its political and social context enhances the rigour of the research. Reflexivity is ongoing through data collection, analysis, interpretation and writing up.

Quality and creativity

There is an essential tension between the focus on method and creativity, which is sometimes neglected by those who endlessly grapple with validity and its equivalents. There is no complete consensus about the quality of qualitative research and the criteria adopted. Whittemore *et al.* (2001) add secondary criteria to those outlined by some of the writers mentioned before.

The obsession of qualitative researchers with validity and related issues is due to a defensive stance in relation to the critics of qualitative research by positivist writers. Sparkes (2001) claims that the topic of validity will remain unresolved and different perspectives on it can coexist because of the variety of epistemological and ontological stances. However, as long as qualitative inquiry is seen as 'not really' valid by quantitative researchers, those who carry out qualitative studies will have to explain why their work is trustworthy, and that there are quality criteria by which to judge it.

Summary

There are several distinct schools of thought about criteria for judging qualitative inquiry.

- Qualitative researchers use either the conventional criteria of validity and reliability or alternatives such as trustworthiness and authenticity. There are a few writers who do not see the need to make it explicit but there is no shared understanding of the concepts.

- Strategies to ensure the quality of the research include member checking, the search for alternative cases, peer debriefing, triangulation, disclosing an audit trail, thick description and reflexivity.
- It is important for researchers to spend time in the setting and immerse themselves in this.

References

Angen, M.J. (2000) Evaluating interpretive inquiry: reviewing the validity debate and opening the dialogue. *Qualitative Health Research*, **10** (3) 378–95.

Aroni, R., Goeman, D., Stewart, K. *et al.* (1999) Concepts of rigour: when methodological, clinical and ethical issues intersect. AQR conference: Issues of Rigour in Qualitative Research. Melbourne, November 1999.

Bryman, A. (2001) *Social Research Methods*. Oxford, Oxford University Press.

Carr, W. & Kemmis, S. (1986) *Becoming Critical: Education, Knowledge and Action Research*. London, The Falmer Press.

Cutcliffe, J.R. & McKenna, H. (1999) Establishing the credibility of qualitative research findings. *Journal of Advanced Nursing*, **30** (2) 374–80.

Dahlberg, K., Drew, N. & Nyström, M. (2001) *Reflective Lifeworld Research*. Lund, SWE, Studentlitteratur.

Denzin, N.K. (1989) *The Research Act: A Theoretical Introduction to Sociological Methods*, 3rd edn. Englewood Cliffs, Prentice-Hall.

Erlandson, D.A., Harris, E.L., Skipper, B.L. & Allen, S.D. (1993) *Doing Naturalistic Inquiry*. Newbury Park, Sage.

Geertz, C. (1973) *The Interpretation of Cultures*. New York, Basic Books.

Geertz, C. (1988) *Works and Lives: The Anthropologist as Author*. Stanford, Standford University Press.

Guba, E.G. & Lincoln, Y.S. (1989) *Fourth Generation Evaluation*. New York, Sage.

Halpern, E.S. (1983) Auditing naturalistic inquiries: the development and application of a model. Unpublished doctoral dissertation. Indiana University (cited by Rodgers and Cowles (1993) qv).

Hammersley, M. (1998) *Reading Ethnographic Research: A Critical Guide*, 2nd edn. London, Longman.

Ingram, R. (1994) Passive euthanasia: a student nurse's perspective. Unpublished BSc study, Bournemouth, Bournemouth University.

Koch, T. (1994) Establishing rigour in qualitative research: The decision trail. *Journal of Advanced Nursing*, **19**, 976–86.

Koch, T. & Harrington, A. (1998) Reconceptualising rigour: The case for reflexivity. *Journal of Advanced Nursing*, **28** (4) 882–90.

Lincoln, Y.S. (1995) Emerging criteria for quality in qualitative and interpretive research. *Qualitative Inquiry*, **1** (3) 275–89.

Lincoln, Y.S. (2000) Personal communication. Conference: Qualitative Research in Health and Social Care. Bournemouth, Bournemouth University.

Lincoln, Y.S. & Guba, E.G. (1985) *Naturalistic Inquiry*. Beverly Hills, Sage.

Maxwell, J.A. (1996) *Qualitative Research Design: An Interactive Approach*. Thousand Oaks, Sage.

Morse, J.M. (1994) Designing funded qualitative research. In *Handbook of Qualitative Research* (eds N.K. Denzin & Y.S. Lincoln), pp. 220–35. Thousand Oaks, Sage.

Morse, J.M. (2001) Qualitative verification: building evidence by extending basic findings. In *The Nature of Qualitative Evidence* (eds J.M. Morse, J.M. Swanson and A.J. Kuzel), pp. 203–20. Thousand Oaks, Sage.

Moustakas, C. (1994) *Phenomenological Research Methods*. Thousand Oaks, Sage.

Murphy, E., Dingwall, R., Greatbatch, D., Parker, S. & Watson, P. (1998) Qualitative research methods in health technology assessment. *Health Technology Assessment*, **2**, 16.

Reason, P. & Heron, J. (1995) Co-operative inquiry. In *Rethinking Methods in Psychology* (eds J.A. Smith, R. Harré & L. Van Langenhove), pp. 122–42. London, Sage.

Rodgers, B.L. & Cowles, V. (1993) The qualitative audit trail: a complex collection of documentation. *Research in Nursing and Health*, **16**, 219–26.

Sandelowski, M. (1986) The problem of rigour in qualitative research. *Advances in Nursing Science*, **8** (3) 27–37.

Sandelowski, M. (1993) Rigor or rigor mortis: the problem of rigour in qualitative research revisited. *Advances in Nursing Science*, **16** (2) 1–8.

Seale, C. (1999) *The Quality of Qualitative Research*. London, Sage.

Silverman, D. (2001) *Interpreting Qualitative Data*. 2nd edn. London, Sage.

Sparkes, A. (2001) Myth 94: Qualitative health researchers will agree about validity. *Qualitative Health Research*, **11** (4) 538–52.

Stake, R.E. (1995) *The Art of Case Study Research*. Thousand Oaks, Sage.

Strauss, A. & Corbin, J. (1998) *Basics of Qualitative Research: Techniques and Procedures for Developing Grounded Theory*, 2nd edn. Thousand Oaks, Sage.

Walker, J., Holloway, I. & Sofaer, B. (1999) In the system: the lived experience of chronic back pain from the perspectives of those seeking help from pain clinics. *PAIN*, **80**, 621–8.

Warren, J., Holloway, I. & Smith, P. (2000) Fitting in: maintaining a sense of self during hospitalisation. *International Journal of Nursing Studies*, **37**, 229–35.

Whittemore, R., Chase, S.K. & Mandle, C.L. (2001) Validity in qualitative research. *Qualitative Health Research*, **11** (4) 522–37.

Wolcott, H.F. (1994) *Transforming Qualitative Data: Description, Analysis and Interpretation*. Thousand Oaks, Sage.

CHAPTER 17

Writing up Qualitative Research

The research report

Researchers submit the results of their work to others, for instance: external examiners, a commissioning or funding agency, or to an academic journal for peer review. It is important to be familiar with the format of a research report or dissertation and with general guidelines for its presentation. The research report mirrors the proposal though it is generally more detailed and, of course, includes the findings and discussion. Although conventions for writing up exist, the format may vary from one institution or agency to another.

Researchers must remember to whom they are addressing the report; there is a clear difference between reports that are written for practitioners in the clinical setting, a report for a major funding body and a research dissertation or thesis. Employers and practitioners are more interested in the results and implications of the research for practice and less concerned with philosophical and theoretical issues, while academics see the latter as important. Occasionally health professionals feel it is more appropriate to write two separate reports on the research, one for the practice setting, the other for the university in which they are taking their degree. In a public report, anonymity and confidentiality of the research participants become major issues.

The format should match research design; there are differences in the writing up between quantitative and qualitative studies. In a qualitative report, the methodology section is of major importance; it provides the audit trail (Lincoln and Guba, 1985). Readers and reviewers will be able to follow all the procedures of the study. This means that the methods and logic of the study are shown to be explicit and open to public scrutiny. The biases of the researcher must be stated and laid open to others. On a practical level it is useful to have a style sheet (similar to the sheet that journal editors present to article writers) where the researcher notes down all the elements that should be consistent, such as certain spellings, the type of referencing both in the chapters and at the end of the dissertation or report, the format for headings and other aspects, so this can be used throughout the report (Wolcott, 2001). Many students lack consistency in style and spelling. Of course, it is also important in academic work to follow the advice of the institution.

Use of the first person

When writing up the introduction and the methodology, it is better to write in the first person. It sounds pompous and arid when they state 'the researcher has found ... the author does ... the writer considers...' etc. (Webb, 1992). Qualitative research – and increasingly quantitative research – does not proceed this way. Wolcott (2001) too, suggests the use of the first person because researcher roles become integrated into the study. They can use the first person when they describe what they themselves chose to do. For instance, researchers would not say when speaking about their own actions 'the author chose a sample, or the researcher used the methods...' etc. They might write 'I chose a purposive sample of ... I collected the data through...' It is, of course, important that the first person is not overused, and the use of 'I think, I feel, I believe' is not appropriate. Those who do not wish to use the first person can choose the passive form; for instance 'a purposive sample was chosen...' etc. Indeed Wolcott confirms:

> 'Recognising the critical nature of the observer's role and the influence of his or her subjective assessments in qualitative research makes it all the more important to have readers remain aware of that role, that presence. Writing in the first person helps authors achieve those purposes. *For reporting qualitative research, it should be the rule rather than the exception.*' (emphasis added)
>
> (Wolcott, 2001: 21)

The format of the report

Generally, writers of qualitative studies organise their dissertation in the following sequence:

- Title
- Abstract
- Acknowledgement and dedication
- Contents
- Introduction
  - Background and justification for the study (including its aim)
  - Initial literature review (or overview of the literature)
- Entry issues and ethical considerations
- Methodology and research design

- Description and justification of methods (including type of theoretical framework such as symbolic interactionism or phenomenology)
  - The sample and the setting
  - Specific techniques and procedures
  - Data analysis
  - Trustworthiness and authenticity (or validity and reliability, depending on the terms used)
- Findings/results and discussion
- Conclusion and implications
- Reflections on the research
- References
- Appendices

Qualitative writing may differ substantially from a quantitative report although commonalities exist. The main distinction lies in the flexibility of the qualitative report. The findings and discussion are the most important elements of the final write-up, and consequently contain more words.

Title

The title of a study is important especially if it is presented as a student project, dissertation or thesis because it is the first and most immediate contact the reader has with the research, and its impact on judging the work can be considerable. We would suggest a concise but informative title which sounds interesting but not facetious. It must be remembered that it is initially a working title and may change when some of the research has been done, so it can encompass emergent ideas. Morse, Bottorf and Hutchinson (1994) chose a title which contains the essence of a qualitative study in nursing or midwifery: *The Phenomenology of Comfort*. Other examples of titles are *Illness narratives: time, hope and HIV* (Ezzy, 2000) or *They know best: women's perceptions of midwifery care* (Bluff and Holloway, 1995). Writers often use explanatory subtitles; Silverman (2000) also prefers two-part titles.

The title gives a clear but succinct picture of the study's content. Novice researchers sometimes include unnecessary redundancies in the title such as 'A Study of...' 'Aspects of...' or 'Inquiry', 'Analysis', 'Investigation'. Although the title should reflect the aim of the research it would be clumsy to give the whole aim in the title. Questions usually do not make good titles.

The title page in a dissertation or thesis contains the title, the name of the researcher, the date of the dissertation, and the name of the educational institution at which the student was enrolled. There is generally a pro forma for the title page at most universities. They specify other details for the finished dissertation such as word allowance or size of margins.

Abstract

The abstract is a summary of the research and is written when the study is completed. It appears on the page behind the title but before the table of contents and the full report. The abstract provides the reader with a quick overview of the research question and aim, methods adopted (very brief) and the main results of the study. From the abstract, readers gain a clear picture of the aim, content, methods and main findings. Depending on the size and type of study, the abstract should contain between 150 and 300 words, usually no more than one sheet of A4 paper in single spacing and written in the past tense. Writers should keep to the word limit specified and be selective about the content. Punch (2000: 69) states 'the title should convey as much information as possible in as few words as possible'.

Example of abstract

This paper aims to show how people with chronic back pain manage the status passage from being a well person to becoming a 'pain afflicted' patient, and how they see their own progression through the pain career path. This is examined through in-depth narrative interviews. The data were processed through thematic analysis. It was found that during the transition, a change in perceived identity occurs, and that people grieve over the loss of their former self, the loss of future, of social relationships and occupational career.

The paper also reflects on the value of narratives in revealing transformations over time. This technique is intended to capture evolving self-understandings of personal identity as persons negotiate the path through complex and critical life events.

Holloway et al., 2000

The above is an abstract for a research article. In a student dissertation it could be a little longer and also include the implications of the study in one or two succinct sentences.

Acknowledgement and dedication

Traditionally writers give credit to those who supported, advised or supervised the research, and they also acknowledge the input of the participants. Sometimes the writing is dedicated to particular individuals such as parents or spouses. (We once had a student who acknowledged the help of her cat.) Wolcott (1990) claims that researchers sometimes overdo dedications, which, he suggests, should only be given in major work, but he does see acknowledgement of others' help as important.

Contents

Most academic studies have a table of contents before its main chapters begin. It cannot, of course, be finished before the whole project is finalised and written. The content is sectioned into chapter headings and subheadings with page numbers. In an undergraduate student project, the table of contents should be concise and need not be too long and detailed.

Some writers provide a glossary of terms and list of abbreviations at the beginning of the research or in an appendix.

Introduction

Background and justification

In the introduction the writer tells the audience about the research question or topic. The introduction consists of the background and context of the research as well as the aim – the overall purpose of the project. Writers explain why they have become interested in the question, how their project relates to the general topic area, and what gap in nursing knowledge might be filled by the new research through linking the question to the possible implications for practice. In the introduction the nurse explains the significance of the study for the clinical setting and how it could improve clinical practice or policy. Edwards and Talbot (1994: 41) tell researchers to give the answers to the following questions in the rationale or justification of their studies: 'Why this (rather than any other topic), why now, why there, why me?' The background section sets the scene for the study. One of our colleagues claims that it is useful for the researcher to ask the 'so what?' question to keep the background section relevant.

Initial literature review (or overview of the literature)

This section can stand on its own, or it can become an integral part of the introduction. The literature in qualitative studies has a different place from that in quantitative research. Of course, it must show some of the relevant research that has been done in the field. The researchers summarise the main ideas from these studies, some of the problems and contradictions found, and show how they relate to the project in hand. It is important in qualitative reports not to use every piece of known research in the field, nor to give a critical review of all the literature but only the main pertinent studies including classic and most recent research (Minichiello et al., 1990) as well as the methodological approaches and procedures that were used for them. Gaps in knowledge become apparent at this point. At this stage, the research question is linked to the literature (see also Chapter 2 for more detail on literature review). By the end of the introductory section, the reader should be in no doubt that qualitative research, in the form suggested by the researcher, was most appropriate to meet the research aim.

Entry issues and ethical considerations

Nurse and midwife researchers describe entry and ethical issues (see Chapters 2 and 3). It must be stated how the participants were approached, for instance whether researchers advertised on a notice board or approached the potential participants personally. How did the researchers gain permission from gate-keepers, those in the position of power to grant access to the setting (managers at various levels, Trust and local research ethics committees)? If patients are involved, their consultants or GPs would have to be asked for their permission too. It is important that individual participants cannot be recognised in the report. Last, but most importantly, nurses should make explicit how the ethical principles were followed in the study and how the participants' rights were protected.

Methodology and research design

The methodology chapter includes several subsections: the research design and methodology; the methods, including data collection, sampling, detailed interviewing or observation procedures; and a description of the data analysis. In qualitative research the methodology takes up more space. It is important because the researcher is the main research tool and has to make explicit the path of the research, so that the reader knows about the details of design, biases, relationships and limitations and is able to follow the decision trail.

Description and justification of methods

The research design usually includes the main methods and the theoretical framework. Researchers briefly describe the methodology they adopt and the reasons and justification for it. They also explain the fit between the research question and the methodology.

The sample and setting

The sample is described in detail. As stated before, in qualitative research the purposive sample is not fixed from the beginning. Concepts rather than people are sampled. The writer describes the informants, who they were, how many were chosen and the reasons for the choice. Researchers tell the reader how they obtained their sample and portray the setting in which the study took place. The inclusion of theoretical sampling must be explained (see Chapters 5 and 10).

Example 1: People and setting

In the study five social workers and five health visitors were interviewed. The social workers originated from the same area office, the health visitors came from the same health authority. They also worked in a locale that was coterminous. This was deemed important in order to reduce the difference between operational styles and policies of both social service office and health authority.

Wheeler (1989)

Example 2: Theoretical sampling

[For instance] The sample was not predetermined but depended on the concepts relevant to the emerging theoretical ideas. It seemed that the twelve women were more compliant than the four men in the sample. Interviewing a larger group of men followed this up.

Specific techniques and procedures

The methodology section gives information about the data collection. The researcher describes the procedures such as interviewing, observation or other strategies that were used and any problems encountered. The outline should not be a general essay on procedures but a step-by-step description of the work in hand so that the reader can follow it closely. It is necessary that researchers give the reasons for using a particular methodology and research strategies and describe the procedures of collecting data. The reader should know how the data were collected and stored.

Example (A dissertation or thesis needs more detail)

The data were collected through unstructured interviews (with an *aide mémoire*) which took place in the informants' own homes and which were tape-recorded with their permission. Interviews lasted between one and three hours. I transcribed the interviews and stored the numbered transcriptions safely away from the list of informants' names. Collection and analysis of data took place simultaneously as is usual in grounded theory.

Data analysis

The data analysis needs to be explained, including the ways in which data were coded and categorised and how theoretical constructs were generated from the data. It is useful, and essential in dissertations, to give examples from the study. A detailed account of the chosen type of analysis is required. The readership is entitled to know whether a computer analysis was used.

Example of data analysis in grounded theory research

Using guidelines based on the initial work by Glaser and Strauss (1967) and modified by Strauss and Corbin (1998) data were collected (a detailed description of the data collection procedures is necessary here) and analysed simultaneously. The method of analysing data by 'constant comparison' is one of the unique features of the GT approach. The data were coded, categorised and constantly compared (detailed examples should be given) to produce concepts grounded in the data. Through theoretical sampling, I followed theoretical concepts that had relevance to the emerging theory. Comparison with the data and the sampling of ideas in the literature was continued until saturation occurred and no new data of relevance emerged.

If this were a dissertation, more detail and examples of each step should have been given, so that the audit trail is clearly demonstrated.

Trustworthiness

See Chapter 16 for a discussion of this topic.

Findings/results and discussion

There are two main ways (and other, alternative strategies) to present qualitative findings and discussion. The first is written in the traditional format in which findings and discussion are separated and follow one another. However, findings without discussion and comments do not make a good storyline. Therefore the findings and discussion are usually integrated. This gives more meaning to the report and shows the storyline more clearly (but again, no rigid rule exists about this). Some writers present a brief summary of the results in a diagram, and then discuss each major category (or construct, or theme) in a few sentences before starting the Findings and Discussion chapter. In each chapter the data the researcher collected are discussed first. The relevant literature is integrated into the discussion where it fits best and serves as additional evidence for the particular category or as a problem for debate.

Telling the tale

In a qualitative report writers tell a story which should be vivid and interesting as well as credible to the reader. This sometimes means writing and rewriting drafts until a story line can be discerned clearly. Although there may be similarities with journalism or fiction, writers have to keep in mind that these stories have a different purpose, namely to give an accurate and systematic analysis of the data and a discussion of the results. This should not be dry and mechanistic, but must reflect the researcher's involvement. The events, the people and their words and actions should be made explicit, so that readers can experience the situation as real, in a similar way to the researcher.

The use of quotes from participants

Direct quotes from the interviews or excerpts from the fieldnotes are inserted at an appropriate place to show some of the data from which the results emerged. Sandelowski (1994) lists some of the uses of quotes in qualitative studies and suggests that they give insight into people's real experiences and illustrate the arguments. The content of the quotes helps the reader to judge how the results were derived from the data and to establish the credibility of the emerging categories and provide the reader with a means of auditing these. The writer, of course, must take care that the quotes convey the meanings and feelings of the participant and are directly connected with the themes they seek to illustrate. Sandelowski gives importance to both content and style of quote. The direct quotation in the participant's words in a study makes the discussion more lively and dynamic. Long rows of quotes from informants or continuous duplication are not needed. Wolcott (1990: 67) suggests: 'Save the best and drop the rest', but frequent very short quotes make the study look fragmented.

The use of quotations from the literature

Trying to give substance to their own arguments, inexperienced nurse researchers often quote the words of experts. This can interrupt the story line of the research. It is better to avoid a quotation when it can be paraphrased or summarised, but the idea should still be credited to the originator.

However, when a specific phrase is critical and written by a well known expert or author of a classic text on the field of study, a quote can be used. Occasionally it does enhance a piece of writing and is appropriate. When using a lengthy quote from books or articles, a page number should be given.

Example

Wolcott (1990: 67) suggests: 'Save the best and drop the rest'.
Or
Wolcott (1990, p. 67) suggests: 'Save the best and drop the rest'.
Or
Wolcott (1990) suggests: 'Save the best and drop the rest' (p. 67).

We must warn researchers of two common mistakes. First, researchers often write in a very complex way and use incomprehensible terminology. In their fear of sounding simplistic and not academic, nurses and midwives often complicate and obscure simple and clear issues. It is important to express ideas in clear and unambiguous terms, although they should not, of course be simplistic. The second flaw is linked to a lack of analysis. It is not enough to simply give a collection of lengthy quotes and summarise their content. This is not analysis. Researchers have to develop their theoretical ideas and interpretations and they can illustrate them with the relevant quotes from the participants.

Conclusion and implications

Generally studies end with a conclusion. The conclusion is a summary of the results in context. It must be directly related to the results of the specific study, and no new elements (or references) should be introduced here. The conclusion reviews what has been learnt in relation to the aim, the theoretical ideas and propositions that emerged from the study. Dramatic and overly assertive conclusions can be dangerous and pretentious in a small project. Novice researchers seldom generate 'formal theory' or come to significant conclusions; in fact, their research is of 'more modest scope and consequence' (Wolcott, 1994: 44). However, this does not mean that the small piece of research has no importance or implications for the clinical area. Woods (1999) has a list of considerations for the conclusion. He asks researchers whether their writing has answered the questions asked, whether there are weaknesses and limitations, and how they can be addressed. Of course, it is also important to demonstrate that that the study has added to knowledge in the field. Sometimes the conclusion might provide a new light on the data.

In health research and other projects in professional settings, the conclusion contains the implications and, occasionally, the recommendations that could be made on the basis of the results. The implications can be integrated into the conclusion, they can be discussed towards its end or they can form a separate section following on from the conclusion. It is important to remember that the implications must be based directly on the results of the study; all too often they seem unrelated to the findings.

To check the quality of their conclusion researchers might ask the following questions:

- Why is this included here? (on reflecting about an issue or a statement)
- What are the main issues arising from the data?
- What were the major aims, and how has the study achieved these?
- What were the answers to the research questions?
- Does the conclusion directly relate to them
- What are the implications for the profession that derive directly from the study?

Reflections on the research

Many academic researchers reflect on their project and take a critical stance to it, usually towards the end of their dissertation or thesis. They demonstrate how the research could be improved, extended or illuminated from another angle. At this point they might point to its limitations and their own biases, which they did not make explicit in the main body of the study, and describe some of the problems they encountered. Not all studies contain this reflective section, and sometimes they are part of the conclusion. Nurses and midwives who take a reflective stance could discuss at this point how they have professionally and personally developed and changed through the research. Wolcott (1994) states that this personal approach, rarely adopted in quantitative research, is seen as appropriate in qualitative research.

A statement about validation of a study by a survey or other quantitative methods might suggest a lack of awareness that a qualitative study can stand on its own, has its own validation procedures and cannot be judged from the quantitative researcher's point of view.

References

For academic studies the Harvard system of referencing is generally used, but other formal systems of referencing may be acceptable to the students' supervisors, journals or funding bodies. It is best to find out about this before the start of the study from supervisors, course leaders or handbooks and journals.

The writer should compare the references in the text with the selected bibliography and make sure that every reference is included. We often find that student referencing is incomplete, incorrect or insufficient. Page (the singular) is shortened to p.; pages – the plural – to pp. but for journals the pp. or p. is usually left out. The title of the book or the name of the journal should be underlined or written in italics. Page numbers are stated in the references when an article in a journal is given, or a chapter in an edited book is referenced.

Examples

Woods, P. (1999) *Successful Writing for Qualitative Researchers*. London, Routledge.

Warren, J., Holloway, I. & Smith, P. (2000) Fitting in: maintaining a sense of self during hospitalisation. *International Journal of Nursing Studies*, 37, 229–35.

Emerson, R.M., Fretz, R.I. & Shaw, L.L. (2000) Participant observation and field-notes. In *Handbook of Ethnography* (eds P. Atkinson, A. Coffey, S. Delamont, J. Lofland & L. Lofland), pp. 352–67. London, Sage.

Educational institutions, within certain parameters, may have their own rules about referencing. Publishers of books and articles, too, use different ways of referencing. In this book for instance we follow the guidelines of our publisher.

Appendices

A list of informants (with pseudonyms) their ages, experience or length of service is sometimes included by writers (making sure, however, that anonymity is preserved, particularly when the participants or informants might easily be recognised). An interview guide and a sample interview transcript (in a study that uses interviews) could be attached as an example for the reader to help in understanding the development of the data collection. Some fieldnotes from observations might be given to demonstrate their use. Appendices depend on the advice given to students and on their own common sense, but there should not be too many sections. Sometimes researchers attach the formal initial letter to participants or an example of the letter of permission. A copy of the letter of approval from the ethical committee should be attached where appropriate without identification of the location of the research. The words in appendices do not count as part of the study.

The appendices (the plural of appendix) are placed at the very end of the study after the bibliography in the order in which they appear in the chronology of the study. For instance, the example of the initial letter to participants would be placed before the exemplar of an interview transcript. Universities have their own rules about this.

Publishing the research

Books

If the findings are significant, the researcher has the responsibility to disseminate them to a wider group such as colleagues and other health professionals. Sometimes nurses or midwives produce a book based on their thesis (Lawler, 1991; Smith, 1992) or a chapter in an edited book such as that by Morse and Johnson (1991). Most publishers have guidelines for writing book proposals. The proposal then goes to their editorial board to decide whether the book is worth publishing, in their view, and commercially viable. Researchers should not be disturbed if their proposal is not accepted. Commercial considerations are the main concern of publishers, and these depend on the general appeal of the piece of research. Editors are, of course, also concerned about the quality of the content and the ability of the researcher to write clearly and in an accessible style.

Articles

More often, students who have carried out research publish an article in a professional or academic journal, often with their supervisor at an early stage of their research. The length and style of the article will depend on the type of journal; for instance, articles in the *Journal of Advanced Nursing* are more academic and generally longer than those in the *Nursing Times*. Articles have higher standing in research circles than chapters in books because articles in important academic journals are refereed by experts in the field and count more in the research assessment exercise.

The detailed guidelines for scripts are laid out at the front or the back of the journal. Some journal editors want a very detailed description of the methods adopted (for instance the journal *Midwifery*), others claim that a well known and widely published methodology, such as grounded theory – can be summarised rather than discussed in great detail (*Sociology of Health and Illness*). Writers must take into account the different styles and guidelines of these journals. As a long research study cannot be fully discussed in article format, researchers choose what to include or exclude. For example, just one chapter, one category or a methodological issue might form the basis of the article.

It is important to write in a lively manner in an article or a book based on qualitative research. This can be achieved through a good storyline and enhanced through vignettes or excerpts from interviews or fieldnotes, taking into account, of course, that individuals should not be recognised in the descriptions. Good diagrams might clarify some of the aspects of the work. Different journals address different audiences.

Types of article

Strauss and Corbin (1998) claim that three types of paper are published in journals, intended for different readership:

(1) For academic colleagues
(2) For practitioners
(3) For lay readers

Articles for academic colleagues

There are those colleagues who have a particular interest in the theoretical and methodological framework as well as in the research topic. The *Journal of Advanced Nursing*, *Midwifery* and *Qualitative Health Research* are good examples for journals publishing this type of article. The journal *Qualitative Inquiry* deals exclusively with methodological issues but is not a nursing publication (this and *Qualitative Health Research* are journals published in the USA while *Qualitative Research* is published in Britain). *Nurse Education Today* covers educational issues and research in nurse and midwifery education. The *Journal of Nursing Management* is concerned with management issues. The academic standard of some journals is very high, and it is more difficult to publish in refereed journals.

Articles for practitioners

Examples of journals intended to assist practitioners are *Nursing Times* or *Senior Nurse*, or the *British Journal of Midwifery*. There are many others. In these journals one can find articles which describe findings and address the implications of these findings. Often the writers of these articles give an overview of procedures or develop ideas that assist in the understanding of patients.

Articles for the lay reader

Some articles are meant for lay readers. Although most nurse and midwife researchers do not write for this readership, occasionally an article in a specialist magazine could actually help members of a group or the general population. For instance, an article on research into hormone replacement therapy in a women's journal might give information to women, though it would have to be short and non-academic. It is necessary that researchers write with integrity and factual accuracy.

All students carrying out PhD or MPhil and even MA/MSc research should attempt some articles; some universities encourage this during the process of the research, others suggest writing after completion of the research degree. There is an academic tradition that these students publish with their supervisors who, of course, have had a major input in the research and will help in refining the article. Nevertheless, supervisors' names should not be first on the list of authors unless they have actually written the article.

It is very useful for undergraduate students to publish, as they not only get used to disseminating their research, but also because it will eventually enhance their status within the profession. They are, however, advised to seek the advice and help of their supervisors.

Critical assessment and evaluation

Researchers must be aware that the readers of a research study or report apply certain criteria to judge the quality and credibility of the research and look for particular components in the final write-up. Not all, but some of these are specific to qualitative research. The checklist below contains important factors readers consider when evaluating the study. It would be useful for researchers to examine their own study in the light of these elements.

The research question

- Is the research problem or question stated clearly?
- What is the topic area, and has it been justified?
- Is the aim of the research suitable and feasible?
- Is the problem appropriate for qualitative research?
- Is the title concise and informative?
- Do the questions show that the researchers have not imposed their own framework, but that the data will have priority?

The abstract

- Does it state the aim and describe the methodology?
- Does it summarise results and state conclusions?

The literature

- Is there an initial overview giving the rationale for the study?
- Has the appropriate literature been integrated into the study?
- Are the references ongoing, comprehensive, relevant and up to date?

Data collection

- What is the type of data collection, and is it appropriate for the study?
- How are the data collected, transcribed and stored?

The sample

- Does the researcher use purposive sampling (including theoretical sampling if appropriate)?
- Are the criteria for sampling made explicit?
- Is the sampling explained adequately?
- Is the type and size of sample justified?
- Are criteria for inclusion and exclusion given?

Entry and ethical issues

- Does the researcher state how he or she gained access to the participants?
- Who was approached for permission to obtain access?
- Were the rights of participants safeguarded (including their right to withdraw from the study)?
- Has the researcher ensured the anonymity of participants?
- Are issues of power taken into account?

- Has the researcher excluded particularly vulnerable clients?
- If vulnerable clients are included in the sample, is this inclusion justified?
- Are major ethical issues discussed?

Data analysis

- Is the method of analysis identified?
- Is the data analysis described (giving examples)?
- Is the data analysis systematic and detailed?
- Is the 'decision trail' traced in detail?
- (In grounded theory: do data collection and analysis interact?)

The findings

- Does the researcher explain the trustworthiness (validity) of the study?
- How have these issues been managed?
- Is the explanation appropriate for a qualitative approach?
- What does the researcher learn from the research?
- Is there a storyline or core category?
- Has the study met its aim?
- Does the conclusion clearly state what was learned from the research?
- Do the conclusions come directly from the data?

Importance to nursing or midwifery

- Are the implications for clinical practice discussed?
- Do they emerge directly from the study?

Blaxter (1995) produced a draft paper for discussion at a conference on medical sociology in which she developed some ideas for the evaluation of qualitative research. She states clearly that the criteria by which to judge qualitative research are different from those of quantitative approaches but also argues for rigour in qualitative research (see Chapter 16 p. 251).

Summary

The main points to remember when writing up research are listed below.

- Qualitative research provides more flexibility in writing up than quantitative approaches.
- The main sections of the write-up are separated into: *introduction* – the rationale for the study; an *overview of the literature* to identify a knowledge gap; a detailed *methodology* including a description of the sample; *data collection* and *analysis*, the main *findings* and *discussion* of these.

- Ethical issues and access must also be described.
- The findings and discussion are the major part of the study in which the literature is integrated.
- The final section of the study contains the conclusions and implications for the clinical setting.
- A lively and interesting storyline is important.
- A research report needs a strong conclusion with implications for the profession.

References

Blaxter, M. (1995) *Workshop on Criteria for the Evaluation of Qualitative Research.* Medical Sociology Conference, York, 22–24 September, British Sociological Association.

Bluff, R. & Holloway, I. (1995) They know best: women's perceptions of midwifery care. *Midwifery*, **10**, 157–64.

Edwards, A. & Talbot, R. (1994) *The Hard-Pressed Researcher*. London, Longman.

Erlandson, D.A., Harris, E.L., Skipper, B.L. & Allen, S.D. (1993) *Doing Naturalistic Inquiry*. Newbury Park, Sage.

Ezzy, D. (2000) Illness narratives: time, hope and HIV. *Social Science and Medicine*, **50**, 605–17.

Glaser, B.G. and Strauss, A.L. (1967) *The Discovery of Grounded Theory*. Chicago, Aldine.

Holloway, I., Sofaer, B. & Walker, J. (2000) The transition from well person to 'pain afflicted' patient: The career of people with chronic back pain. *Illness, Crisis and Loss*, **8** (4) 373–87.

Lawler, J. (1991) *Behind the Screens: Nursing, Somology and the Problem of the Body*. Melbourne, Churchill Livingstone.

Lincoln, Y. & Guba, E. (1985) *Naturalistic Inquiry*. Beverly Hills, CA, Sage.

Minichiello, V., Aroni, R., Timewell, E. & Alexander, L. (1990) *In-Depth Interviewing: Researching People*. Melbourne, Longman Cheshire.

Morse, J.M. & Johnson, J.L. (1991) *The Illness Experience*. Newbury Park, Sage.

Morse, J.M., Bottorf, J.L. & Hutchinson, S. (1994) The phenomenology of comfort. *Journal of Advanced Nursing*, **20**, 184–95.

Punch, K.F. (2000) *Developing Effective Research Proposals*. London, Sage.

Sandelowski, M. (1994) The use of quotes in qualitative research. *Research in Nursing and Health*, **17** (6) 479–83.

Silverman, D. (2000) *Doing Qualitative Research: A Practical Handbook*. London, Sage.

Smith, P. (1992) *The Emotional Labour of Nursing*. Basingstoke, Macmillan.

Strauss, A. & Corbin, J. (1998) *Basics of Qualitative Research: Techniques and Procedures for Developing Grounded Theory*, 2nd edn. Thousand Oaks, Sage.

Webb, C. (1992) The use of the first person in academic writing: objectivity, language and gatekeeping. *Journal of Advanced Nursing*, **17**, 747–52.

Wheeler, S. (1989) Health visitors' and social workers' perceptions of child abuse. Unpublished BSc project. Bournemouth, Bournemouth University.

Wheeler, S.J. (1992) Perceptions of child abuse. *Health visitor*, **65** (9) 316–19.

Wolcott, H.F. (1990) *Writing up Qualitative Research*. Newbury Park, Sage.

Wolcott, H.F. (1994) *Transforming Qualitative Data: Description, Analysis, and Interpretation*. Thousand Oaks, Sage.

Wolcott, H.F. (2001) *Writing up Qualitative Research*, 2nd edn. Thousand Oaks, Sage.

Woods, P. (1999) *Successful Writing for Qualitative Researchers*. London, Routledge.

Glossary

Abstract: A concise summary or synopsis of the research which appears at the beginning of the report stating the aim, nature and scope of the study and its implications.

Action research: A cyclical approach to research in which researchers are, or collaborate with, practitioners to effect change or use an intervention; they then modify their practices and the whole process starts again until the optimum situation has been achieved.

Aide mémoire: Key words or short questions that aid the memory of the researcher and focus on areas of interest or importance for the researcher during in-depth interviewing.

Analytic induction: An approach to analysis that involves inductive processes and which makes inferences from the specific to find general rules or theories.

Appendix (pl: appendices): Additional material at the end of the study. It is not included in the word limit and is located either before or after the bibliography (depending on institutional rules).

Assumption: A belief or assertion which is taken for granted by the researcher but has not been verified.

Auditability: Research is auditable if readers or other researchers are able to follow the methodological processes of the first researcher.

Audit trail (or decision trail): A detailed explanation of the decision-making processes of the researcher to demonstrate the logic and development of the research path.

Authenticity: A term used to demonstrate that the findings of a research project are representative of the participants' perspectives, that the study is fair and helps participants to understand their social world and improve it.

Bias: A distortion or error in the data collection, analysis or interpretation which has its origin in strongly held values or feelings of the researcher or an individual participant.

Bracketing (in phenomenology): The focus of the research is placed in brackets and everything else, such as assumptions and presuppositions about the phenomenon, is set aside.

Case study: Research with and on a single unit of study such as an organisation, a person or a subculture which is bounded by time and location.

Category: A group of concepts and ideas with similar characteristics that form a unit of analysis.

Causality: A link between cause and effect.

Code: A label given to specific data.

Coding (in analysis): Examining and breaking down the data. Assigning a name (or a number) to a specific datum.

Concept: An abstract or generalised idea that describes a phenomenon.

Concept mapping: Linking and relating concepts and presenting the interrelationship in a diagram.

Constant comparison (in grounded theory): Qualitative data analysis where each datum is compared with every other piece.

Construct: A construct encompasses a number of concepts or categories and has a high level of abstraction. The term is often used for a major category that has evolved from the reduction of a number of smaller categories.

Constructionism: An approach in social science based on the assumption that human beings construct their social reality, and that the social world cannot exist independently of human beings. In research terms this means that participants and researcher construct meaning together.

Contextualisation: Researchers link the data and findings to their context.

Core category (in grounded theory): A concept that links with all other categories in the project and integrates the data.

Criterion (pl criteria): A standard by which something is evaluated.

Criterion-based sample: See purposive sample.

Critical incident technique: A data collection and analysis technique focusing on critical situations, events and incidents in the research setting.

Critical theory: The view that people can critically evaluate social phenomena and change society in order to become emancipated.

Data (plural): The information collected for the research.

Data analysis: Organisation, reduction and transformation of the data by exploring meanings of research participants. Researchers search the data for concepts and categories.

Deduction: The procedure of testing a general principle or hypothesis to explain specific phenomena or cases.

Delimitations: The boundaries of the research such as inclusion or exclusion.

Description: A detailed account of the significant phenomenon or phenomena in the research to generate a picture of the world as seen by the participants.

Design: The overall plan of the research, including methods and procedures for collecting, analysing and interpreting data.

Dross rate: Information obtained from participants which is irrelevant to the outcome of a particular study.

Emic perspective (anthropological term): The 'insider's' point of view (see also etic perspective).

Epiphany: A sudden revelation or turning point in a person's life.

Epistemology: The theory of knowledge concerned with the ways in which human beings know the world.

Ethnography: Research that is concerned with a description of a culture or group and its members' experiences and interpretations. It is both the research process and the completed product, that is, the research report.

Etic perspective: The outsider's view, the perspective of the researcher (see also emic perspective).

Exhaustive description (in phenomenology): Writing that aims to capture and describe the intensity and depth of the participants' experience.

External validity: Generalisability (see generalisability).

Fieldnotes: A record of observations in the field.

Fieldwork (initially a term from anthropology): The collection of data outside the laboratory, in the field.

Focused interview: An interview in which questions are focused on emerging and relevant issues (see also funnelling).

Focus group: A group of people with similar experiences or common traits who are interviewed as a group in order to obtain their thoughts and perceptions about a particular topic.

Funnelling: The process of interviewing that starts with a broad basis and becomes progressively more specific during the interview process (see also focused interview).

Gatekeepers: Those individuals who have the power to permit or restrict access to an organisation, a setting or people.

Generalisability: The extent to which the findings of the study can be applied to other events, settings or groups in the population.

Grounded theory: A research method which generates theory from the data through constant comparison.

Hermeneutics: A branch of phenomenology that focuses on the interpretation rather than the description of a phenomenon.

Heterogeneity: The extent to which units of a sample are dissimilar in characteristics important for the study.

Homogeneity: The extent to which units of a sample are similar in traits important for the research.

Hypothesis: An assumption or statement of a relationship between variables which can be tested, verified and falsified.

Idiographic methods: Methods focused on the unique and individual. These differ from nomothetic methods (qv) that seek law-like generalities subsuming individual cases.

Immersion: The process whereby researchers stay in, learn about and become completely familiar with the field.

Induction: A reasoning process in which researchers proceed from the specific and concrete to general and abstract principles.

Informant: A person as a member of the group under study participates in the research and helps the researcher to interpret the culture of the group (see also key informant).

Informed consent: A voluntary agreement made by participants after having been informed of the nature and aim of the study.

Interpretivism: An approach in social science that focuses on human beings and the way in which they interpret and make sense of their reality.

Interviewer effect (see also observer effect): The effect of the researcher's presence on the research.

Interview guide: Loosely formed questions which are used flexibly by the interviewer in in-depth interviews.

Interview schedule: Standardised questions which are used by the quantitative researcher who uses the same sequence and wording for each respondent. (NB: Often used inappropriately in qualitative research.)

In vivo *code* (in grounded theory): Codes in which the researcher uses the words of the participant as a label.

Iteration: Continuous movement between parts of the research text and the whole, between raw data and analysed data.

Key informant: (in ethnography): A long-standing member of a culture or group who has expert knowledge of its rules, customs and language.

Limitations: Weaknesses, restrictions and incompleteness of the research (not always used in a negative way).

Member check: Checking and verification of the data or interpretations by participants.

Memoing: Notes of varying degrees of abstraction when carrying out fieldwork.

Method: Procedure and strategy for collecting, analysing and interpreting data.

Methodology: The framework of theories and principles on which methods and procedures are based.

Narrative: The description of experiences by the participants. The reconstruction of their lives or experiences.

Nomothetic methods: The search for law-like generalities or rule-following behaviour that subsumes individual cases (see also idiographic methods).

Objectivity: A neutral and unbiased stance.

Observer effect: See interviewer effect.

Ontology: A branch of philosophy concerning the nature of being. It is related to assumptions about the nature of reality.

Paradigm: A theoretical perspective or approach to reality recognised by a community of scholars. A position that provides the researcher with a set of beliefs to guide the research.

Participant observation: Observation in which the researcher becomes a participant in the setting or culture under study.

Phenomenon: The central concept to be researched: in phenomenology (qv), the meaning of the experiences in the life world of the participant in a study.

Phenomenology: A philosophy which explores the meaning of individuals' lived experience through their own description. The research approach adopted is based on this philosophy.

Pilot study: A small-scale trial run of a research interview or observation.

Positivism: A direction in the philosophy of social science which aims to find general laws and regularities based on observation and experiment parallel to the methods of the natural sciences.

Premature closure: Arriving too early at explanation or theoretical ideas.

Progressive focusing: See funnelling.

Proposition: A working hypothesis which consists of linked concepts. It establishes some regularities and relationships between categories.

Pseudonym: Fictitious names given to informants to protect their anonymity.

Purposive (or purposeful) sample: A judgemental sample of individuals chosen by certain pre-determined criteria relevant to the research question (also called criterion-based sample, qv).

Reactivity: Participants react to the presence of the researcher. The researcher also reacts to the responses of the participants.

Reflexivity: Reflecting on and critically examining the research process. Consideration of researcher's subjectivity and experiences brought to the research.

Reliability: The ability of a research tool to achieve consistent results.

Research aim: The intention of the researcher to uncover something about the phenomenon under study in order to answer the research question.

Research question: The problem or statement that guides a study and establishes the baseline for other questions.

Rigour: High standard in research which seeks detail, accuracy, trustworthiness and credibility.

Saturation: A state where no new data of importance to the study emerge and when the elements of all categories are accounted for.

Serendipity: A chance and unexpected discovery during data collection.

Storyline: An analytic description and overview of the story told in the research.

Subjectivity: A personal view influenced by personal background and traits.

Symbolic interactionism: An interpretive approach in sociology that focuses on meaning in interaction.

Tacit knowledge: Implicit knowledge that is shared but not openly articulated.

Theoretical sampling (in grounded theory, qv): Sampling which proceeds on the basis of emerging, relevant concepts and is guided by developing theory.

Theoretical sensitivity (concept developed by Glaser): Sensitivity and awareness of the researcher to detect meaning in the data.

Theory: A set of interrelated concepts and propositions that explain social phenomena.

Thick description (concept developed by Geertz): Dense detailed and conceptual description which gives a picture of events and actions within the social context.

Triangulation: The combination of different methods of research, data collection approaches, investigators or theoretical perspectives in the study of one phenomenon (e.g. qualitative and quantitative methods, interviews and observation etc.).

Validity: The extent to which the researcher's findings are accurate, reflect the purpose of the study and represent reality (validity in qualitative research differs from that in quantitative research).

Verification: Empirical validation after testing a hypothesis; in qualitative research, testing a proposition or a working hypothesis.

Index